YOGA
THE TECHNOLOGY OF ECSTASY

The impulse toward transcendence is intrinsic to human life. Nowhere has this drive found a more consistent and versatile expression than in India. The civilization of India has spawned an overwhelming variety of spiritual beliefs, practices, and approaches. The goal of Yoga, the most famous and globally widespread of India's spiritual traditions, is to take us beyond ourselves to the Absolute Reality, to the utterly blissful union of the individual self with the transcendental Divine.

In recent decades the practice of Yoga, once known only in the East, has spread across the world, and this great Indian tradition has now become a household word in the West. In spite of the wealth of books published on the subject, the historical origins and philosophical underpinnings of this rich and varied spiritual technology have remained obscure even to its millions of Western practitioners. Yoga: The Technology of Ecstasy *is a work of unparalleled scope which at last weaves the daunting complexity of five thousand years of Yoga into a single tapestry. Here, for the first time, is a clear, comprehensive, and systematic overview of the history, philosophy, and practice of every major branch of Yoga, including Hatha-Yoga and Tantra, which have gained wide followings in the West.*

This book features a lucid explanation of Yoga's roots in Indian culture, outlines its relationship to other important Indian traditions, and discusses the diverse forms it has taken in Hinduism, Buddhism, and Jainism. Yoga: The Technology of Ecstasy *contains illuminating diagrams and illustrations as well as an invaluable glossary of Sanskrit terms, many original translations of primary source material, and a comprehensive chronology. This work combines heartfelt eloquence and practical understanding with the kind of intellectual clarity that could be provided only by an author who is both an impeccable scholar and a dedicated practitioner. Speaking always to the contemporary reader, Georg Feuerstein offers a compelling and relevant articulation of Yoga's profound life-transforming value for modern men and women.*

Select other books by Georg Feuerstein:

The Essence of Yoga
The Philosophy of Classical Yoga
The Bhagavad-Gita: Its Philosophy and Cultural Setting
Structures of Consciousness
Enlightened Sexuality
Encyclopedic Dictionary of Yoga
The Yoga-Sutra of Patanjali

योग आनन्दकल्पनः

YOGA

The

TECHNOLOGY

of

ECSTASY

Georg Feuerstein

FOREWORD BY
Ken Wilber

Jeremy P. Tarcher, Inc.
Los Angeles

Library of Congress Cataloging in Publication Data

Feuerstein, Georg.
    Yoga : the technology of ecstasy / Georg Feuerstein.
        p.   cm.
    Bibliography.
    Includes index.
    ISBN 0-87477-525-6. — ISBN 0-87477-520-5 (pbk.)
    1. Yoga. I. Title.
    B132.Y6F488 1989
    181'.45—dc20

Jeremy P. Tarcher, Inc.
9110 Sunset Blvd.
Los Angeles, CA 90069

Distributed by St. Martin's Press, New York

Design by Robert Tinnon

Manufactured in the United States of America
10 9 8 7 6 5 4 3 2 1
First Edition

Contents

v

Foreword

It is a great pleasure, indeed honor, to write this Foreword. I have been a fan of Georg Feuerstein ever since I read his classic *Essence of Yoga*. His subsequent works simply reinforced my belief that in Georg Feuerstein we have a scholar-practitioner of the first magnitude, an extremely important and valuable voice for the perennial philosophy, and arguably the foremost authority on Yoga today.

In the East, as well as in the West, there tend to be two rather different approaches to spirituality—that of the scholar and that of the practitioner. The scholar tends to be abstract, and studies world religions as one might study bugs or rocks or fossils—merely another field for the detached intellect. The idea of actually practicing a spiritual or contemplative discipline rarely seems to dawn on the scholar. Indeed, to practice what one is studying is held to interfere with one's "objectivity"—one has become a believer and therefore nonobjective.

Practitioners, on the other hand, although admirably engaged in an actual discipline, tend to be very uninformed about all the various facets of their tradition. They may be naive about the cultural trappings of their particular path, or about its actual historical origins, or about how much of their path is essential truth and how much is simply cultural baggage.

Rare, indeed, to find a scholar who is also a practitioner. But when it comes to writing a book on Yoga, this combination is absolutely essential. A treatise on Yoga can be trusted neither to the scholars nor the practitioners alone. There is an immense amount of information that must be mastered in order to write about Yoga, and therefore a scholar is needed. But Yoga itself is born in the fire of direct experience. It must be engaged, and lived, and practiced. It must come from the head, but equally from the heart. And this very rare combination is exactly what Georg brings to this remarkable topic.

The essence of Yoga is very simple: it means *yoking* or *joining*. When Christ said, "My yoke is easy," he meant "My yoga is easy"—whether East or West,

Yoga is the technique of joining or uniting the individual soul with absolute Spirit. It is a means of liberation. And it is therefore fiery, hot, intense, ecstatic. It will take you far beyond yourself; some say it will take you to infinity.

Therefore, choose your guides carefully. The book you now hold in your hands is, without a doubt, the finest overall explanation of Yoga now available, a book destined to become a classic. And for a simple reason: it comes from both the head and the heart, from impeccable scholarship and dedicated practice. In this sense, it is much more perceptive and accurate than the works of, say, Eliade or Campbell.

Enter now the world of Yoga, which is said to lead from suffering to release, from agony to ecstasy, from time to eternity, from death to immortality. And know that on this extraordinary tour, you are indeed in good hands.

KEN WILBER

Preface

My first encounter with India's spiritual heritage occurred at the age of fourteen or fifteen, through the works of Paul Brunton, whom I regard as one of the finest Western mystics of this century.[1] Brunton, who died in 1971, ranks among the pioneers of the East-West dialogue, and his writings have been widely influential. I still vividly remember the yearning I experienced when reading about Brunton's remarkable encounter with Sri Ramana Maharshi, the great sage of Tiruvannamalai in south India, whose spontaneous and effortless enlightenment at the age of sixteen became an archetypal symbol for me. I would gladly have abandoned school, which I found utterly boring, to follow in the footsteps of the great saints and Self-realizers of India.

It was in 1965 that I encountered the spirit of India more concretely in the person of a Hindu swami who was making headlines in Europe for his astounding physical feats. He was able to bear the weight of a steamroller on his chest, pull a loaded wagon with his long hair, and stop his pulse at will. While I was duly impressed by these spectacular accomplishments, they fascinated me far less than the secret behind this physical prowess.

I felt mysteriously attracted to this miracle worker with an impressive physique and a great deal of charisma. I found a way to make contact with him and ended up as his disciple, as I had intuited I would. In the year I spent with him at his hermitage in the Black Forest (West Germany), I learned a great deal about Hatha-Yoga but more about self-discipline and persistence. In the middle of winter, he had me move into a sparsely furnished room, without carpet or wallpaper and with a broken window that I was not to repair. In the early morning, I was expected to break the ice in the well and wash myself outdoors. I quickly learned that to keep warm and well, I had to stay active and do a lot of breathing. It was all rather exhilarating.

Step by step I learned about the teacher-disciple relationship, which involves trust, love, and the constant willingness to be tested. I benefited from the wonderful opportunity for self-transcendence this circumstance presents. But later I also experienced its drawbacks. Gradually I discovered that my teacher was not only an accomplished master of Hatha-Yoga but also suffered from an inflated ego—something not unheard-of in yogic circles, as I was to find out.

When I tried to break loose from that close-knit relationship, I learned another invaluable lesson: Psychic powers are a reality to be reckoned with, and some teachers will use them to hold their disciples. Although I had severed my external ties to my teacher, he continued to influence my life through psychic means, which proved most disturbing. Two clairvoyants, who knew nothing about me, independently described his bearded face with strong eyes and prominent nose, saying that he was the cause of a lot of my inner turmoil and physical troubles.

Fortunately, I never suffered the terrible agonies of a fully awakened but misconducted life-force (kundalini), as was the case, for instance, with the late Pandit Gopi Krishna. Nevertheless, I experienced firsthand some of the disturbing side effects of a kundalini that had been tampered with, particularly states of dissociation from the body. It took many years, and the benign help of another spiritual personage, before the link was finally broken and I could get on with my life. Although the experience had been rewarding on the whole, it left me disappointed, and for a good many years I steered clear of any Eastern teachers.

In the meantime I had developed an interest in learning Sanskrit and studying the great religious and philosophical writings of the Hindus in the original. I channeled my frustrated spiritual impulse into a professional career in Indology, especially Yoga research. Occasionally I dabbled with this or that yogic technique and meditative practice. However, not until 1980 did I make a more decisive spiritual gesture again. A series of life crises freed up my attention to ponder the great question *Who am I?* more seriously.

It was then that I started to scout for practical help with my inner life. I was looking for a competent teacher and a supportive environment. Since 1966 I had enjoyed the spiritual friendship of Irina Tweedie, a Sufi practitioner in England whose invaluable diary has meantime been published, and now I renewed that relationship. She helped me immensely in those days of reorientation, and thanks to her I experienced my first real spiritual break-throughs. Also, unbeknownst to me, she groomed me for a greater spiritual adventure.

In 1982 I had my first meeting with the American adept Da Free John, whose teaching had both excited and touched me deeply. This time around, with fifteen years' worth of learning behind me, it was more difficult to follow my instincts and entrust myself to the spiritual process that had mysteriously come alive in me. Da Free John fitted none of the stereotypes I had come to associate with spiritual teachers. He was not a mild-mannered, gentle sage but, by his own admission, a "wild character" and a "fire." His Dionysian quality was a shock to the Apollonian tendencies of my mind.

Yet, once I allowed my heart to make a response, this new relationship proved enormously beneficial, opening up vistas of spiritual understanding and experience for me that I had only dreamed of previously. It has also taught me just how demanding and challenging a life of self-transcendence is, especially when it is not lived in the seclusion of forest or cave but in the thick of a culture that places little value on spiritual matters. Now, seven years later, I look back with enormous gratitude for a discipleship that was difficult but also extraordinarily rewarding. Among other things, I was constantly confronted by my tendency to think about spiritual life rather than to engage it in concrete, practical terms. Whereas previously my meditations were more relaxed musings, the spiritual transmission of my teacher added an experiential depth to this process that I knew existed but had almost ceased to hope for. Although my formal pupilage under Da Free John came to an end two years ago, I continue to discover the pervasive effects of the "guru-function" in my life, for which I am profoundly grateful.

Over the years, I came to enjoy many different states of consciousness that in the past I had only read and speculated about. Now when I study the ancient Sanskrit scriptures of Yoga, I have a far more bodily sense of the meaning of their teachings and certainly a far greater appreciation of how little Western scholars, myself included, understand of the esoteric processes with which the Yoga writers were thoroughly familiar.

I felt it was necessary to begin this volume with a brief autobiographical note, because even the most "objective" treatment is shot through with personal qualities: I approach the history, philosophy, and psychology of Yoga not as an antiquarian but as someone who has the deepest appreciation for what the Indian spiritual genius has created over the millennia. I have witnessed some of its effectiveness on my own person and in the case of others who were spiritually more adept than I.

I am in basic sympathy with the spiritual traditions of India, which are authentic efforts at transcending the self. My practical experience of them encourages me to assume that their fundamental insights are genuine and worthy of serious consideration. I further maintain that anyone who wishes to disclaim any of these insights or goals must do so on the basis of personal experimentation rather than mere theoretical consideration.

In some cases, however, my own experience and knowledge oblige me to differ from the authorities of Yoga. For instance, I no longer regard the temporary state of unqualified ecstasy (nirvikalpa-samadhi), the flawless mystical merging of subject and object, as the climax of spiritual life. Such states are indeed extraordinary accomplishments, which come more naturally to some people than others, but they are inherently no more spiritual than our everyday awareness.

I have come to believe that what really matters is how we use the perspective gained in such uncommon states in our daily relationship with others and in life in general. As my twenty-one-year-old son put it to me: It all boils down to whether we love or we don't. I wish I had arrived at this insight when I was his age. The fulcrum of spiritual life is self-transcendence (which can be called "love") as a constant orientation. As I understand it, self-transcendence is not merely the pursuit of altered states of consciousness. It also implies a constant willingness to be transformed and, in Meister Eckehart's sense, to be "superformed" by the larger Reality whose existence and benignity is revealed to us in meditative and ecstatic states of awareness.

This volume is the distillate of two decades of scholarly and practical preoccupation with the tradition of Yoga. It has grown out of my earlier and long out-of-print *Textbook of Yoga,* published in 1975 by Rider & Co., London. I had borrowed three months from my postgraduate research at Durham University to write that book in the summer of 1974. Even though the volume was well received and has since been translated into several languages, I was from the beginning diffident about its many shortcomings, which I saw perhaps more clearly than most readers. Ever since then, I had been waiting for an opportunity to revise and expand the text. Then it became apparent that a completely new book was called for. So, when the present publisher expressed an interest in a comprehensive handbook on Yoga, I jumped at the opportunity —and wrote an entirely new and substantially larger book.

The objective of this volume is to give the lay reader a systematic introduction to the many-faceted phenomenon of Indian spirituality, especially in its Hindu guise, while at the same time summarizing, in broad outlines, what scholarship has discovered about the evolution of Yoga so far. This presentation should enable the reader to grasp and appreciate not only the astonishing complexity of Yoga but also its intricate relationship to other aspects of Indian culture. Inevitably I have had to deal with some rather involved ideas that will be foreign to those who have no background in philosophy, especially Eastern thought. Without watering down anything, I have tried to introduce such ideas in as graduated a fashion as possible.

To facilitate the reader's access to the wealth of material, I decided to adopt a dual approach, proceeding both by subject (in Part One) and through history (in Part Two). Because this method introduced a small amount of overlap, I have taken pains to furnish cross-references in each section as well as to supply an exhaustive index. In order to add a touch of immediacy, I have included my own translations of numerous passages from the Sanskrit scriptures that are important to a better understanding of different aspects or phases of Yoga. My translations attempt to be as literal as possible, because I believe this is the best way of doing justice to the intentions of the original text. All too often, renderings from the Sanskrit that read smoothly fail to preserve the meaning of the original work.

Originally, I had hoped to include my renderings of several key works of Yoga, such as the Yoga-Sutra of Patanjali, the Goraksha-Paddhati, and the Bhakti-Sutra of Narada. This proved infeasible, however, because it would have swelled this already substantial volume even more. I plan to make my renderings available in a future publication.

For the benefit of the nonspecialist, I have appended a chronology and a short glossary of key terms.

The emphasis throughout this work is on comprehensiveness and intelligibility. While I did my best to give each facet of Yoga a fair hearing depending on its significance in the overall picture, I could treat many issues only to a certain depth, given the purpose and scope of this volume as well as the limited number of pages available. My other publications and the works of other scholars will fill some of the gaps. However, I want to emphasize that our knowledge of the Yoga tradition is still incomplete, in some cases pitifully so. This is particularly true of Tantric Yoga, which has developed an elaborate esoteric technology and symbology.

While this volume is specifically geared toward a lay readership, I believe that its efficiency as an orientational tool also extends to specialists in the history of religion, intellectual history, theology, the study of consciousness, and transpersonal psychology. Obviously, it was not possible to proffer detailed treatments of all the different aspects of the Yoga tradition, but I have endeavored to make my portrayal as balanced as possible. It was not always easy, however, to resist the temptation of providing more detailed explanations of those aspects for which I have a special affinity and which I have studied more closely, such as Classical Yoga and the crazy wisdom tradition.

To write this book was a rewarding experience, because I was able to integrate materials that had been gestating in me for many years and because I was obliged to make my ideas as intelligible as possible, which always forces one to think and write clearly. To what degree I have succeeded in this will be determined by my readers. I hope that they will find this book as enjoyable to read as I have found it to write.

Georg Feuerstein
August 1989
Lake County, California

Acknowledgments

It remains for me to thank some of those who, in one way or another, have made this book possible. First I wish to express my heartfelt gratitude to the spiritual teachers mentioned previously, particularly Da Free John, whose teaching has revolutionized my practical understanding of spiritual matters, and Irina Tweedie, who has repeatedly demonstrated to me the immense advantage of "good company" (sat-sanga). I dedicate this volume to both teachers.

The person who encouraged me the most in my writing career, possibly without suspecting it, is Dr. Daniel Brostoff, a former editor-in-chief of Rider & Co. He adopted my first four books, when I was still struggling with the English language and publishing etiquette. Unfortunately, I have lost contact with him. Wherever you are, Daniel, I am greatly in your debt.

It is impossible to mention all the friends and colleagues who over the years have contributed to my understanding of Yoga. I particularly benefited from the fine scholarly works of Prof. J. W. Hauer and Prof. Mircea Eliade, two giants of Yoga research who are unfortunately no longer among us. The vast scholarship of Dr. Ram Shankar Bhattacharya of Varanasi, India, has also been an inspiration. More than any other researcher known to me, he is sensitive to the fact that scholars engaged in Yoga research need to be informed by Yoga practice. His always prompt and informed advice has been invaluable. Another person whose intellectual labors have inspired me for the past fifteen years is my friend Jeanine Miller. In her own field of Vedic studies, she also seeks to combine scholarship with spiritual sensitivity. I have drawn on her pioneering works for my treatment of Yoga in ancient Vedic times.

This book would not exist without the farsightedness of its publisher, Jeremy Tarcher. I am very grateful to him for his faith in my work and in making this project possible. My gratitude extends to Dan Joy, whose enthusiasm for this book knew no bounds and whose astute editorial input definitely helped make this a far more readable book. He is everything an author could hope for in an editor.

I would also like to record my gratitude to Stephan Bodian, editor of *Yoga Journal,* for having given me the opportunity over the past several years to exercise my skills in writing for a nonacademic audience.

I am beholden to Ken Wilber for his complimentary foreword. My gratitude extends to his many seminal works that have stimulated my own thinking over the years. His great gift for synthesis has been both inspiration and encouragement.

While I was working on this manuscript, two close friends volunteered much-appreciated practical help. I want to express my cordial thanks to Claudia Minkin and Stacey Koontz for assisting with some of my concurrent projects, allowing me to spend more time completing the present work. My thanks are also due to Lydia dePole for executing most of the line drawings.

Finally, I wish to record my gratitude to, and love for, my wife, Trisha. She has been my traveling companion on the spiritual path for the past seven years and my business partner for two. Her kindnesses throughout the day are numerous and her steadfastness is exemplary.

Transliteration and Pronunciation of Sanskrit Words

For the convenience of the lay reader, I have used a simplified transliteration of Sanskrit expressions, and each term is explained at its first occurrence. The expert will easily recognize the technical terms and can supply the correct diacritical marks by consulting a Sanskrit dictionary. I have also translated most titles of the Sanskrit texts mentioned. Those left untranslated either defied translation or had meanings that were obvious from the context.

Academic Transliteration	**Simplified Transliteration**
(as used in most scholarly works on the subject)	(as used in the main body of this volume)

(I) Vowels

a, ā, i, ī, u, ū, ṛ, ṝ, ḷ	a, i, u, ri, li
e, ai, o, au	e, ai, o, au

(II) Consonants

Gutturals: k, kh, g, gh, ṅ	k, kh, g, gh, n
Palatals: c, ch, j, jh, ñ	c, ch, j, jh, n
Cerebrals: ṭ, ṭh, ḍ, ḍh, ṇ	t, th, d, dh, n
Dentals: t, th, d, dh, n	t, th, d, dh, n
Labials: p, ph, b, bh, m	p, ph, b, bh, m
Semivowels: y, r, l, v	y, r, l, v
Spirants: s, ś, ṣ, h	s, sh, sh, h
Visarga: ḥ	h
Anusvara: ṃ	m

Pronunciation

The vowels *ā, ī, u̇,* and the rare *r̥* as well as the diphthongs *e, ai, o,* and *au* are long; all aspirated consonants, like *kh, gh, ch, jh,* etc., are pronounced with a distinctly discernible aspiration; e.g., *kh* as in "ink-horn," *th* as in "pot-house," etc.; *ṅ* sounds like *ng* in "king"; the palatals *c* and *j* sound like the *ch* in "church" and the *j* in "join" respectively; cerebrals are pronounced with the tongue curled back against the roof of the mouth; *s* sounds like *s* in "sin," *ṣ* like sh in "shun," and *ś* is pronounced midway between the two; *v* is pronounced like *v* in "very."

Preview

The tradition of Yoga is as complex as it is ancient. The present volume seeks to do justice to this fact. At the same time, however, this book attempts to make a potentially difficult subject matter accessible to the nonspecialist. I have always believed it is possible and desirable to combine authentic scholarship with communication to a large audience. In fact, disciplines that fail to foster such broad communication are prone to overspecialize to the point of irrelevance and barrenness. In this spirit, then, the present volume is intended as a contribution to both Yoga research and the popular understanding and appreciation of one of the great psychospiritual traditions of the world.

The chapters of Part One furnish the reader unacquainted with the subject with the necessary background and basic definitions.   Chapter 1, "Building Blocks," introduces some of the prominent features of all forms of Yoga. Thus, its first section, "The Essence of Yoga," provides an understanding of the primary purpose of Yoga, which is to transcend the ego-personality in order to recover our original Identity, the transcendental Self (atman, purusha), or Spirit.

"What's in a Name?— The Term *Yoga*" defines the Sanskrit word *yoga* more precisely and shows just how rich the traditional connotations are.

In "Degrees of Self-Transcendence: The Practitioner (Yogin)," we will look at the variety of yogic practitioners and levels of spiritual practice.

"Guiding Light: The Teacher (Guru)" introduces the important figure of the spiritual preceptor, or guru. The reader will begin to appreciate that Yoga is an initiatory tradition that places great emphasis on proper discipleship and, above all, practical experimentation.

In "Learning Beyond the Self: The Disciple (Shishya)," we will examine this theme from the perspective of the disciple (shishya), who must discover himself before he can hope to recover the transcendental Self-Identity, or Spirit.

"Giving Birth to a New Identity: Initiation (Diksha)," looks at the secret process of initiation (diksha), which is the heart of the relationship between the guru and the disciple. The reader will learn about the different types of initiation, which are all a matter of grace, transmitted by one's spiritual teacher. They open up the hidden dimension of existence and, in some cases, even reveal the Self to the spiritual aspirant.

"Crazy Wisdom and Crazy Adepts" introduces the fascinating topic of crazy wisdom, a particular style of teaching found in all the major religious traditions of the world. It affords the reader a glimpse into the work done by the guru.

Each of the eight sections of Chapter 2, which is entitled "The Wheel of Yoga," surveys one of the main schools of Yoga. Patanjali's Royal Yoga, which is discussed in section two, ("Raja-Yoga: The Resplendent Yoga of Spiritual Kings"), is the high road of meditation as taught by the adept Patanjali. His model of the eightfold path is widely known in yogic circles.

Most modern practitioners of Yoga, especially in the West, are adherents of Hatha-Yoga, the "forceful" Yoga of bodily transformation. Section three, "Hatha-Yoga: The Yoga of the Adamantine Body," can serve as an introduction to the basic philosophy and goals of this school, which is treated in more detail in Part Two, Chapter 13 ("Yoga as Spiritual Alchemy"). Perhaps the best-known modern representatives of this type of Yoga are B. K. S. Iyengar (who has trained many Western practitioners), Swami Vishnudevananda, and Swami Rama of the Himalayan Institute in Pennsylvania. That even Westerners can aquire considerable mastery in this approach to Truth was demonstrated by Theos Bernard, who underwent a traditional pupilage in the Himalayas and has been missing since 1947. His book *Hathayoga* documents, in words and telling pictures, his own story.

Section four ("Jnana-Yoga: Cultivating the Eye of Wisdom") deals with the Yoga of Wisdom, which in our century has been epitomized so well in the sagely figure of Ramana Maharshi, who was made famous by the works of Paul Brunton. Other well-known adepts of this path from our time are Sri Nisargadatta Maharaj, a contemporary sage and merchant of Bombay; Swami Jnanananda of Jyotir Mutt, a sage and yogi well known in modern south India; and (not least) Swami Vivekananda, the illustrious disciple of Sri Ramakrishna, whose missionary work is responsible for much of the contemporary Western interest in Hinduism and Yoga.

The path of love and devotion is discussed in section five ("Bhakti-Yoga: The Self-Transcending Power of Love"). This is the approach exemplified by Swami Ramakrishna, the great nineteenth-century mystic and the guru of Vivekananda; the beloved Swami Ramdas, who renounced the world in 1922 and who, until his death in 1963, constantly recited the name *Ram* (signifying the Divine); as well as the widely venerated woman saint Anandamayi Ma, who lived and taught in modern Bengal, a region that since pre-Christian times has spawned a never-ending stream of spiritual heroes.

The Yoga of Action is dealt with in section six ("Karma-Yoga: Freedom in Action"). Its best-known practitioner in modern times is undoubtedly Mahatma Gandhi. Today we may add another (Christian) name recognized worldwide—Mother Teresa.

In section seven ("Mantra-Yoga: Sound as a Vehicle of Transcendence"), we take a look at the Yoga of sacred power-sounds, which is often presented as the easiest of all spiritual paths. This approach has won tens of thousands of Western followers, especially in the form of Transcendental Meditation as taught by Maharshi Mahesh Yogi.

Finally, Laya-Yoga, which can be equated with Kundalini-Yoga, is discussed in section eight ("Laya-Yoga: Dissolving the Universe"). This Yoga is not easily understood. Some of its technicalities are introduced in Chapters 12 and 13 of Part Two, which deal with Tantrism and Hatha-Yoga. Perhaps the widely known teaching of Swami Muktananda can serve as a reference point for understanding the nature of this highly esoteric path. Also, the works of Gopi Krishna, in particular his spectacular autobiography, furnish the reader with the flavor of the Tantric or Kundalini-Yogic approach.

In Chapter 3 ("Yoga and Other Hindu Traditions"), we will examine the relationship of the proliferous Yoga movement to other schools of thought within the fold of Hinduism. This will give the reader a deepening appreciation of the degree to which Yoga has inspired, and been inspired by, other systems. Part Two, which forms the core of this volume, is a comprehensive outline of the historical unfolding of the Yoga tradition within Hinduism.

This part begins with a brief statement about the importance of knowing history.

Then, in Chapter 4 ("Yoga in Ancient Times"), readers will travel back in time to the very earliest beginnings of Indian culture. They will learn about the splendid civilization that once thrived along the Indus river, the invasion of the Sanskrit-speaking tribes that brought with them much sacred knowledge, ancient Indian magic, and the mysterious brotherhoods that were in part responsible for the creation of Yoga.

Chapter 5 ("The Whispered Wisdom of the Early Upanishads") deals with the most ancient Upanishads, the oldest repositories of nondualist esoteric teachings. It was during the time of these Upanishads that the great Vedanta doctrine of the identity of the self with the transcendental Reality was first announced. Aham brahma asmi, "I am the Absolute," said the Upanishadic sages.

Yogic ideas and practices are not confined to Hinduism. They can also be found in India's two other great spiritual traditions, Buddhism and Jainism. Chapters 6 ("Jaina Yoga") and 7 ("Yoga in Buddhism") provide an introduction to the yogic teachings in those two traditions. They will give the reader a sufficient basis for independently launching into a study of Buddhist and Jaina Yoga.

The ten sections of Chapter 8 ("The Flowering of Yoga") deal with an exciting phase in the evolution of Yoga—the centuries immediately preceding the Christian era. They produced, among other things, the greatest and most popular of all Yoga scriptures, the Bhagavad-Gita. It was during this time that Yoga emerged as a truly independent tradition within Hinduism.

In the five sections of Chapter 9 ("Yoga as Philosophy and Religion"), the reader will be introduced to the philosophy of Raja-Yoga, or Classical Yoga, with its eight limbs. Each limb is carefully explained according to the Yoga-Sutra of Patanjali.

The yogic developments subsequent to Patanjali can conveniently be labeled Post-Classical Yoga. They show an astounding richness and diversity. The six sections of Chapter 10 ("The Nondual Approach to God") are an attempt to capture some of this wealth of yogic experimentation and thought on paper. Chapter 11 ("God, Visions, and Power"), which deals with the medieval Yoga-Upanishads, continues the investigation started in the preceding chapter.

With Chapter 12 ("The Esotericism of Medieval Tantra Yoga") we arrive at the climax of the unfolding story of Yoga. It treats Tantrism, which represents one of the most misunderstood chapters in the history of Indian spirituality. Tantrism is an approach that seeks to incorporate the primary fact of our human embodiment into the spiritual quest, leading to a positive evaluation of bodily existence. Because of this body- and sex-positive orientation, Tantrism has undergone a certain renaissance in the West. Largely, however, this neo-Tantrism falls short of the original Indian tradition, which has nothing to do with hedonism but everything to do with transcending the ego-personality, even (and especially) when sexual intercourse is used in a sacred context.

In Hatha-Yoga, which is discussed in more detail in Chapter 13 ("Yoga as Spiritual Alchemy"), the esoteric Tantric work of uniting Male (shiva) and Female (shakti) is pursued not so much through sexual means but through processes of psychosomatic integration.

Our historical survey ends with Hatha-Yoga. The Chronology at the back of this volume provides readers with a quick overview of these 3000-year-long developments.

Apart from the Integral Yoga of Sri Aurobindo, there have been no major innovative developments in Yoga during the past 200 years. However, Yoga is what the late Mircea Eliade has called a "living fossil," and it continues to grow and unfold—now also in Western countries. The dialogue between East and West has only just begun. There is no telling how Western attitudes and insights into reality will shape the evolution of Yoga, or how yogic wisdom will help transform our Occidental world-view. What is certain is that the traditions of India, especially Yoga, have already made a tremendous impact on our Western culture. They have been responsible, along with other influences, for the spiritual renaissance that we are witnessing today. This book is intended as a contribution to this promising beginning.

Introduction: The Impulse Toward Transcendence

REACHING BEYOND THE EGO-PERSONALITY

The desire to transcend the human condition, to go beyond our ordinary consciousness and personality, is a deeply rooted impulse that is as old as humanity. We can see it at work in the magically charged cave paintings of southern Europe and, earlier still, in the Stone Age burials of the Middle East. In both cases, the desire to connect with a larger reality is expressed. We also encounter that desire in the animistic beliefs and rites of archaic shamanism, and we see its flowering in the religious traditions of the neolithic age—of Sumer, Egypt, India, and China.

But nowhere on earth has the impulse toward transcendence found more consistent and creative expression than on the Indian peninsula. The civilization of India has spawned an almost overwhelming variety of spiritual beliefs, practices, and approaches. These are all targeted at a dimension of reality that eclipses our individual human lives and the orderly cosmos of our human imagination. That dimension has variously been called God, the Absolute, the (transcendental) Self, the Spirit, the Unconditional, and the Eternal.

Different thinkers, mystics, and sages—not only of India but from around the world—have given us a plethora of images or explanations of the ultimate Reality and its relation to the manifest universe. All, however, are in agreement that God, or the Self, transcends both language and the mind. With few exceptions, they are also unanimous in making three related claims, namely that the Ultimate

1. is *single*—that is, an undivided Whole complete in itself, outside which nothing else exists;

1

2. is of a higher degree of *reality* than the world of multiplicity reflected to us through our senses; and

3. is our highest good—that is, the *most desirable* of all possible values.

Additionally, many mystics claim that the ultimate Reality is utterly blissful. This bliss is not merely the absence of pain or discomfort, nor is it a brain-dependent state. It is beyond pain and pleasure, which *are* states of the nervous system. This goes hand in hand with the insistence of mystics that their realization of the transcendental Identity is not an experience, as ordinarily understood. Such adepts simply *are* that Reality. Therefore, I prefer to speak of God- or Self-*realization* as opposed to mystical *experience*.

India's spirituality is undoubtedly the most versatile in the world. In fact, it is hard to think of any metaphysical problem or solution that has not already been thought of by the sages and pundits of ancient or medieval India. The "sacred technicians" of India have experienced and analyzed the entire spectrum of psychospiritual possibilities—from paranormal states to the unitive consciousness of temporary God-realization to permanent enlightenment (known as sahaja-samadhi, "spontaneous ecstasy").

The methods and lifestyles developed by the Indian philosophical and spiritual geniuses over a period of at least three millennia all have one and the same purpose: to help us break through the habit patterns of our ordinary consciousness and to realize our identity (or at least union) with the perennial Reality. India's great traditions of psychospiritual growth understand themselves as paths of liberation. Their goal is to liberate us from our conventional conditioning and hence also free us from suffering, because suffering is a product of our unconscious conditioning. In other words, they are avenues to God-realization, or Self-realization, which is an utterly blissful condition.

God, in this sense, is not the Creator-God of deistic religions like Judaism, Islam, and Christianity. Rather, God is the transcendental totality of existence, which in the nondualist schools of Hinduism is styled the brahman, "Absolute." That Absolute is regarded as the essential nature, the transcendental Self, underlying the human personality. Hence, when the unconscious conditioning by which we experience ourselves as independent egos is removed, we realize that at the core of our being we are all that same One. And this singular Reality is considered the ultimate destination of human evolution. As the modern yogin-philosopher Sri Aurobindo put it:

> We speak of the evolution of Life in Matter, the evolution of Mind in Matter; but evolution is a word which merely states the phenomenon without explaining it. For there seems to be no reason why Life should evolve out of material elements or Mind out of living form, unless we accept the Vedantic[1] solution that Life is already involved in Matter and Mind in Life because in essence Matter is a form of veiled Life, Life a form of veiled Consciousness. And then there seems to be little objection to a farther step in the series and the admission that mental consciousness may itself be only a form and a veil of higher states which are beyond Mind. In that case, the unconquerable impulse of man towards God,

Light, Bliss, Freedom, Immortality presents itself in its right place in the chain as simply the imperative impulse by which Nature is seeking to evolve beyond Mind, and appears to be as natural, true and just as the impulse towards Life which she has planted in certain forms of Matter or the impulse towards Mind which she has planted in certain forms of Life. . . . Man himself may well be a thinking and living laboratory in whom and with whose conscious co-operation she wills to work out the superman, the god. Or shall we not say, rather, to manifest God?[2]

The idea that the impulse toward transcendence is a primary and omnipresent, if mostly hidden, force in our lives has lately been vocalized by a number of eminent transpersonal psychologists, notably Ken Wilber. He speaks of this force as the "Atman project":

Development is evolution; evolution is transcendence; . . . and transcendence has as its final goal Atman, or ultimate Unity Consciousness in only God. All drives are a subset of that Drive, all wants a subset of that Want, all pushes a subset of that Pull—and that whole movement is what we call the Atman-project: the drive of God towards God, Buddha towards Buddha, Brahman towards Brahman, but carried out initially through the intermediary of the human psyche, with results that range from ecstatic to catastrophic.[3]

The impulse toward transcendence is thus intrinsic to human life. It manifests itself not only in humanity's religiospiritual search but also in the aspirations of science, technology, philosophy, theology, and art. This may not always be obvious, especially in those areas that, like contemporary science, are anxious to deny any associations with metaphysical thought and instead pay homage to the twin idols of skepticism and objectivity. Nevertheless, as perceptive critics of the scientific enterprise have pointed out, in its passionate quest for knowledge and meaning, science is merely usurping the supreme place that was once accorded to religion and theology.

Today, the metaphysical roots of science are rendered visible especially by quantum physics, which undermines the materialistic ideology that has been the creed of many, if not most, scientists for the past 200 years. In fact, avant-garde physicists like David Bohm, Fritjof Capra, and Fred Alan Wolf have formulated broad quantum-physical interpretations of reality that converge in many respects with traditional Eastern ideas about the fundamental structure of the world: The universe is a single and ultimately unimaginable sea of energy in which differentiated "forms" appear and disappear, possibly forever. Quantum physicist Gary Zukav writes:

Quantum mechanics, for example, shows us that we are not as separate from the rest of the world as we once thought. Particle physics shows us that the "rest of the world" does not sit idly "out there". It is a sparkling realm of continual creation, transformation, and annihilation. The ideas of the new physics, when wholly grasped, can produce extraordinary *experiences*. The study of relativity theory, for example, can produce the remarkable experience that space and time are only mental constructions![4]

It is clear from the work of such creative scientists as those mentioned above that science, like every other human endeavor, harbors within itself the impulse toward transcendence.

If we look upon science and technology as forms of the same impulse toward transcendence that has motivated the Indian sages to explore the inner universe of consciousness, we can see many things from a radically new perspective. We need not regard science and technology as *perversions* of the spiritual impulse, but rather as *unconscious expressions* of it. No moral judgment is implied here, and we can simply set about introducing a more comprehensive and self-critical awareness into the scientific and technological enterprise. In this way, we can hope to transform what has become a runaway obsession of the rational mind into an authentic and legitimate pursuit in service of the whole human being and the whole of humankind.

In Rabindranath Tagore's delightful work *Gitanjali,* there is a line that sums up our modern attitude, which is one of dilemma: "Freedom is all I want, but to hope for it I feel ashamed."[5] We feel ashamed and awkward because we feel that the pursuit of spiritual freedom, or ecstasy, belongs to a bygone age, a lost world view. But this is only a half-truth. While certain conceptions of and approaches to spiritual freedom are clearly antiquated, freedom and its pursuit are as important and relevant today as they have ever been. The desire to be free is a timeless urge and concern. We want freedom, or abiding happiness, but we seldom acknowledge this deep-seated wish. It remains on the level of an unconscious program, secretly motivating us in all our undertakings— from scientific and technological ingenuity to artistic creativity, to religious fervor, to sports, to sexuality, to socializing, and, alas, also to drug and alcohol addiction. We seek to be fulfilled, made whole or happy by all these pursuits. Of course, we find that whatever happiness or freedom we gain is frustratingly ephemeral, and we take this as an incentive to continue our ritual quest for self-fulfillment by seeking further stimulation.

Today, however, we can take encouragement from the new vision embodied in quantum physics and transpersonal psychology and boldly raise this urge to the level of a conscious need. In that event, the unrivaled wisdom of the liberation teachings of India and the Far East will assume a new significance for us, and the present-day encounter between East and West can fulfill itself.

TECHNOLOGIES OF EAST AND WEST

Material technology has changed human life and the face of our home planet more than any other cultural force, but its gifts to humanity have not always proven to be benign. Since the 1970s the public attitude toward technology, and indirectly toward science, has become increasingly ambivalent. In the words of Colin Norman, an editor of *Science* magazine, technology is "the God that limps."[6] It is a God that thrives on logic but suffers from a dearth of wisdom. The consequences of a technology that is destitute of balanced judgment need no spelling out; they are everywhere apparent in our planet's ecology.

A different attitude prevails in the "counter"-technology of India, which is essentially a matter of wisdom and personal growth. It has evolved over millennia on the rich humus of hard-won inner experience, psychospiritual maturation, nonordinary states of consciousness, and (not least) the condition of liberation itself. The discoveries and accomplishments of the Indian spiritual virtuosos are at least as remarkable as electric motors, computers, space flight, organ transplants, or gene splicing. Their practical teachings can indeed be considered a type of technology that seeks to achieve control over the inner universe, the environment of consciousness.

Psychospiritual technology is applied knowledge and wisdom that is geared toward serving the larger evolutionary destiny of humankind by fostering the psychospiritual maturation of the individual. It avoids the danger of runaway technology by placing at its center a deep concern not merely for what is *possible* but for what is *necessary*. It is thus an ethical technology that views the human individual as a multidimensional and, above all, *self-transcending* being. It is, by definition, a technology that revolves around human wholeness. In the last analysis, psychospiritual technology is not even anthropocentric but theocentric, having Reality itself as its final reference point. If technology is,

Destruction of the Ecology and the Human Race	**Individual and Collective Wholeness**
↑	↑
Psychic Imbalance	Recognition of the Need for Integration
↑	↑
Dehumanization through the Materialistic Denial of Spiritual Values	Dehumanization through the "Psychification" of Spiritual Values
↑	↑
Material Technology	Psycho-Spiritual Technology
↑	↑
Desire to Conquer Nature	Desire to Master the Ego-Personality

Hidden Impulse toward Self-Transcendence

Two kinds of technology and their possibilities.

in the words of physicist Freeman J. Dyson, "a gift of God,"[7] psychotechnology is a way to God. The former technology can, if used rightly, liberate us from economic want and social distress. The latter can, if applied wisely, free us from the psychic proclivity of living as self-encapsulated beings at odds with ourselves and the world.

Psychospiritual technology is more than applied knowledge and wisdom. It is also an instrument of knowledge, insofar as its use opens up new vistas of self-understanding, which include the higher dimensions of the world that form the reaches of inner space.

The Indian liberation teachings—the great Yogas of Hinduism, Buddhism, and Jainism—clearly represent an invaluable resource for contemporary humankind. We have barely scratched the surface of what they have to offer us. It is obvious, however, that in order to find our way out of the tunnel of materialistic scientism, we require more than knowledge, information, statistics, mathematical formulas, sociopolitical programs, and technological solutions.

We are in need of wisdom. And what better way is there to rejuvenate our hearts and restore the wholeness of our being than to look to the wisdom of the East, especially the great, lucid insights and realizations of the Indian seers, sages, mystics, and holy folk?

REALITY AND MODELS OF REALITY

It is important to remember that India's spiritual technology, like Western exotechnology, is also based on *models* of reality only. The ultimate realization, known as enlightenment or awakening, is ineffable: It transcends thought and speech. Hence the moment the God-realized adept opens his or her mouth to speak of the nature of that realization, he or she must resort to metaphors, images, and models—and models are intrinsically limited in their capacity to communicate that condition.

In some respects, the models proposed in the consciousness disciplines of the East have greater fidelity to reality than those proposed by modern science. The reason for this is that the yogic models are grounded in a more comprehensive sensitivity to what there is. The yogins use means of cognition that are barely acknowledged to exist by Western scientists, such as clairvoyance and higher states of identification with the object of contemplation, which are called samadhi. In other words, Yoga operates with a more sophisticated theory of knowledge (epistemology) and theory of being (ontology), recognizing levels or dimensions of existence that are barely suspected to exist by science. At the same time, however, those traditional spiritual models are not as rigorously formulated as their modern Western counterparts. They are more intuitive-hortatory than analytical-descriptive. Their purpose is not to accumulate knowledge about the world but to transcend all knowledge and every possible model. Manifestly, each approach has its distinct field of application and usefulness, and both can learn from each other.

The reigning paradigm of Western science is Newtonian materialistic dualism, which affirms that there are real subjects (observers) confronting real objects "out there." This view has of late been challenged by quantum physics, which suggests that there is no reality entirely divorced from the observer. India's psychospiritual technology is likewise subject to a ruling paradigm, which can be described as verticalism: Reality is thought to be realizable by turning attention inward and then manipulating the inwardly focused consciousness to ascend into ever-higher states in the inner hierarchy of experience, until everything is transcended. Thus, the typical motto of Indian Yoga is "in, up, and out."

This vertical model of spirituality is founded in archaic mythical imagery that pictures Reality in polar opposition to conditional existence: heaven above, earth below. As the contemporary adept Da Free John has shown, this model is a conceptual representation of the human nervous system. As he put it succinctly:

> The key to mystical language and religious metaphor is not theology or cosmology but anatomy. All the religious and cosmological language of mysticism is metaphorical. And the metaphors are symbols for anatomical features of the higher functional structures of the human individual.
>
> Those who enter deeply into the mystical dimension of experience soon discover that the cosmic design they expected to find in their inward path of ascent to God is in fact simply the design of their own anatomical or psycho-physical structures. Indeed, this is the secret divulged to initiates of mystical schools.[8]

The most severe limitation of the verticalist paradigm is that it involves an understanding of spiritual life as a progressive inward journey from unenlightenment to enlightenment. This gives rise to the misconception that Reality is to be found only within, away from the world, and that, consequently, to renounce the world means to abandon it.

It is to the credit of India's adepts that this paradigm did not remain unchallenged. For instance, in the tradition of Tantrism, which straddles both Hinduism and Buddhism, a different understanding of spirituality is present. As I will elaborate in a later chapter, Tantrism is founded in the radical assumption that if Reality is anywhere, It must be everywhere and not merely inside the human psyche or beyond the world.[9] The great dictum of Tantrism is that the transcendental Reality and the conditional world are coessential — nirvana equals samsara. In other words, transcendental ecstasy and sensory pleasure are not finally incompatible. Upon enlightenment, pleasure reveals itself to be ecstasy. In the unenlightened state, pleasure is simply a substitute for the ecstasy that is its abiding ground. This insight has led to a beginning integration between spiritual concerns and material existence, which is particularly relevant today.

YOGA AND THE MODERN WEST

We need not, of course, become converts to any path, or accept yogic ideas and practices without questioning. Carl Gustav Jung's warning that we should not attempt to transplant Eastern teachings into the West holds true *in principle;* mere imitation does more harm than good.[10] The reason is that if we adopt ideas and lifestyles without truly assimilating them emotionally and intellectually, we run the risk of living inauthentic lives. In other words, our role playing gets the better of us.

Yet, in our struggle for self-understanding and psychospiritual growth, we can benefit immensely from a liberal exposure to India's spiritual legacy. Jung was pessimistic about people's ability to sift the wheat from the chaff, or to learn and grow whole even from their negative experiences.

Moreover, his insistence that Westerners differ radically in their psychic constitution from Easterners is plainly incorrect. There are indeed psychoconstitutional differences between the Eastern and the Western branches of the human family—differences that are readily apparent to seasoned travelers and to those who cross the cultural divide between "East" and "West" or "North" and "South" in order to do business. These differences are, admittedly, even considerable when we compare ancient Easterners and contemporary Westerners, but they are not radical or unbridgeable. With the possible exception of a few isolated tribal peoples, humanity has shared the same structures of consciousness ever since what the German philosopher-psychiatrist Karl Jaspers has called the "axial age," the great transformative period around the middle of the first millennium B.C. During the axial age, the world of antiquity went beyond the dreamlike quality of thought of the earlier mythological age. Pioneering spirits like Pythagoras, Socrates, Gautama the Buddha, Mahavira, Lao Tzu, and Confucius embodied a new cognitive capacity—the ability to think rationally rather than in purely mythological terms.[11] Hence we can resonate with the ancient teachings of Yoga, even though they are the product of a psychic constitution and culture that did not yet suffer from the unbalanced growth of left-brained thought, or reason, which is the hallmark of our own epoch.[12]

The dialogue between East and West is one of the most significant events of our century. If, as Jung confidently asserted, the West will create its own Yoga in the centuries to come, it will not be on the foundations of Christianity alone, which was his contention, but rather on the new foundations laid as a result of that dialogue between the two halves of planetary humankind. At any rate, it is important to understand that this dialogue is necessarily a *personal* matter, which occurs on the stage of the individual's heart and mind. That means we—you and I—must initiate and nurture it. This undertaking is an enormous challenge and obligation but also an unparalleled opportunity for assisting the "Atman project," as it moves us toward our own awakening in the larger Reality.

PART ONE

FOUNDATIONS

योग आनन्दकल्पनः

chapter 1
Building Blocks

THE ESSENCE OF YOGA

Yoga is a spectacularly multifaceted phenomenon, and as such is very difficult to define because there are exceptions to every conceivable rule. What all branches and schools of Yoga have in common, however, is that they are concerned with a state of being, or consciousness, that is truly extraordinary. One ancient Yoga authority captures this essential orientation in the following equation: "Yoga is ecstasy."[1]

In this context, the Sanskrit word for "ecstasy" is *samadhi*. This term will be encountered again and again in this volume, and therefore it seems appropriate to explain it more carefully. Sanskrit, the language in which most Yoga scriptures are written, is particularly suited for philosophical and psychological discourse. It allows the concise expression of nuances in thought that in English often require several terms. The word *samadhi*, for instance, is composed of the prefixes *sam* (similar to the Latin *syn*) and *a*, followed by the verbal root *dha* ("to place, put") in its feminine form *dhi*. The literal meaning of the term is thus "placing, putting together."

What is put together, or unified, is the conscious subject and its object or objects. Samadhi is both the *technique* of unifying consciousness and the resulting *state* of ecstatic union with the object of contemplation. Christian mystics speak of this condition as the "mystical union" *(unio mystica)*. As the world-renowned historian of religion Mircea Eliade observed, samadhi is really "enstasy" rather than "ecstasy."[2] The Greek-derived word *ecstasy* means to stand *(stasis)* outside *(ex)* the ordinary self, whereas *samadhi* signifies one's standing *(stasis)* in *(en)* the Self, the transcendental Essence of the personality. But both interpretations are correct, because we can only abide in and as the Self (atman) when we transcend the ego-self (ahamkara). For convenience, I will therefore render the term *samadhi* consistently as "ecstasy," asking the reader to bear in mind the other connotation. Yoga, then, is the technology of ecstasy, of self-transcendence. How this ecstatic condition is interpreted and what means are proposed for its realization differ, as we will see, from school to school.

The Sanskrit term *yoga* is most frequently interpreted as the "union" of the individual self (jiva-atman) with the transcendental Self (parama-atman). This definition is at home in the nondualist tradition of Vedanta, the dominant branch of Hindu philosophy, which has also greatly influenced the majority of Yoga schools. Vedanta originated with the ancient esoteric scriptures known as the Upanishads, which first taught the "inner ritual" of meditation on, and absorption into, the unitary Ground of all existence.[3]

According to Vedanta, the individual self is alienated from its transcendental Core, the supreme Self, which is none other than the Absolute (brahman). How this alienation is understood varies from school to school. Some regard the finite self, together with the phenomenal universe, as merely illusory or a superimposition on Reality; others consider it to be quite real but caught in the "dis-ease" of estrangement from the ultimate Reality. Because of these differing notions about the true existential status of the individual self, there are also a variety of interpretations of the nature of its re-union with the transcendental Reality. Some schools of thought even deny that there can be such a re-union, because we are never separated from the Ground, and our discovery of this fact is more a kind of remembering our eternal status as the ever-blissful transcendental Self.

While the notion of union makes some sense within the tradition of Vedanta, it is not representative of all forms of Yoga. It is valid in regard to the earlier (Pre-Classical) schools of Yoga belonging to the pre-Christian era, and it also applies to the later (Post-Classical) schools of Yoga, which subscribe to a type of Vedantic nondualist philosophy. However, the metaphor of union does not at all fit the system of Classical Yoga, as formulated by Patanjali in the second century A.D. In Patanjali's Yoga-Sutra, the basic scripture of Classical Yoga, there is no mention of a union with the transcendental Reality as the ultimate target of the yogic endeavor. Given Patanjali's dualistic metaphysics, which strictly separates the transcendental Self from Nature (prakriti) and its products, this would not even make any sense.

One of Patanjali's aphorisms (II.44) merely refers to a coming in "contact" with one's "chosen deity" (ishta-devata) as a result of intense self-study. This chosen deity is not the Absolute itself but a specific deity of the Hindu pantheon, like Shiva, Vishnu, Krishna, or the Goddess Kali.[4] The yogin, in other words, may have a vision of his adopted *representation* of the transcenden-

अथ योगानुशासनम् ॥१॥

Patanjali's introductory aphorism (sutra) defining Yoga.

tal Reality, just as a devout Christian may have a visionary encounter with his favorite patron saint. No more is implied in that aphorism.

Patanjali defines Yoga simply as "the restriction of the whirls of consciousness" (citta-vritti-nirodha). That is to say, Yoga is the focusing of attention to whatever object is being contemplated to the exclusion of all others. Ultimately, attention must be focused on the transcendental Self. This is not merely a matter of preventing thoughts from arising. It is a whole-bodily focusing in which one's entire being is quieted. As is clear from a study of the Yoga-Sutra, the terms *citta* and *vritti* are part of Patanjali's technical vocabulary and therefore have fairly precise meanings. We learn, for instance, that the process of restriction reaches far deeper than the verbal mind, because in the end one's entire conditional being must be held in a state of balance and transparency. We can readily appreciate the difficulty of this undertaking when we try to stop the conveyor belt of our own thinking even for thirty seconds.

Patanjali explains that when this psychomental stoppage has been successfully accomplished, the transcendental Witness-Consciousness shines forth. This Witness-Consciousness, or "Seer" (drashtri), is the pure Awareness (cit) that abides eternally beyond the senses and the mind, uninterruptedly apperceiving all the numerous and changeable contents of consciousness. All schools of Hinduism agree that the ultimate Reality is not a condition of stonelike stupor but superconsciousness.

This assertion is not mere speculation but is based on the actual realization of thousands of yogins, and their great discovery is corroborated by the testimony of mystics in other parts of the world. The immutable Essence, or Spirit, of the human being is Being-Consciousness. All else is, according to Patanjali's philosophy, insentient matter that pertains to the realm of Nature, the counterpole to the Witness-Consciousness.

Classical Yoga avows a strict dualism between Spirit (purusha) and Matter (prakriti), which is reminiscent of Gnosticism, the esoteric movement that rivaled Christianity and flourished in the Mediterranean around the same time that Patanjali composed his aphorisms. On the strength of this uncompromising dualism, King Bhoja of the eleventh century A.D., who wrote a learned commentary on the Yoga-Sutra, was able to propose that *yoga* really means *viyoga*, "separation": The basic technique of Classical Yoga, argued King Bhoja, is the "discernment" (viveka) between the transcendental Self and the "nonself" (anatman), which is the entire psychophysical personality, belonging to the realm of matter.

Having understood this all-important difference between Spirit and mind, the yogin next attempts to withdraw, step by step, from that which he has recognized as not constituting his essential nature, namely from the body-mind in its entirety. This gradual separation from the phenomenal reality is completed when the yogin has recovered his true Identity, *as* the transcendental Witness-Consciousness.

Interestingly, this procedure is adopted even in the nondualist schools of

Yoga and Vedanta, where it is known as apavada ("annulment"). It is the method of neti-neti ("not thus, not thus"), as invented by the sages whose innovative teachings are recorded in the ancient Upanishads. This method consists in a progressive withdrawal of attention from the various aspects of psychophysical existence, thereby leading to a gradual dismantling of the false sense of identity with a particular body-mind-ego. This approach is strikingly illustrated in the Nirvana-Shatka, a well-known didactic poem ascribed to Shankara, who lived in the late eighth century A.D. and is widely recognized as the greatest authority of nondualist Vedanta:

> Om. I am not reason, intuition (buddhi), egoity (ahamkara), or memory. Neither am I hearing, tasting, smelling, or sight; neither ether nor earth; fire or air. I am Shiva, in the form of Consciousness-Bliss. I am Shiva. (1)

This describes the *via negativa* of Hindu spirituality. At the same time it affords a good example for the alternative, and often complementary, method recommended by the authorities of Vedanta: Rather than "dismembering" himself, the yogin presumes his fundamental Identity as the transcendental Being-Consciousness. Thus, he affirms "I am the Absolute" (aham brahma asmi) or, as in the above-quoted text, "I am Shiva" (shivo'ham). Shiva is here not a personal deity but the Absolute itself. This affirmative procedure is extolled in the Tejo-Bindu-Upanishad (III.1–43), a work of post-Christian origin, where God Shiva himself at some length instructs the sage Kumara in the highest realization. Here is an excerpt of Shiva's ecstatic confession-instruction:

> I am the supreme Absolute. I am supreme Bliss. I am of the form of unique Knowledge. I am unique and transcendental. (1)
>
> I am of the form of unique tranquillity. I am made of unique Awareness (cit). I am of the form of unique eternity. I am everlasting. (2)
>
> I am of the form of unique Being (sattva). Having relinquished the I, I am. I am of the essence of That which is devoid of all. I am made of the ether of Awareness. (3)
>
> I am of the form of the unique "Fourth" (turya).[5] I am the unique [Reality] transcending the Fourth. I am ever of the form of Consciousness (caitanya). (4)

We may assume that Shankara, the famous sage who composed the above passage, did so in the ecstatic or enlightened disposition. He was not in an "altered" state of consciousness, nor was he simply making a pious declaration. He was not merely submerged in the condition of unqualified ecstasy (nirvikalpa-samadhi), for in that condition no body-awareness and therefore no speech is possible. Rather, he spoke *as* that singular Being-Consciousness.

His enlightenment was not a momentary flash but a permanent plateau realization. He spoke as an enlightened or liberated adept, a self-transcender of the highest order.

Liberation (mukti, moksha) is the continuous ecstatic enjoyment of the transcendental Self-identity. It is the *raison d'être* of all authentic Yoga. The technology of Yoga fulfills itself in its own transcendence. For liberation is not a technique but a way of being in the world. After climbing to the topmost rung on the ladder of Yoga, the accomplished yogin kicks off the ladder and abandons himself to the infinite play of Reality.

WHAT'S IN A NAME?—THE TERM *YOGA*

Our world, the sages of ancient India tell us, is but a wonderfully bewitching collage of name (nama) and form (rupa). In this they anticipated contemporary philosophy. Reality is a continuum that we divide up into a multitude of discrete phenomena, and we do so by means of language. Our naming of things in a way creates them. Our words reify, or "thingify," reality. For the most part, this is of practical usefulness when we want to find our way about in our rather complex universe. However, it can also be a handicap, because our words may set up barriers that block understanding and stifle love. Nevertheless, so long as we remember that words are not identical with the reality they are meant to denote, they can be useful.

Thus, it seems appropriate to inquire into the meaning of the word *yoga*. in its technical sense, *yoga* refers to that enormous body of spiritual values, attitudes, precepts, and techniques that have been developed in India over three millennia and that may be regarded as the very foundation of the ancient indian civilization. *Yoga* is thus the generic name for the various Indian paths of ecstatic self-transcendence, or the methodical transmutation of consciousness to the point of liberation from the spell of the ego-personality. It is the psychospiritual technology specific to the great civilization of India.

By way of extension, the word *yoga* has also been applied to those traditions that have been directly or indirectly inspired by the Indian sources, such as tibetan Yoga (Vajrayana Buddhism), Chinese Yoga (ch'an), and Japanese Yoga (Zen). It is, however, somewhat misleading to speak of a Hebrew Yoga or a Christian Yoga, unless the word *yoga* is employed as a straightforward

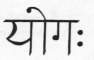

The Sanskrit word "yoga" in the devanagari script.

substitute for "mysticism" or "spirituality." Both Jewish and Christian mysticism have sprung up independent of the Indian spiritual adventure, and only in this century has there been some attempt to utilize yogic ideas and practices within the Judeo-christian tradition.[6]

In its restricted sense, the term *yoga* stands for the system of Classical Yoga as propounded by Patanjali in the early post-christian era. It is counted among the six great traditions or viewpoints (darshana) of Hinduism. The other five orthodox traditions are Nyaya, Vaisheshika, Samkhya, Mimamsa, and Vedanta. The relationship of Yoga to these systems is treated in Chapter 3 ("Yoga and other Hindu Traditions").

It should also be noted that the term *yoga* is used at times in the Sanskrit scriptures to denote the actual goal of Yoga—that is, the condition of liberation. In rare instances, the word is even used to refer to the adherent of the Yoga tradition—the yogin, to whom I will turn next.[7]

The term *yoga* is frequently used in the Sanskrit literature. The word is already employed in many ways in the ancient Rig-veda, which is to the pious hindu what the Old Testament is to the Christian. It is a collection of archaic hymns, many of which date back to about 1500 B.C., and as such is the oldest literary signpost of the Indo-europeans. The word *yoga* is etymologically derived from the verbal root *yuj*, meaning "to bind together, to yoke," and can have many connotations, such as "union," "conjunction of stars," "grammatical rule," "endeavor," "occupation," "team," "equipment," "means," "trick," "magic," "aggregate," "sum," and so on. It is related to English *yoke*, french *joug*, german *joch*, greek *zugos*, latin *iugum*, russion *igo*, spanish *yugo*, and Swedish *ok*, which all have similar meanings.

In the ninth century A.D., Vacaspati Mishra composed a scholarly subcommentary, entitled Tattva-Vaisharadi, on Patanjali's aphorisms. At the outset of this work, he notes that the term *yoga* should be derived from the root *yuja* (in the sense of "concentration") and not from *yuji* (in the sense of "conjunction"). Perhaps Vacaspati Mishra felt called to make this comment because, as we have seen, in the nondualist tradition of Vedanta, the term *yoga* is frequently explained as the union (samyoga) between the individual self and the transcendental Self. This definition does not strictly apply to Classical yoga, which is dualistic, distinguishing as it does between the transcendental self and multiform Nature.

In the Mahabharata (XIV.43.24), one of India's two national epics, the characteristic mark of Yoga is said to be "activity" (pravritti). This reminds one of the definition in the Bhagavad-gita (II.50), the Hindu equivalent of the new Testament, according to which "yoga is skill in action." This means that the yogin performs his allotted work and discharges his obligations without hankering for any reward. This attitude is further explained in the "karma-yoga" section of Chapter 2.

The Bhagavad-gita (II.48) also defines *yoga* as "equanimity" (samatva). this Sanskrit word means literally "sameness" or "evenness" and has all kinds of overtones. Essentially it is the attitude of looking dispassionately at life and being unruffled by its ups and downs.

DEGREES OF SELF-TRANSCENDENCE: THE PRACTITIONER (YOGIN)

The word *yogin* (in the nominative: *yogi*) is derived from the same verbal root as *yoga* and denotes the practitioner of Yoga, who may be a novice, an advanced student, or even a full-fledged, God- or Self-realized adept. A female practitioner is called *yogini*.[8] The designation *yogin* is generally loosely applied to all spiritual practitioners. Sometimes a distinction is made—for instance, between the yogin and the samnyasin (renouncer), or between the yogin (as a practitioner of a particular discipline) and the jnanin (knower), who purports to follow no ideology or method but lives on the basis of spontaneous spiritual understanding, or higher intuition. For example, in the Mandukya-Karika, a seventh-century authoritative work on Advaita Vedanta, we find the following stanza:

> The intangible Yoga (asparsha-yoga) [of nondualism] is difficult to realize by all yogins. The yogins are afraid of it, perceiving fear in [That which is really of the essence of] fearlessness. (III.39)

Here the author Gaudapada, who was the teacher of Shankara's teacher, distinguishes between yogins and jnanins—those who have realized the intangible, nondual Reality. The distinction is somewhat biased, because there are also realized adepts among the followers of Yoga. But then, what is in a name? Gaudapada simply wanted to establish the superiority of the jnanins, free of self and fear, over those who anxiously strive to realize God or the ultimate Reality, not understanding that their very search is their stumbling block. For as long as there is a goal there is also a seeker—and thus an ego-personality trapped in the condition of unenlightenment.

The spiritual maturation of the yogin is thought to take place in a series of distinct phases. Thus, in the third chapter of the Jivanmukti-Viveka ("Discrimination on Living Liberation"), the medieval scholar and Yoga practitioner Vidyaranya speaks of two classes of yogins: those who have transcended the self and those who have not—a simple and effective classification. The famous Vedanta philosopher Vijnana Bhikshu, who lived in the sixteenth century, distinguishes in his Yoga-Sara-Samgraha ("Compendium on the Essence of Yoga") between the following grades:

योगी योगिनी

The Sanskrit words "yogi" and "yogini."

1. Arurukshu—one who is desirous of spiritual life.
2. Yunjana—one who is actually practicing.
3. Yoga-arudha—one who has ascended in Yoga; he is also called yukta ("yoked one") or sthita-prajna ("one of steady wisdom").

The Bhagavad-Gita ("Lord's Song"), the earliest and undoubtedly most popular work on Yoga, characterizes the aspirant (arurukshu and yunjana) and the adept (yoga-arudha) in these words:

For the sage who desires to ascend in Yoga, action is stated to be the means. For him who has ascended in Yoga, serenity (sama) is said to be the means. (VI.3)

When he does not cling to the sense-objects or to deeds and has renounced all desires, then he is called "one who has ascended in Yoga." (VI.4)

When he has controlled the mind and is established in the Self (atman) only, devoid of all desires, then he is said to be a "yoked one." (VI.18)

The perfected man, who is of "steadied wisdom" (sthita-prajna), is described in the second chapter of the Bhagavad-Gita as follows:

He whose mind is not affected in sorrow and is free from desire in pleasure and who is without attachment, fear, or anger—he is called a sage of "steadied insight" (sthita-dhi). (II.56)

In the literature of the vast spiritual movement of medieval India known as Tantrism,[9] a distinction is made between the realizing aspirant (sadhaka, or sadhika if female) and the perfected adept (siddha), who has attained emancipation or perfection (siddhi), the pinnacle of the path-to-Realization (sadhana). Other classifications are employed in the various Puranas (popular quasi-religious encyclopedias) and the Agamas and Samhitas (sectarian works of encyclopedic scope), as well as in the scriptures of Hatha-Yoga (the "forceful" Yoga of physical discipline). Furthermore, the great religious traditions of Buddhism and Jainism, which have incorporated and contributed to Yoga, also have their own scales of spiritual achievement and adepthood.

An interesting fourfold division is found in the Yoga-Bhashya. The legendary author, Vyasa, makes these distinctions:

1. Prathama-kalpika—the neophyte in the first stage.
2. Madhu-bhumika—"he who is in the delightful (lit. 'honey') stage."
3. Prajna-jyotis—"he who has attained the light (jyotis) of wisdom."
4. Atikranta-bhavaniya—"he who is about to transcend [all of conditioned existence]."

Vyasa sheds some light on these four orders of spiritual attainment. He explains:

The first is the practitioner (abhyasin), for whom the light is just dawning. The second has [attained to] "truth-bearing" transcendental wisdom. The third is he who has subjugated the elements and sense organs and who has developed means for securing all that has been and is yet to be cultivated [by him]. . . . While the fourth, who has passed beyond that which may be cultivated, has as his sole aim the resolution (pratisarga) of the mind [into the primordial World-Ground, whereupon the Self shines forth in its original purity.] (III.51)

The last stage of transcendence leads directly to the realization of the supreme goal of Classical Yoga—"aloneness" (kaivalya). This is the rediscovery of the transcendental Self (purusha), the eternal Essence of the human being, beyond the ever-changing dimension of the cosmos. Kaivalya is the highest degree of spiritual perfection and the consummation of the life of the yogin who follows the path taught by Patanjali.

In his Yoga-Bhashya (I.21), Vyasa also explains that there are nine classes of yogins, according to the intensity of their quest, which may be mediocre or extremely vehement. The renowned ninth-century scholar Vacaspati Mishra elucidates that the degree of intensity depends on previously acquired subliminal impressions as well as on invisible (karmic) influences, called adrishta. In other words, our commitment to Yoga practice is not entirely under our control. The depth of our attraction to God, or the transcendental Self, is not subject to our will but is preconditioned by our karmic past: Our actions and intentions in past lives determine our future state or states of being (our genetic makeup and to some degree even our psychosocial personality). This explains why sometimes our best intentions on the spiritual path are foiled, especially at the beginning of our practice, and why we must continue to persist in disciplining ourselves.

A frequent synonym of *yogin* is *yoga-vid,* meaning "knower of Yoga," which is widely employed particularly in the literature of Hatha-Yoga. The advanced practitioner is, as we have seen, sometimes referred to as a yukta, "yoked one," whereas the novice is occasionally known as a yoga-yuj, "Yoga-joined." The perfected yogin is often styled "king of Yoga" (yoga-raj) and "lord of yogins" (yoga-indra, contracted for euphonic reasons to yogendra).

The term "yogist" is of modern coinage and describes the Western enthusiast who is primarily interested in the physical aspect of Yoga–especially the postures (asana)—rather than in Yoga as a spiritual discipline of Self-realization.

GUIDING LIGHT: THE TEACHER (GURU)

As Mircea Eliade pointed out in his well-known study on Yoga, "What characterizes Yoga is not only its practical side, but also its initiatory structure."[10] Yoga, like all forms of esotericism, presupposes the guidance of an initiate, a master who has firsthand experience of the phenomena and realizations of the yogic path. Ideally, he should have reached the ultimate spiritual destination of all yogic endeavor—enlightenment (bodha), or liberation (moksha). Thus, contrary to the "pop" Yoga espoused by a large number of Westerners, authentic Yoga is never a do-it-yourself enterprise. "One does not learn Yoga by oneself," observed Eliade.[11] Rather, Yoga involves, as do all other traditional Indian systems, an actual pupilage during which a master imparts his secrets to the worthy disciple or devotee. And those secrets are not exhausted by the kind of knowledge that can be expressed in words or printed in books.

Much of what the teacher (guru) imparts to the disciple falls under the category of spiritual transmission (sancara). Such transmission, in which the guru literally empowers the student through a transference of spiritual energy (corresponding to the Holy Ghost of Christian baptism), is the fulcrum of the initiatory process of Yoga. By means of it, the practitioner is blessed in his or her struggle for transcendental realization. As a result, the initiated yogin or yogini experiences the necessary conversion or "turnabout" (paravritti) that is crucial to the spiritual process: He or she begins to find the Real, or the Self beyond the ego, more attractive than the numerous possibilities of worldly experience. The basis for that attraction is a tacit intuition of the Self, which grows stronger in the course of practice.

The initiatory nature of Yoga is expressed in a variety of symbols, the most striking being that of rebirth. For example, in the Atharva-Veda ("Atharvan's Knowledge"), composed about 1000 B.C., we find this verse:

Initiation takes place in that the teacher carries the pupil in himself as it were, as the mother [bears] the embryo in her body. After the three days of the [initiation] ceremony, the disciple is born. (XI.5.3)

A similar archaic "gynecological" metaphor is used, more than a millennium later, in the Buddhist Hevajra-Tantra:

The school is said to be the body. The monastery is called the womb. Through freedom from attachment, one is in the womb. The yellow robe is the membrane [around the embryo]. And the preceptor is one's mother. The salutation is the head-first position (mastaka-anjali). Discipleship is one's worldly experience. (II.4.61–62)

Through the teacher's grace, the deserving disciple is initiated into the great alternative of existence—the reality of the Spirit, or transcendental Being-Consciousness-Bliss. Therefore, it is important that the teacher should be a fully realized master, an adept. Only then is the practitioner assured of complete passage across the ocean of phenomenal existence. For, as the legendary author of the Shiva-Purana (VII.2.15.38) observes, if a preceptor is only nominal, so is the "liberation" he will bestow on his disciple.

The initiatory teacher/disciple system dates back to the early Vedic period

(c. 1200–900 B.C.), where a young boy would spend his youth and adolescence in the home of a teacher of the sacred scriptures, the repository of the epoch's deepest wisdom and finest knowledge. Study of the sacred Veda ("Knowledge") was the sacred duty of all "twice-born" (dvija) members of society—that is, the priestly estate (brahmana), the military estate (kshatriya), and the agricultural estate (vaishya). The servile estate (shudra) was excluded from this time-honored tradition, though exceptions were occasionally made for unusual individuals. The Vedic lore was transmitted to the student by word of mouth and had to be carefully memorized. It was the teacher's obligation to guide the disciple in his study and understanding of the wisdom of the Vedas and to look after his welfare.

The student, in return for the teacher's guidance and paternal supervision, was expected to honor and obey the guru as he would his father and to invest considerable energy in diligent study and service (seva) to the teacher's household. In the Shiva-Samhita ("Shiva's Collection"), an eighteenth-century Hatha-Yoga text, this ideal is expressed as follows:

> There is no doubt that the guru is father; the guru is mother; the guru is God. Therefore he should be served by all in deed, speech, and thought. (III.13)

Much of the contact between teacher and pupil was strictly formalized. For the disciple, it included the daily rituals of begging for alms (bhiksha) and the ceremonial offering of fuel sticks to the guru. The student was expected to stay with his teacher until completion of his course of study; those who, like so many Western acolytes, wandered from teacher to teacher were derogatorily called "crows at a sacred place" (tirtha-kaka).[12]

Apart from the actual study of the sacred tradition, the disciple's foremost obligation was to live a chaste life (brahmacarya)—hence the general appellation of *brahmacarin* for the student. The term means literally "one whose conduct is brahmic"—that is, one who behaves in consonance with the rules laid down for a priest (brahma-brahmana), or whose behavior imitates the condition of the Absolute (brahman), which is asexual. Chastity was traditionally considered imperative for a moral life and for the cultivation of the life-force (prana) in the body-mind, aiding concentration, memory, and health.

The institutionalized relationship between teacher and disciple is known as the guru-kula, "teacher's household," system. Its rationale is given in the Taittiriya-Upanishad, composed perhaps in the eighth century B.C., thus:

> The teacher is the first letter [of the alphabet]. The student is the last letter. Knowledge is the meeting-place. Instruction is the link. (III.1.1)

Fortunate was the student who found a teacher who was not only well-versed in the scriptures but who had also realized their esoteric import. Out of this emerged the equation of the guru with scriptural authority. Both scripture and teacher came to be regarded as having revelatory and salvific power. The teacher, in a way, is the embodiment of the living Truth that is indicated in the sacred texts. The ancient Vedic system of living in the teacher's household (guru-kula) continued to be the traditional model of education in India.

The Upanishads, the ancient esoteric works on nondualist Vedanta, have preserved examples of some of the more profound teacher/disciple relationships, in which the excellence of wisdom and God-realization, not merely intellectual knowledge, was pursued. The enlightened master, having fulfilled the scriptural revelation, is uniquely equipped to prepare others for the same realization. Hence the Shiva-Samhita declares:

> [Only] knowledge imparted by way of the teacher's mouth is productive; otherwise it is fruitless, weak, and causes much affliction. (III.11)

Hinduism distinguishes between different types of teachers, who belong traditionally to the brahmana estate: the guru ("weighty one"); the acarya ("preceptor," who performs the ceremony of investiture, or upanayana, with the sacred thread worn by all "twice-born," and also conveys to the student the appropriate rules of conduct, or acara); the upadhyaya ("tutor," who teaches a portion of the sacred lore for a fee); the adhvanka ("mentor"); the pradhyapaka ("seasoned instructor," who may instruct other teachers); the pracarya ("senior preceptor"); the raja-guru ("royal teacher"); and the loka-guru ("world teacher")—all of whom embody a particular teaching role and spiritual status. There is even a generic term for the various kinds of teachers, namely *pravaktri*, "communicator."

The God-realized teacher grants "divine knowledge" (divya-jnana), as the Yoga-Shikha-Upanishad (V.53) puts it. It is knowledge that springs from enlightenment and attracts to enlightenment. The Advaya-Taraka-Upanishad (16) gives an esoteric explanation of the word *guru*, deriving it from the syllable *gu* indicating ("darkness") and *ru* (indicating "dispeller"). Thus, the guru is he who dispels the devotee's spiritual benightedness.

Of all the teachers, the God-realized adept is even today given a special place in Hindu society. He alone is capable of initiating the spiritual seeker into the supreme "knowledge of the Absolute" (brahma-vidya). He alone is a sad-guru, or "teacher of the Real" or "true teacher." He is celebrated as a potent agent of grace. As the Shiva-Samhita (III.14) states, "By the teacher's grace, everything auspicious for oneself is obtained." And the Hatha-Yoga-Pradipika (IV.9) declares that without a true teacher's compassion (karuna), the state of transcendental Spontaneity (sahaja) is difficult to attain.

Because of his realization, the guru is considered to be an embodiment (vigraha) of the Divine itself. "The guru alone is Hari [=Vishnu] incarnate," announces the Brahma-Vidya-Upanishad (31). The teacher is not *a* specific deity but the all-encompassing Divine, here named Hari. This "deification" of the God-realized master must not be misunderstood. He is not God in any exclusive sense. He is, rather, thought to be coessential with the transcendental Reality. That is to say, he has abrogated the ordinary person's misidentification with a particular body-mind. He abides purely as the transcendental Identity of all beings and things. There is no trace of egoity in him, for his ego has been replaced by the Self. His body-mind and personality continue for their allotted time, but he is no longer implicated by their automaticities. The unenlightened being, by contrast, believes himself to be a particular entity or individual consciousness, somehow lodged within a body and associated with, possibly even driven by, a particular personality complex.

In the thirteenth chapter of the Kularnava-Tantra, God Shiva, addressing his divine spouse Devi, has this to say about realized masters as opposed to ordinary teachers:

> There are many gurus, like lamps in house after house, but hard to find, O Devi, is the guru who lights up all like the sun. (104)

> There are many gurus who are proficient in the Vedas [revealed sacred knowledge] and the Shastras [textbooks], but hard to find, O Devi, is the guru who has attained to the supreme Truth. (105)

> There are many gurus on earth who give what is other than the Self, but hard to find in all the worlds, O Devi, is the guru who reveals the Self. (106)

> Many are the gurus who rob the disciple of his wealth, but rare is the guru who removes the afflictions of the disciple. (108)

> He is the [true] guru by whose very contact there flows the supreme Bliss (ananda). The intelligent man should choose such a one as his guru and none other. (110)

The Kularnava-Tantra (XIII) also speaks of six types of gurus, who are classified according to their function:

1. Preraka—the "impeller" who stimulates interest in the would-be devotee, leading to his initiation.
2. Sucaka—the "indicator" who points out the form of spiritual discipline (sadhana) for which the initiate is qualified.
3. Vacaka—the "explainer" who expounds the spiritual process and its objective.
4. Darshaka—the "revealer" who shows the details of the process.
5. Shikshaka—the "teacher" who instructs in the actual spiritual discipline.
6. Bodhaka—the "illuminator" who, as the text has it, "lights up in the disciple the lamp of mental and spiritual knowledge."

There are many other functional types of gurus, and the Yoga scholar M. P. Pandit, in his translation of the Kularnava-Tantra, mentions no fewer than twelve.[13] But it is always the God-realized master who is extolled in the yogic scriptures above all others.

LEARNING BEYOND THE SELF: THE DISCIPLE (SHISHYA)

Traditionally, when a person—usually a male—had resolved seriously to take up spiritual life, he approached a master of Yoga "with fuel in hand," hoping that he would be accepted. The fuel sticks that he ceremoniously presented to his prospective teacher were an outward sign of his inner readiness to submit himself to the guru, to be burned up by the fire of spiritual practice. Yoga, or the spiritual process in general, has always been compared to a purificatory conflagration that consumes the ego-personality, until the transcendental Self-Identity alone is left. Therefore, only the foolhardy would approach an adept unprepared—and were apt to be rejected, though perhaps not without having been taught some useful lessons about self-transcendence, love, obedience, or nonattachment.

Once an aspirant presented himself to a master of Yoga, he was carefully scrutinized by the teacher for signs of emotional and spiritual maturity. The esoteric lore must never be passed on to an unqualified individual, lest it cause him harm or be abused by him to the detriment of others. Spiritual pupilage is always a demanding affair and, ultimately, a matter of life and death. As we can read in the Mahabharata epic:

> This great path of the wise priests is arduous. No one can tread it easily, o bull of Bharata [India]! It is like a terrible jungle creeping with large snakes, filled with pits, devoid of water, full of thorns, and quite inaccessible. (XII.300.50)

What is at stake in the spiritual process is the conditional ego-personality itself, which fiercely struggles to survive but which must be surrendered in order for the transcendental Self to shine forth. Spiritual life demands a rebirth that is as dramatic as the transformation of a caterpillar into a butterfly. This transmutation does not happen without pain, and not all aspirants are able to complete the process. Some even get lost en route, succumbing to insanity or terminal disease.

Because the spiritual path is like a razor's edge, a responsible teacher will not accept an unprepared individual for discipleship. He will, rather, apply certain traditional (and commonsense) criteria of competence (adhikara). Nonetheless, a teacher may decide to take on an ill-prepared aspirant if he detects in him a certain spiritual potential. Such a student (shishya) must not expect to receive more than exoteric teachings until he has been purified of his personal weaknesses through much service and study.

The Shiva-Samhita (V.10ff.) distinguishes four types of aspirant, classifying them according to the intensity of their commitment. The weak (mridu) practitioner is characterized as unenthusiastic, foolish, fickle, timid, ill, dependent, rude, ill-mannered, and unenergetic. He is only fit for Mantra-Yoga, consisting in the meditative repetition of a sacred syllable or phrase given to him and empowered by the teacher.

The mediocre (madhya) practitioner, who is capable of practicing Laya-Yoga—the path of meditative absorption—is said to be endowed with even-mindedness, patience, a desire for virtue, kind speech, and the tendency to practice moderation in all undertakings.

The exceptional (adhimatra) practitioner, who qualifies for the practice of Hatha-Yoga, is expected to demonstrate the following qualities: firm understanding, an aptitude for meditative absorption (laya), self-reliance, liberal-mindedness, bravery, vigor, faithfulness, the willingness to worship the teacher's lotus feet (both literally and figuratively), and delight in the practice of Yoga.

For the extraordinary (adhimatratama) practitioner, who may practice all forms of Yoga, the Shiva-Samhita lists no fewer than thirty-one qualities: great energy, enthusiasm, charm, heroism, scriptural knowledge, the inclination to practice, freedom from delusion, orderliness, youthfulness, moderate eating habits, control over the senses, fearlessness, purity, skillfulness, liberality, the ability to be a refuge for all people, capability, stability, thoughtfulness, the willingness to do whatever is desired by the teacher, patience, good manners, observance of the moral and spiritual law (dharma), the ability to keep his struggle to himself, kind speech, faith in the scriptures, the willingness to worship God and the guru (as the embodiment of the Divine), knowledge of the vows pertaining to his level of practice, and, lastly, the practice of all types of Yoga.

After a person has been accepted by a teacher, he can expect to be tested again and again. There are traditional prescriptions for such testing, although the teacher who is a Self-realized adept is unlikely to need any guidelines for ascertaining his disciple's seriousness about spiritual life. At this point, a student may begin to live with or close to his teacher, serving and attending him constantly. Such a student is known as an antevasin, "one who abides near." In the company of the God-realized master, the practitioner is continuously exposed to the realizer's spiritualized body-mind, and by way of "contagion" his own physical and psychic being is gradually transformed. This can be understood, in modern terms, as a form of rhythm entertainment, where the guru's faster vibratory state gradually speeds up the disciple's vibration.

For this spontaneous process to be truly effective, the disciple must consciously cooperate with his guru. He accomplishes this by making the teacher his focus of attention. This is the great principle of sat-sanga. The word means literally "company of the True" or "relationship to the Real." Sat-sanga is the supreme means of liberation in guru-yoga. And since the guru has from ancient times been deemed essential to yogic practice, sat-sanga is at the core of all schools of Yoga. It would not be wrong to say that all Yoga is guru-yoga.

In practice, the aspirant must move from the stage of the student to that of the disciple and, finally, to that of the devotee (bhakta). At the student level, the aspirant still has an exoteric understanding of, and relationship to, the teacher. The student is inspired by listening to his teacher's discourses but has not yet seriously taken up spiritual life. He wavers in his commitment to the yogic process, and worldly life still exerts a strong pull on him. The disciple, by contrast, is more sensitive to the esoteric relationship between the guru and himself, understanding that there is a continuous psychospiritual link to the teacher that must be honored and cultivated. The devotee, finally, *experiences* the guru as a spiritual reality rather than as a human personality and is therefore naturally inclined to assume a devotional attitude that acts as a powerful conduit between the guru and himself.

To enter into conscious relationship to the Real, in the form of the teacher, means more than to pay the guru attention in the conventional sense. What the scriptures call for is devotion to, or love for, the adept-teacher. Thus, in the Mandala-Brahmana-Upanishad (I.1.4), perhaps composed in the fourteenth century A.D., "devotion to the teacher" (guru-bhakti) is listed as one of the constituents of the ninefold moral code (niyama) for yogins. And the Yoga-Shikha-Upanishad, which is of a similar age, declares:

> There is no one greater in the three worlds than the guru. It is he who grants "divine knowledge" (divya-jnana) and should [therefore] be worshipped with supreme devotion. (V.53)

Similarly, the Tejo-Bindu-Upanishad (VI.109) regards devotion to the teacher as indispensable for the serious aspirant. And according to the Brahma-Vidya-Upanishad (30), devotion to the teacher should always be practiced, because the teacher is none other than the Divine. The equivalence of guru worship and worship of the Divine is emphasized in the Shiva-Purana (I.18.95) and in numerous other Sanskrit texts—far too many to list here.

However, there are at least two scriptures exclusively dedicated to the theme of devotion to the spiritual master. The first stems from the tradition of Hinduism. This is the Guru-Gita, which is widely circulated in India as an independent composition but which belongs to the latter part of the Skanda-Purana.[14] It consists of 352 stanzas, delivered in the form of a didactic dialogue between Shiva and his divine spouse Uma (or Parvati). The second scripture is a favorite Buddhist text—Ashvaghosha's Guru-Panca-Shikha, which is extant only in a Tibetan translation.[15] Ashvaghosha (c. A.D. 80) was a celebrated poet and eminent teacher of Mahayana Buddhism, who achieved fame through his artistic biography of Gautama the Buddha, called the Buddha-Carita ("Buddha's Conduct"), and a philosophical exposition entitled Shraddha-Utpada-Shastra ("Scripture on the Awakening of Faith").

During the antevasin period the devotee discovers the potency of the mutual love between himself and the adept-teacher, creating profound trust in the guru and faith in the spiritual process itself. His service (seva, sevana) becomes more demanding as his ability to take responsibility increases. According to the Kularnava-Tantra (XII.64), such service (the text uses the word *sushrusha*, meaning "obedience") is fourfold: service through one's bodily self (atman), through material means (artha), through respect (mana), and through a good disposition (sad-bhava). It is made clear that service is for the benefit of the devotee rather than the teacher.

Meantime the guru constantly monitors his disciple's progress, waiting for the right moment at which initiation (diksha) can take place. As soon as he judges his disciple ready, the guru will begin to impart to him the secrets of his esoteric lineage, as handed down to him by his own teacher and as tested in his own life. Only the fully qualified disciple, called *adhikarin,* is eligible for formal spiritual initiation. Only the fully Self-realized adept is capable of empowering that initiation, so that the disciple's life is mysteriously guided toward the fulfillment of the "Atman project"—the impulse toward realizing the Whole that makes whole.

GIVING BIRTH TO A NEW IDENTITY: INITIATION (DIKSHA)

According to the Kularnava-Tantra (X.1), it is impossible to attain enlightenment, or liberation, without initiation (diksha, abhisheka), and there can be no real initiation without a qualified teacher.

In anthropological contexts the term "initiation" stands for a person's rite of passage into a new social grade or status, usually induction into a privileged group such as adult society or a secret brotherhood. Such initiation is frequently marked by special mandatory ceremonies involving tests and trials of courage for the initiate—from seclusion and mutilation to the observance of special vows. Often the initiatory process is symbolized as the initiate's death and subsequent rebirth. While these formal aspects of tribal initiation may also be associated with yogic initiation, the crux of diksha is something more profound.

Rather than an induction into a new social status, the yogic diksha is primarily a form of spiritual transmission (sancara) by which the disciple's bodily, mental, and spiritual condition is changed through the adept's transference of spiritual energy. Diksha is first and foremost "enhallowment," which is captured in the synonym *abhisheka,* meaning "sprinkling," which refers to the ceremonial spraying of consecrated water on the devotee—a form of baptism. By means of initiation, which may occur informally or in a more ritual setting, the spiritual process is either awakened or magnified in the practitioner. It is always a direct empowerment, in which the teacher effects in his disciple a change of consciousness, a turnabout, or metanoia. It is a moment of conversion from ordinary worldliness to a hallowed life, which alters the initiate's state of being.

From then on the disciple's spiritual struggle has a new depth. The

Kriya-Samgraha-Panjika ("Concise Compendium on Action"), a Buddhist Tantric scripture, quotes the following saying:

> The yogin who aspires to "yogihood" (yogitva) but has not been initiated is [like a person who] strikes out at the sky with fists and drinks the water of a mirage. (manuscript, p. 5)

Initiation creates a special link between the guru and his devotee—a spiritual connection that represents a unique responsibility on the teacher's part and a significant challenge for the practitioner. Through initiation, the aspirant becomes an integral part of his teacher's lineage (parampara), which is understood as a chain of empowerment that exceeds the world of space-time, insofar as it continues after the death of both the teacher and the disciple. Admission to this chain must be earned through self-surrender. This has been made clear by the well-known Tibetan teacher Chogyam Trungpa:

> Without abhisheka our attempts to achieve spirituality will result in no more than a huge spiritual collection rather than real surrender. We have been collecting different behavior patterns, different manners of speech, dress, thought, whole different ways of acting. And all of it is merely a collection we are attempting to impose upon ourselves. Abhisheka, true initiation, is born out of surrender. We open ourselves to the situation as it is, and then we make real communication with the teacher. In any event, the guru is already there with us in a state of openness; and if we open ourselves, are willing to give up our collections, then initiation takes place.[16]

Thus, the disciple's emotional vulnerability, or openness, forms the basis for spiritual transmission. He must become like an empty vessel to be filled by the teacher's gift of transmission.

What is passed on from teacher to disciple on this initiatory occasion? The Tantric term for this process of transference is *shakti-pata*, which literally means "descent of the power," and it encapsulates the central occurrence in the initiatory event. Shakti-pata is the event and the experience of the descent of a powerful energy current into the body, usually starting from the crown of the head or the upper torso and moving down into the pelvic area (which is the location of an important psychophysical center, the muladhara-cakra) and sometimes into the lower extremities.

By virtue of his enlightenment, or at least his advanced spiritual state, the adept-teacher has become a locus of concentrated psychophysical energy. Whereas the ordinary body-mind represents a low-energy system, the adept's body-mind is like a powerful radio beacon. This statement is not a mere metaphor. Rather, it is an experiential fact that is recognized in many esoteric traditions. There is a remarkable passage in Plato's works where a conversation is recorded between Socrates and his pupil Aristeides. The latter confesses to Socrates that his philosophical understanding increases whenever he associates with the great philosopher, and that this effect is most pronounced when he sits close to him and touches him.

In Aristeides' case, it was intellectual insight that was deepened by sheer proximity to that great lover of wisdom, the saintly Socrates. In the case of the yogic initiate, a different transmission occurs. He is inducted into the secret dimension of existence: He discovers experientially that the apparent material cosmos, including his own body, is a vast sea of psychophysical energy. He begins to understand and experience the reality behind the mathematical models of modern quantum physics. The initiate's body-mind and the universe reveal themselves as indefinable patterns of light and energy, imbued with superconsciousness.

Shakti-pata can be inaugurated by the adept through a verbal command, his touch, his glance, or, in the case of an enlightened master, even his mere presence. In the last-mentioned case, when the aspirant is graced with a temporary state of ecstasy, the initiation is known as shambhavi-diksha (see, e.g., the Kularnava-Tantra XIV.56). The word *shambhavi* means "belonging to Shambhu," and Shambhu is a form of Shiva, the ultimate Being.

This type of instant initiation is generally contrasted with shaktika-diksha on the one hand and anavi-diksha on the other. In the former type of initiation the teacher activates by esoteric means the disciple's innate capacity (shakti) for God-realization so that, after a period of time, enlightenment is spontaneously attained. The latter kind of diksha involves spiritual instruction, including the imparting of a mantra, a sacred word or phrase, which the devotee then recites as directed. Thus, both shambhavi-diksha and shaktika-diksha are initiations that lead to realization spontaneously, but whereas the one is instant, the other represents a delayed reaction due to the gradual effect of the awakened shakti. Only anavi-diksha calls for a course of application on the devotee's part. He is given the teacher's empowerment but has to cooperate with the psychic forces set in motion in him through the esoteric process of initiation. The word *anavi* means "pertaining to *anu*," while *anu*, "atom," is a designation for the individual psyche.

The Kularnava-Tantra (XIV.34ff.) distinguishes three principal forms of initiation, namely initiation by touch (sparsha-diksha), initiation by sight (drig-diksha), and mental initiation (manasa-diksha). The first form of initiation is compared to the slow nurturing by a bird that grants its fledgling the warmth of its wings. The second form is likened to the nurturing by a fish that protects its offspring through watchful eyes. The third form is said to be similar to the nurturing by a tortoise that simply thinks of its young—a simile that may mean more to an indologist than a biologist.

The same scripture mentions other classificatory schemes. Thus, it states (XIV.39ff.) that initiation, capable of bestowing liberation, comprises seven types:

1. Kriya-diksha, "initiation through ritual," is said to be of eight forms, depending on the type of ceremonial implements used.

2. Varna-diksha, "initiation through the alphabet," has three versions, according to whether the alphabet used has forty-two, fifty, or sixty-two letters. Sanskrit letters are visualized by the teacher on the aspirant's body and are then gradually dissolved until the state of ecstatic unification with the Divine is attained. Visualization is not ordinary mental picturing but a powerful tool that, on the level of energy, actually creates objects perceivable by yogic means.

3. Kala-diksha, "initiation through the kala," is threefold, though the text offers no explanation. The kala ("part") is the power-of-manifestation, a subtle form of energy thought to be the matrix of visible forms. It is referred to by different names according to its appearance in different bodily regions. Thus, it is called nivritti ("cessation") from the soles of the feet to the knees, pratishtha ("foundation") from the knees to the navel, vidya ("knowledge") from the navel to the neck, shanti ("peace") from the neck to the forehead, and shanty-atita ("peace-transcending") from the forehead to the crown of the head. These areas of the disciple's body are visualized by the teacher as gradually dissolving, until the pupil's consciousness reaches the zero-point of the manifest world itself, whereupon it flips over into the transcendental state.

4. Sparsha-diksha, "initiation through touch," where the teacher makes physical contact with the devotee.

5. Vag-diksha, "initiation through speech," occurs when the teacher, with his attention firmly implanted in the Divine, utters a mantra or sacred verse from the scriptures.

6. Drig-diksha, "initiation through sight," where the teacher closes his eyes and, in a meditative mood, gazes into the very being of his disciple.

7. Manasa-diksha, "initiation through thought," involves projection or visualization practices similar to those in varna-diksha and kala-diksha.

Many more intriguing facts about the ceremonial aspects of diksha can be found in the tenth chapter of the Mahanirvana-Tantra, a seventh- or eighth-century scripture greatly venerated by the practitioners of Tantric Yoga.

Beyond the yogic technique of shakti-pata there is also the spontaneous spiritual transmission of the enlightened adept. This is the continuous initiatory "presence" that emanates from the God-realized master. For the devotee it represents a constant confrontation with Reality. This transmission does not consist in any special psychophysical energy; it is essentially a magnification of the individual's native Intelligence, or intuition of Reality, whereby a crisis in consciousness is provoked: Through his intensified sensitivity to the transcendental Condition, the devotee understands more deeply the mechanisms by which he maintains himself in the state of unenlightenment. He experiences the basic dilemma or suffering of his ordinary existence, seeing how everything he does, thinks, and feels is governed by the principle of egoic separation.

Under the impact of the God-realized adept's transmission, he goes through spiritual crisis after crisis, awakening more and more to the sublime principle that he is presently free, enlightened, and blissful. As this recognition grows in him, the devotee finds that his egoic impulses, motivations, and obsessions are becoming increasingly obsolete. The teacher's grace (prasada) draws him, step by step, into a different disposition—the disposition of enlightenment.[17] It is for this reason alone that initiation is given such prominence in the esoteric schools of India.

> Diksha, verily, releases [the aspirant] from the extensive bondage impeding [the realization of] the supreme Abode, and it leads [him] upward to Shiva's Domain.[18]

CRAZY WISDOM AND CRAZY ADEPTS

In Tibet there is a tradition known as "crazy wisdom." The phenomenon for which this term stands is found in all the major religions of the world, though it is seldom acknowledged as a valid expression of spiritual life by the religious orthodoxy or the secular establishment. Crazy wisdom is a unique mode of spiritual teaching, which avails itself of seemingly irreligious or unspiritual means in order to awaken the conventional ego-personality from its spiritual slumber.

The unconventional means used by adepts who teach in this risky manner seem crazy or mad in the eyes of ordinary people, who seldom look beyond appearances. Crazy-wisdom methods are designed to shock, but their purpose is always benign: to reflect to the ordinary worldling the "madness" of his or her existence, which, from the enlightened point of view, is an existence rooted in a profound illusion. That illusion is the ingrained presumption that the individual is an ego-identity bounded by the skin of the human body, rather than the all-pervasive Self-Identity. Crazy wisdom is a logical extension of the deep insights of spiritual life in general, and it is at the core of the relationship between adept and disciple—a relationship that has the express function of undermining the disciple's ego-illusion.

The crazy-wisdom message and method are understandably offensive to both the secular and the conventionally religious establishments. Hence crazy adepts have generally been suppressed. This was not the case in traditional Tibet and India, however, where the "holy fool" or "divine madman" has been recognized as a legitimate figure in the compass of spiritual aspiration and realization. Thus, the "saintly madman" (Tibetan: lama myonpa) has been venerated throughout the history of Tibet. The same is true of the Indian avadhuta, who has, as the word suggests, "cast off" all concerns and conventional standards in his God-intoxication.

The equivalent to the saintly madman of Tibet and the Hindu avadhuta is found even in the Christian world, in the form of the "fool for Christ's sake." Yet the large conservative faction among both the Christian clergy and the laity has long driven the unorthodox figure of the "fool" (Greek: salos) into oblivion. The modern Christian knows next to nothing about such remarkable "holy idiots" as St. Simeon, St. Isaac Zatvornik, St. Basil, or St. Isadora, the last being one of the few female examples. It was the apostle Paul who first used the phrase "fool for Christ's sake" (1 Cor. 4:10). He spoke of the wisdom of God that looks like folly to the world, whereas the world's wisdom is founded in pride. When Mark the Mad, a desert monk of the sixth century A.D., came to the city to atone for his sins, the townspeople considered him insane. But Abba Daniel of Skete instantly recognized his great sanctity, shouting to the crowd that they were all fools for not seeing that Mark was the only reasonable man in the entire city.

St. Simeon, another sixth-century fool for Christ's sake, was a skilled simulator of insanity. Once he found a dead dog on a dung heap. He tied his cord belt to the dog's leg and dragged the corpse behind him through town. The people were outraged, failing to understand that the mad monk's burden was a symbol of the excess baggage they themselves carried around with them—the ego, or conventional mind lacking love and wisdom. The very next day, St. Simeon entered the local church and threw nuts at the congregation when the Sunday liturgy began. At the end of his life, the saint confessed to his most trusted friend that his eccentric behavior had been solely an expression of his indifference (apatheia) to things of the world. Its purpose was to denounce hypocrisy and hubris.

The mad saint, who in his God-intoxication fearlessly steps beyond the mores of his era, made his appearance also in the stern religions of Islam, among the masters of Sufism, and Judaism, among the Hasidic mystics.

These holy fools represent a wide spectrum of spiritual attainment, ranging from the religious eccentric to the enlightened adept. The common denominator between them is that in their lifestyle, or at least in their occasional behavior, they invert or reverse the standards and conventions of society.

The most pristine manifestation of crazy wisdom is found in the myonpa and the avadhuta traditions of the Indian subcontinent. The Tibetans distinguish different kinds of madness, including what one might call religious neurosis (Tibetan: chos-myon) with sociopathic and paranoid symptoms. These are carefully held apart from saintly madness. Some of the characteristics of saintly madness are not dissimilar to the symptoms of secular and religious madness. However, their nature and causes are quite distinct. The crazy adept's eccentric behavior is a direct expression not of any personal psychopathology, but of his spiritual status and attainment.

Crazy wisdom is the articulation in life of the realization that the phenomenal world (samsara) and the transcendental Reality (nirvana) are coessential. Seen from the perspective of the unillumined mind, operating on the basis of a sharp separation between subject and object, perfect enlightenment is a paradoxical condition. The enlightened adept exists as the ultimate spaceless, timeless Being-Consciousness but appears to animate a particular body-mind in space-time—a body-mind that, moreover, inheres in that all-encompassing Reality that he is. In the nondualist terms of Advaita Vedanta, enlightenment is the fulfillment of the two axioms that the innermost self (atman) is identical with the transcendental Self (parama-atman), and that the ultimate Ground (brahman) is identical with the cosmos in all its levels of manifestation, including the self.

Thus, the enlightened adept lives as the Totality of existence, which, from the narrow perspective of the finite personality, is a veritable chaos. While this is the immediate "experience" of all enlightened masters who live consummately spontaneous (sahaja) lives, there are those whose appearance and behavior reflect more directly their divine madness. These are the crazy adepts who do not care to make sense and who, for the sake of instructing others, disregard conventional expectations, norms, and obligations.

They feel free to reject customary behavior and to be subversive, criticizing and poking fun at the worldly and religious establishment, dressing in bizarre ways or even going about naked, ignoring the niceties of social contact, ridiculing the narrow concerns of scholars and scholastics, cursing and using obscene language, employing song and dance, consuming stimulants and intoxicants (like alcohol), and engaging in sexuality. They incarnate the esoteric principle of Tantrism that liberation (mukti) is coessential with enjoyment (bhukti); that Reality transcends the categories of transcendence and immanence; that the spiritual is not inherently separate from the world.

In their wild and eccentric behavior, the crazy adepts constantly challenge the limitations that unenlightened individuals presume and thus confront them with the naked truth of existence: that life is mad and unpredictable, except for the inescapable fact that man is thrown into the chaos of manifestation for only a brief span of time. They are a perpetual reminder that our whole human civilization is an attempt to deny the inevitability of death, which makes nonsense out of even the noblest efforts to create a symbolic order out of the infinite plastic that is life.

Unlike conventional wisdom, which is meant to create a higher order or harmony, crazy wisdom has the primary function of disrupting humankind's model-making enthusiasm, its impulse to create order, structure, and meaning. Crazy wisdom is enlightened iconoclasm. What it smashes, in the last analysis, is the egocentric universe and its creator, the subjective sense of being a separate entity—the ego. Thus, crazy wisdom is spiritual shock therapy.

The crazy adept's "naturalness" must be carefully distinguished from the mere impulsiveness of the child or the emotionally labile adult, just as it must be differentiated from the kind of spontaneity that is pursued in various humanistic therapies. Spontaneity (sahaja) implies more than enhanced awareness or integration of the body-mind, as part of a comprehensive psychohygiene. The realized adept is not just a particularly successful ego. He is an ego-transcender, and his spontaneity is not an acquired skill. His spontaneity is absolutely pure. It coincides with the world-process itself. He acts out of the Whole, as the Whole.

The best-known crazy adept of the Tibetan tradition is undoubtedly Tibet's folk hero Milarepa (A.D. 1040–1123), yogin and poet extraordinaire. His hard years of pupilage under Marpa "the translator" exemplify the ego-grinding tribulations of all authentic spiritual discipleship. Who would not be touched by the traditional Tibetan biography of Milarepa in which we see him rebuild the same tower again and again, fighting physical pain, anger at the futility of it all, doubt about his guru, and spiritual despair? Already an accomplished magician and miracle worker by the time he met his guru, Milarepa became an adept-teacher in his own right through Marpa's guidance and grace. Clad only in a white cotton robe, he traversed the borderland between Tibet and Nepal, teaching by way of his poems and songs. Occasionally Milarepa would be found naked, and in one of his songs he observes that he knows no shame, since his genitals are natural enough. His disposition of crazy wisdom is indicated by the fact that, though living the life of a wandering renunciate, he is known to have initiated several of his female devotees into esoteric sexuality. To the common mind, sex and spirituality do not mix. Tantrism, as we will see in Chapter 12, contradicts this popular assumption.

Marpa (A.D. 1012–1097) himself, the founder of the Kagyupa school of Vajrayana Buddhism (Tibetan Tantrism), was a crazy-wisdom master. A generous and humorous personage, he would often animate an angry disposition toward Milarepa to provoke in his beloved devotee the spiritual crisis that alone could lead to Milarepa's liberation. In addition to his chief wife, Marpa also associated with eight Tantric consorts.

The most exaggerated and outrageous crazy adept of Tibet was undoubtedly Drukpa Kunley (A.D. 1455–1570). Like many other saintly madmen, he started out as a monk but upon Realization adopted the life of a mendicant. His Tibetan biography, which contains much symbolic and legendary material, claims that he initiated no fewer than 5000 women into the sexual secrets of Tantrism. Portrayed as a fond consumer of chung, the Tibetan beer, and an accomplished raconteur, Drukpa Kunley's humorous but pointed commentary on his monastic contemporaries and his fearless confrontations with authority are still related today in Himalayan roadside taverns.

The crazy-wisdom tradition of India revolves largely around the figure of the avadhuta. This Sanskrit word means literally "cast off," referring to him who has abandoned all the cares and concerns that burden the ordinary mortal. He is an extreme type of renouncer (samnyasin), a "supreme swan" (parama-hamsa) who, as the title indicates, drifts freely from place to place like a great swan, depending on nothing but the Divine. The designation *avadhuta* came into vogue during the post-Christian period, which saw the rise of Tantrism.

Possibly one of the earliest references to the avadhuta is found in the Mahanirvana-Tantra (VIII.11). This work states that the "crazy" lifestyle of the avadhuta is to the kali-yuga—the present "dark age"—what the lifestyle of the renouncer was to the preceding epoch, where the moral fiber was still strong. In the kali-yuga, more drastic means of awakening people are required because of their general insensitivity to the sacred order. The "shock therapy" of crazy wisdom is thus preferable to the quiet example of the world-renouncing ascetic.

The Mahanirvana-Tantra distinctly associates the avadhuta with Shaivism, the religiospiritual tradition that has God Shiva as its focus. This scripture (XIV.140ff.) speaks of four classes of avadhutas. The shaiva-avadhuta has received full Tantric initiation, while the brahma-avadhuta employs the brahma-mantra "Om, the One Existence-Consciousness, the Absolute" (om sac-cid-ekam brahma). Both categories are subdivided into those who are as yet imperfect—"wanderers" (parivraj)—and those who have attained perfection—"supreme swans" (parama-hamsa).[19]

One of the earliest Hatha-Yoga scriptures, the Siddha-Siddhanta-Paddhati, contains many verses that describe the avadhuta. One stanza (VI.20) in particular refers to his chameleon-like capacity to animate any character or role. Thus, he is said to behave at times like a worldling or even like a king and at other times like an ascetic or naked renunciant.

The appellation *avadhuta*, more than any other, came to be associated with the apparently crazy modes of behavior of some parama-hamsas who dramatize the reversal of social norms, a behavior characteristic of their spontaneous lifestyle. Their frequent nakedness is perhaps the most symbolic expression of this reversal. In the Avadhuta-Gita, a medieval work celebrating the crazy adept, the avadhuta is depicted as a spiritual hero who is beyond good and evil, beyond praise and blame, indeed beyond any of the categories that the mind can construct. One stanza speaks of his transcendental status:

As a yogin devoid of "union" (yoga) and "separation" (viyoga) and as an "enjoyer" (bhogin) devoid of enjoyment and nonenjoyment—thus he wanders about at leisure, filled with spontaneous Bliss [innate in his own] mind. (VII.9)

The same scripture explains the designation *avadhuta* as follows:

The significance of the letter *a* is that [the avadhuta] abides eternally in Bliss (ananda), freed from the fetters of hope and pure in the beginning, middle, and end. (VIII.6)

The significance of the syllable *va* is that he dwells [always] in the present and that his speech is blameless, [and it applies to him] who has conquered desire (vasana). (VIII.7)

The significance of the syllable *dhu* is that he is relieved of [the practice of] concentration and meditation, that his limbs are grey with dust, that his mind is pure and he is free from disease. (VIII.8)

The significance of the syllable *ta* is that he is freed from [spiritual] darkness (tamas) and the I-sense (ahamkara) and that he is devoid of thought and purpose, with his mind steadfast on Reality (tattva). (VIII.9)[20]

The whole text, which belongs perhaps to the fifteenth century A.D., is written from a lofty nondualist point of view. It is similar to the Ashtavakra-Gita ("Ashtavakra's Song") which, significantly, is also known as Avadhuta-Anubhuti ("Realization of the Crazy Adept") and which has been placed in the late fifteenth century A.D.[21] Both scriptures are ecstatic outpourings, and both celebrate the highest form of nondualist realization.

The Avadhuta-Gita is ascribed to Dattatreya, which may be the name of a real person but more likely refers to the semilegendary spiritual master by that name who later came to be elevated to the status of a deity.[22] Sage Dattatreya's story is told in the Markandeya-Purana (XVI), in a section that belongs perhaps to the fourth century A.D. It describes the miraculous birth of one of the great crazy-wisdom adepts of India.

According to this account, a certain brahmin named Kaushika lived a profligate life, losing both wealth and health as a result of his infatuation with a courtesan. His wife, Shandili, however, was utterly faithful to him. One night she even carried her sick husband to the courtesan's house. On the way, with her husband riding on her shoulders, Shandili accidentally stepped on Sage Mandavya, who was feared for his potent curses. Mandavya promptly condemned the pair to die at sunrise. The chaste woman prayed with all her might, appealing to the sun not to rise at all so that her husband might live. Her pure-hearted prayer was answered. Now all the deities were in uproar, and they enlisted the help of Anushuya, wife of the famous Sage Atri, to convince Shandili to allow the universal order to be restored. Anushuya, herself a paragon of womanly virtue, won Shandili over, on the condition that Kaushika's life would be spared when the sun rose.

In appreciation of her timely intercession, the gods granted Anushuya a boon. She asked for her husband's and her own liberation and then for the principal deities—Brahma, Vishnu, and Shiva—to be born as sons to her. After a period of time, while Anushuya was bowing to her husband, a light shone forth from Sage Atri's eyes and served as the seed for the three divine sons Soma, Durvasa, and Datta—partial incarnations of Brahma, Shiva, and Vishnu, respectively.

Other Puranas (popular encyclopedias) contain different narratives, but all involve the figure of Atri—hence the name Dattatreya, "Datta, son of Atri." It is clear from some of the incidents in Dattatreya's life that he was a rather unconventional figure. For instance, he is said to have immersed himself in a lake, from which he emerged after many years in the company of a maiden. Knowing of Dattatreya's perfect nonattachment, his disciples thought nothing of it. In order to test their faith in him, he began to consume wine with the maiden, but his devotees were not disturbed even by this.

Then again, various Puranas, including the Markandeya-Purana (XXX–XL), say that Dattatreya taught the eight-limbed Yoga of Patanjali, which favors an ascetic lifestyle. Thus, Dattatreya is associated both with ascetic motifs and with situations involving sexuality and alcohol—the two great ingredients of Tantric ritual.[23]

Dattatreya is the archetypal crazy adept. It is not clear how, from a quasi-Tantric sage, he was made into a full-blown deity. Nevertheless, both sage and deity are intimately connected with the avadhuta tradition. Even though mythology remembers Sage Dattatreya as an incarnation of God Vishnu, the preserver of the universe, his name is as closely associated with the cultural sphere of Shiva, the Lord of yogins. It would appear that this great spiritual hero was claimed by both Vishnu and Shiva worshippers. Sage Atri's illustrious son served both traditions as a symbol of the God-realizer whose state transcends all beliefs and customs. Hence it is not surprising that Dattatreya should also be credited with the authorship of the Jivanmukta-Gita ("Song of Living Liberation"), a short tract of twenty-three stanzas that extols the jivan-mukta, the adept who is liberated while still in the embodied condition. Likewise the Tripura-Rahasya ("Tripura's Secret Teaching") is traditionally credited to Dattatreya; considering the focus of this scripture on the supreme mind-transcending disposition of enlightened spontaneity (sahaja), this attribution seems singularly appropriate.

Crazy wisdom is found to varying degrees in most schools of Yoga, because the guru's prescribed task is to undermine the disciple's illusion of being an island unto himself. Most teachers, especially if they are fully enlightened, will on occasion resort to unconventional behavior to penetrate the disciple's protective armor. Few teachers, however, tend to teach in the full-fledged mode of crazy wisdom as did, for instance, Marpa and Drukpa Kunley. Today individuals maintain more carefully defined ego-boundaries than in the past, and so crazy-wisdom methods tend to be experienced as interfering with the personal integrity of the disciple. Hence few teachers are willing to adopt a crazy-wisdom style of teaching. There also remains the broader question of whether this ancient way of teaching is still useful and morally justifiable today.[24]

This brief review of the crazy-wisdom dimension of Hindu and Buddhist spirituality completes this introductory chapter, which explains the fundamental categories involved in the spiritual process of Yoga. The next chapter outlines the major approaches or schools within the yogic tradition.

योग आनन्दकल्पनः

chapter 2
The Wheel of Yoga

OVERVIEW

In its oldest known form, Yoga appears to have been the practice of disciplined introspection, or meditative focusing. In this form we meet with Yoga in the sacrificial ritualism of the Vedas, the 3000-year-old collection of hymns containing the revealed or "superhuman" knowledge of the archaic Sanskrit-speaking settlers in northern India. The rites of the Vedic priests had to be performed with perfect exactitude, demanding the sacrificer's utmost concentration. A similar yogic orientation is found in the consciousness technology of the Upanishads, the esoteric teachings of those who had made meditation their principal approach to God-realization. Out of this rather amorphous approach evolved in the course of centuries an immense body of practices, with more or less elaborate explanations aimed at the transcendence of ordinary human consciousness and even at the literal transmutation of the body-mind into a body of subtle energy or light.

The heritage of Yoga was handed down from teacher to pupil by word of mouth. The Sanskrit term for this transmission of esoteric knowledge is *parampara,* which means literally "one after another" or "succession." As time progressed, much was added, much was left out or changed. Soon numerous schools had sprung up that represented distinct traditions, within which new splits and reformations took place. As we have seen in the preceding chapters, Yoga is by no means a homogeneous whole. Views and practices vary from school to school or teacher to teacher and sometimes cannot even be reconciled with each other. So, when we speak of Yoga, we speak of a multitude of paths and orientations with contrasting theoretical frameworks and occasionally incompatible goals. For instance, the ideal of Raja-Yoga is to recover one's true Identity as the transcendental Self standing eternally apart from the round of Nature, whereas the proclaimed ideal of Hatha-Yoga is to create an immortal body. To give another example, some schools favor the cultivation of paranormal powers (siddhi), whereas others advise practitioners to ignore them altogether.

Historically speaking, the most significant of all schools of Yoga is the classical system of Patanjali, which is also known as *the* "view of Yoga" (yoga-darshana). This system, which came to be equated with Raja-Yoga, is the formalized résumé of many generations of yogic experimentation and culture. Besides this philosophical school there are numerous nonsystematic Yogas, which are often interwoven with popular beliefs and practices. There are also Yogas within the Buddhist and Jaina spheres of teaching, which are briefly discussed in later chapters.

Within the Hindu realm, six major forms of Yoga have gained prominence. They are Raja-Yoga, Hatha-Yoga, Jnana-Yoga, Bhakti-Yoga, Karma-Yoga, and Mantra-Yoga, which will be introduced shortly. To these must be added Laya-Yoga and Kundalini-Yoga, which are closely associated with Hatha-Yoga but are often mentioned as independent approaches.

The Indian Yoga tradition has not ceased to change and grow, adapting to new sociocultural conditions. This is borne out by Sri Aurobindo's Integral Yoga, a unique modern approach that is based on traditional Yoga but goes beyond it by incorporating our contemporary understanding of biological evolution.

Additionally, we find in the Sanskrit scriptures numerous compound words that end in *-yoga*. For the most part, these do not stand for independent schools. Rather the word *yoga* has here the more general significance of "practice." For instance, the compound *buddhi-yoga* means the "practice or application of discriminative knowledge," and *samnyasa-yoga* denotes "the practice of renunciation." Other instances are: *dhyana-yoga,* "practice of meditation"; *samadhi-yoga,* "practice of ecstasy", and *guru-yoga,* "practice in relation to the spiritual teacher". Other compounds can arguably be said to represent a specific orientation, such as *nada-yoga* (Yoga of the inner sound), which is a form of Mantra-Yoga; *kriya-yoga* (Yoga of ritual action); and the Vedantic *asparsha-yoga* (intangible Yoga). The last-mentioned Yoga is so called because it consists in the direct contemplation of the intangible Absolute, which is the ever-present foundation of all existence.

If we liken Yoga to a many-spoked wheel, then the spokes can represent the diverse schools and movements of Yoga, the tire can symbolize the ethical requirements shared by all types of Yoga, while the hub can stand for the ecstatic experience (samadhi) by virtue of which the yogin transcends not only his own limited consciousness but cosmic existence itself. All authentic forms of Yoga are ways to a single center, the transcendental Reality, which may be defined differently by different schools. The genuine yogin is thus always motivated by self-transcendence or Self-realization.

There are also, however, yogins who aspire to the realization of states of consciousness that fall short of ultimate transcendence, or who seek to attain paranormal powers. Their orientations and teachings are magical rather than psychospiritual, as understood here. There is a strong magical component in the archaic tradition of tapas and also in Tantrism, which will both be

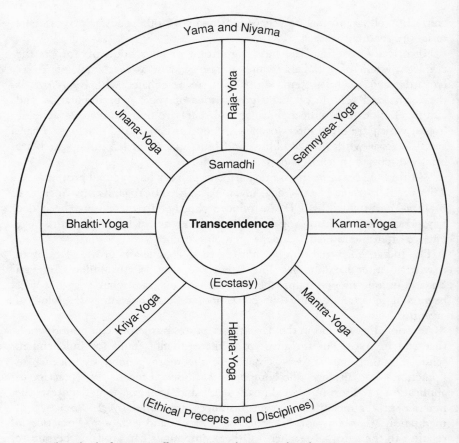

The wheel of Yoga: Different approaches to God-realization in Hinduism.

discussed in due course. Modern students are apt to dismiss the magical dimension of Yoga, but it is an integral aspect of yogic experience. Why else did Patanjali devote an entire chapter to paranormal powers (siddhi) in his Yoga-Sutra? It is important, though, that we remain sensitive to the distinction between magical purposes and the great work of spiritual transformation, which goes beyond the attainment of paranormal experiences and abilities, just as it goes beyond mere mystical states of consciousness. The goal of authentic spirituality, as I have repeatedly pointed out, is Self- or God-realization founded in self-transcendence.

RAJA-YOGA: THE RESPLENDENT YOGA OF SPIRITUAL KINGS

The designation *raja-yoga,* meaning "royal Yoga," is a comparatively late coinage that came in vogue in the sixteenth century A.D. It refers specifically to the Yoga system of Patanjali, created in the second century A.D., and is most commonly used to distinguish Patanjali's eightfold path of meditative introversion from Hatha-Yoga. The idea behind the appellation *raja-yoga* is that this type of Yoga is superior to Hatha-Yoga, which is thought to be for those who cannot dedicate themselves exclusively to the sacred ordeal of meditative practice and renunciation. In other words, Raja-Yoga touts itself as the Yoga for the true heroes of the spirit.

As Westerners, ill-practiced in prolonged contemplation, we can readily appreciate this qualification. At the same time, we cannot fail to note that this qualification is not altogether true to fact. For Hatha-Yoga, too, has its intense meditative practices and can certainly be as much of an ordeal as Raja-Yoga. Unfortunately, both Indian and Western practitioners of Hatha-Yoga do not always respect its ethical foundation or its spiritual goals and often tend to pursue it as a kind of calisthenics or body cosmetics.

Other explanations of the phrase *raja-yoga* are possible. It could refer to the fact that Patanjali's Yoga was practiced by kings, notably the eleventh-century King Bhoja, who even wrote a well-known commentary on the Yoga-Sutra of Patanjali. Switching over to a more esoteric level of explanation, we could also see in the word *raja* a hidden reference to the transcendental Self, which is the ultimate ruler of the body-mind and which is "resplendent" (rajate). Or the word could refer to the "Lord" (ishvara), or God, who is recognized by Patanjali as a special Self among the countless transcendental Selves.

Finally, the Yoga-Shikha-Upanishad, composed perhaps in the fourteenth century A.D., gives a completely esoteric interpretation:

> In the middle of the perineum (yoni), the great place, dwells well-concealed rajas, the principle of the Goddess, resembling the japa and bandhuka [flowers in color]. Raja-Yoga is so called owing to the union (yoga) of rajas and semen (retas). Having attained the [different powers] such as miniaturization through Raja-Yoga, [the yogin] is resplendent (rajate). (I.136–138)

The rajas principle mentioned in the above quote is sometimes identified as menstrual blood, sometimes as ovum. The latter interpretation makes better sense here, because the joining of semen and ovum leads to a new creature—in this case, metaphorically, the condition of enlightenment. Metaphysically speaking, retas and rajas are the male and the female principle respectively, whose perfect harmonization (samarasa) is thought to bring about the leap into unqualified ecstasy. But this esoteric explanation belongs to the realm of Tantric symbolism rather than to Patanjali's philosophical school.

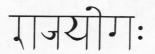

The Sanskrit term "Raja-Yoga" in the devanagari script.

Raja-Yoga, or Classical Yoga, is treated at length in Chapter 9 ("Yoga as Philosophy and Religion"). Since its creation in the second century A.D., it has been one of the most influential schools of Yoga. It is the high road of meditation and contemplation. As Swami Vivekananda declared enthusiastically, "Raja-Yoga is the science of religion, the rationale of all worship, all prayers, forms, ceremonies, and miracles."[1]

Swami Vivekananda added that the goal of Raja-Yoga is "how to concentrate the mind, then how to discover the innermost recesses of our own minds, then how to generalize their contents and form our own conclusions from them."[2] In the end this meditative quest is intended to lead to the discovery of the transcendental Reality beyond thought and image.

HATHA-YOGA: THE YOGA OF THE ADAMANTINE BODY

The "forceful Yoga," or Hatha-Yoga, is a medieval development. Its fundamental objective is the same as that of any authentic form of Yoga: to transcend the egoic consciousness and to realize the Self, or God. Yet the psychospiritual technology of Hatha-Yoga is particularly focused on developing the body's potential so that it can withstand the onslaught of transcendental realization. We are prone to think of ecstatic states like samadhi as purely mental events, which is not the case. Mystical states can have a profound effect on the nervous system and the rest of the body. After all, the experience occurs in or through the body. The hatha-yogin, therefore, seeks to steel the body—to "bake" it well, as the texts say.

Most importantly, enlightenment itself is a whole-body event. This has been made nowhere more clear than in the work of the contemporary spiritual teacher Da Free John, who writes:

> The Enlightenment of Man is the Enlightenment of the whole and entire body-mind. It is literal, even bodily Enlightenment, or Translation of the whole and entire body-mind of the individual into the absolute Radiance, Intensity, Love, or Light that is prior and superior to all the speeds of manifest or invisible light and all the forms or beings that cycle in manifest light, whether subtle or gross.[3]

Thus, the disciplines of Hatha-Yoga are designed to help manifest the

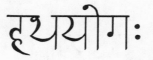

The term "Hatha-Yoga" in Sanskrit.

ultimate Reality in the finite human body-mind. In this, Hatha-Yoga expresses the ideal of Tantrism, which is to live in the world out of the fullness of Self-realization rather than to withdraw from life in order to gain enlightenment.

The hatha-yogin wants to construct a "divine body" (divya-sharira) or "diamond body" (vajra-deha) for himself, which would guarantee him immortality in the manifest realms. He is not interested in attaining enlightenment when this requires prolonged ascetic neglect of the body, which can lead to physical frailty and even death. He wants it all: Self-realization *and* a transmuted body in which to enjoy the manifest universe in its different dimensions. Who would not sympathize with this desire? Yet, as can be imagined, the practitioners of Hatha-Yoga have sometimes sacrificed their spiritual aspirations and settled for lesser, perhaps magical, goals. Magic, like exotechnology, is a way of manipulating the forces of Nature, whereas spirituality is about the transcendence of the manipulative ego-personality.

Narcissism, or body-oriented egocentrism, is as great a danger among hatha-yogins as it is among modern body-builders. A strong will is necessary in all spiritual traditions, but it can never be a substitute for discernment and renunciation. This has led some scholars to characterize Hatha-Yoga as a decadent teaching. Thus, the German Sanskritist J. W. Hauer made this harsh judgment:

> A typical product of the period of decline of the Indian mind, which, in spite of all assurances to the contrary, is far from the ruthlessly honest urge toward full clarification, the liberation of the soul, and the experience of the ultimate Reality . . . Hathayoga has a strong touch of coarse suggestion and is intimately linked with magic and sexuality.[4]

This condemnation certainly applies to the vulgarized versions of Hatha-Yoga practiced in India, but it is unjustifiable in regard to the authentic teachings and teachers of this tradition.

Genuine Hatha-Yoga always demands that it should be understood as psychospiritual technology in service of transcendental realization. In the Hatha-Yoga-Pradipika, the most popular manual of this school, this fact is expressed as follows: "All means of Hatha[-Yoga] are for [reaching] perfection in Raja-Yoga. A person rooted in Raja-Yoga [truly] conquers death" (IV.102). What this stanza suggests is that Hatha-Yoga and Raja-Yoga should be looked upon as a unit, and that the desire to conquer death is fulfilled only in Self-realization, for the transcendental Self is the only deathless, immortal thing there is. Even a specially manufactured body, composed of subtle matter or energy, must sooner or later disintegrate, since all products of Nature are subject to the law of change, or entropy.

Hatha-Yoga reminds one of the many body-oriented therapies that have sprung up in recent years. But the discoveries made by yogins centuries ago about the esoteric or subtle anatomy still need to be fully appreciated. Especially the phenomenon of the kundalini-shakti, the psychospiritual force dormant in the body-mind, is barely understood. Yet, as I will show, it is central to the hatha-yogin's inner work and to his perceptions and insights into dimensions of existence that are just beginning to be of interest to modern science.

The metaphysics and the practical path of Hatha-Yoga are dealt with in some detail in Chapter 13 ("Yoga as Spiritual Alchemy").

JNANA-YOGA: CULTIVATING THE EYE OF WISDOM

The word *jnana* means "knowledge," "insight," or "wisdom" and in spiritual contexts has the sense of what the Greeks called *gnosis,* a special kind of liberating knowledge or intuition. Jnana-Yoga is virtually identical with the spiritual path of Vedanta, the tradition of nondualism. Jnana-Yoga is the path of Self-realization through the exercise of gnostic understanding, or, to be more precise, the wisdom associated with discerning the Real from the unreal.

The term *jnana-yoga* is first mentioned in the Bhagavad-Gita, where Krishna, the God incarnate, declares to his pupil Prince Arjuna: "Of yore I proclaimed a twofold way of life in this world, o guileless [Arjuna]—Jnana-Yoga for the samkhyas and Karma-Yoga for the yogins" (III.3).

Karma-Yoga, as we will see, is the Yoga of self-surrendered action, which is said here to be for the yogins. The samkhyas are the followers of the once powerful Samkhya tradition, which is the contemplative path of distinguishing between the products of Nature and the transcendental Self, until the Self (purusha) is realized. The Samkhya path is discussed in the fourth section of Chapter 3 ("Yoga and Other Hindu Traditions"). The Bhagavad-Gita's characterization of the paths of yogins and samkhyas appears arbitrary. The anonymous author may have felt this, for he tries to bridge the gap between the two by having Krishna reject the view that Yoga and Samkhya are completely separate approaches:

> "Samkhya and Yoga are different" say the simpletons, not the learned. Resorting properly to one [or the other], one obtains the fruit of both. (V.4)

> That state which is obtained by the samkhyas is also reached by the yogins. He who sees Samkhya and Yoga as one, sees indeed. (V.4)

It is clear from the context that Krishna equates Jnana-Yoga with Buddhi-Yoga. In my rendering of the Bhagavad-Gita, I have translated the term *buddhi* as "wisdom-faculty." It signifies illumined reason. Buddhi-Yoga is the path of Self-realization that applies discriminative wisdom to all situations and conditions of life. For this reason, it goes hand in hand with Karma-Yoga. In the words of Krishna:

Renouncing in thought all actions to Me, intent on Me, resorting to Buddhi-Yoga, be constantly "Me-minded." (XVIII.57)

"Me-minded," you will transcend all obstacles by My grace. But if out of egotism (ahamkara) you will not listen, you will perish! (XVIII.57)

The "Me-mindedness" spoken of here is of course not a form of egotism but the practice of placing one's attention on the Divine. The "Me," in other words, is God Krishna, not the human personality.

In contrast to Raja-Yoga, which operates on the basis of a dualistic metaphysics that distinguishes between the transcendental Selves and Nature, the metaphysics of Jnana-Yoga is strictly nondualistic (advaita). As I have mentioned already, it is the path of the Vedanta tradition par excellence. It is the way taught in the Upanishads and is also known as the "road of wisdom" (jnana-marga). In the opinion of the Indian scholar N. K. Brahma, Jnana-Yoga

is fundamentally different from all other forms and stands really unique in the history of the world. It is not the worship of God as an object different from the self and is not a discipline that leads to the attainment of anything distinct from one's own self. It may be described as *atma-upasana* (the worship of God as one's Self).[5]

The practitioner of Jnana-Yoga, who is known as a jnanin, can be said to treat willpower (iccha) and inspired reason (buddhi) as the two guiding principles by which he can attain enlightenment. The Tripura-Rahasya (XIX.16ff.), a late but important work on Jnana-Yoga, distinguishes between three types of aspirants of Jnana-Yoga, depending on the predominant psychic disposition (vasana): The first type suffers from the fault of pride, which stands in the way of a proper understanding of the teachings of Jnana-Yoga. The second type suffers from "activity" (karma), by which is meant the illusion of being an active subject, an ego-personality engaged in acts, which prevents equanimity and clarity as the basis of true wisdom. The third and most common type suffers from the "monster" of desire — that is, from motivations that run counter to the primal impulse toward liberation. A person of this type, for instance, loses himself or herself in the hunger for power, the desire for fame, or in designs of sexual possession.

The prideful type of Jnana-Yoga practitioner overcomes his fault by cultivating trust in the teaching and the teacher. The type who thinks of himself or herself as a doer of actions is simply in need of grace. The third, impulsive type must make a concerted effort to cultivate dispassion and discrimination through study, worship, and frequenting the illumined presence of the sages. Most practitioners of Jnana-Yoga fall into this third group: those who are still confronting the desires and motivations that conflict with the impulse toward emancipation.

The Tripura-Rahasya (XIX.35) further states that the single most important factor of success is the actual urge toward emancipation. Philosophical study on its own is said to be like "dressing up a corpse." It comes alive only through the desire for liberation, and that desire must be deeply felt and not merely based on casual fascination or delusions of grandeur. Above all, the urge toward Self-realization must translate into consistent daily practice in order to bear fruit.

Depending on the practitioner's efforts and personality, Jnana-Yoga can manifest differently in different individuals; although, as the unknown author of the Tripura-Rahasya (XIX.71) is quick to point out, these differences do not mean that wisdom itself is manifold. Rather, jnana admits of no distinction. Jnana is not different from the transcendental Reality.

This marvelous Sanskrit scripture next speaks of those jnanins who are liberated even while continuing to be present in the physical body. These great beings, called jivan-muktas ("living liberated"), are quite unaffected by whatever dispositions or desires may arise in their conditional personalities. A second category comprises those advanced practitioners of Jnana-Yoga who are so focused on the sacred work of self-transcendence that, in their single-mindedness, they appear to be mindless. These are the illustrious sages. Their mindlessness manifests in a childlike quality that reflects their utter inner simplicity. They have no concerns or worries and no interest in acquiring knowledge or in displaying cleverness. The mind is useful to them only insofar as it allows them to handle the practicalities of their lives. Gradually it is superseded by flawless spontaneity in all circumstances, without the intervening circuitry of the mind.

The path of Jnana-Yoga, which has been described as "a straight but steep course,"[6] is outlined with elegant conciseness in the Vedanta-Sara of Sadananda, a fifteenth-century text. Sadananda lists four principal means for attaining emancipation:

1. Discrimination (viveka) between the permanent and the transient; that is, the constant practice of seeing the world for what it is—a finite and changeable realm that, even at its most enjoyable, must never be confused with the transcendental Bliss.
2. Renunciation (viraga) of the enjoyment of the fruit (phala) of one's actions; this is the ideal of Karma-Yoga, which asks students to engage in appropriate actions without expecting any reward.
3. The "six accomplishments" (shat-sampatti), which are detailed below.
4. The urge toward liberation (mumukshutva); that is, the cultivation of the spiritual impulse.

The six accomplishments are:

1. Tranquillity (shama), the art of remaining calm even in the face of

adversity.

2. Sense-restraint (dama), the curbing of one's senses, which are habitually hankering after stimulation.
3. "Cessation" (uparati), abstention from actions that are not relevant either to the maintenance of the body or to the pursuit of enlightenment.
4. Endurance (titiksha), specifically understood as the stoic ability to be unruffled by the play of opposites (dvandva) in Nature, such as heat and cold, pleasure and pain, or praise and censure.
5. Mental collectedness (samadhana), or concentration, the discipline of single-mindedness in all situations but specifically during periods of formal meditation.
6. Faith (shraddha), a deeply inspired, heartfelt reverence for the sacred and transcendental. Faith must not be confused with mere belief, which operates only in the mind.

In some works a sevenfold path is expounded. A good example is Shankara's brilliant commentary on the Brahma-Sutra (I.1.4), which together with the Upanishads and the Bhagavad-Gita is considered the philosophical mainstay of the Vedanta tradition. This sevenfold path includes the above-mentioned practices with the exception of mental collectedness, and additionally has the following means: "listening" (shravana), or reception of the sacred teachings, and pondering (manana) on their import, as well as meditation (nididhya-sana).[7]

Jnana-Yoga, then, is the disciplined cultivation of the eye of wisdom (jnana-cakshus), which alone can lead us, in the words of an ancient Hindu prayer, "from the unreal to the Real."

BHAKTI-YOGA: THE SELF-TRANSCENDING POWER OF LOVE

Raja-Yoga and Jnana-Yoga approach Self-realization chiefly through the transcendence and transformation of the mind, whereas Hatha-Yoga aspires to the same goal through the transmutation of the body. In Bhakti-Yoga, however, the emotional force of the human being is channeled toward the Divine. Therefore, in their discipline of ecstatic self-transcendence, the bhakti-yogins tend to be more openly expressive than the typical raja-yogins or jnanins. The followers of Bhakti-Yoga do not, for instance, shy away from shedding tears of longing for the Divine. In this approach, the transcendental Reality is usually conceived as a supreme Person rather than in impersonal terms as in the Vedanta tradition.

The term *bhakti*, derived from the root *bhaj* ("to share or participate in") is generally rendered as "devotion" or "love." Bhakti-Yoga is thus the Yoga of loving self-dedication to the divine Person. It is the way of the heart.

Shandilya, the author of the Bhakti-Sutra (I.2), defines *bhakti* as "supreme attachment to the Lord." It is the only kind of attachment that does not reinforce the egoic personality and its destiny. Attachment is a combination of placing one's attention on something and investing it with great emotional energy. When we confess that we are attached to a person or a pet, we mean that we enjoy their company or even simply thinking about them, so that when we contemplate their absence or loss, we become saddened. The loss of a loved individual, animal, or even inanimate object seems to diminish our own being.

It is such energized love-attachment (asakti) that the bhakti-yogin harnesses in his quest for communion or union with the Divine. At times when we are emotionally estranged from the Ground of existence, we similarly feel diminished in our being. In fact, the masters of Bhakti-Yoga would say that the confusion and unhappiness prevalent in the world are caused precisely by our alienation from the Divine. St. Augustine undoubtedly intuited this when he exclaimed that "our heart is restless until it rests in Thee."[8]

In Bhakti-Yoga, the practitioner is always a devotee (bhakta), a lover. There are different degrees of devotion, and the Bhagavata-Purana, composed in the ninth century A.D., describes nine stages. These have been formalized as follows:

1. Listening (shravana) to the names of the Divine Person; each of the hundreds of names highlights a different quality of God, and hearing them creates a devotional attitude in the receptive listener.
2. Chanting (kirtana) songs of praise in honor of the Lord; such songs generally have a simple melody and are accompanied by musical instruments. Again, the singing is a form of meditative remembrance of the Divine and can lead to ecstatic breakthroughs.
3. Remembrance (smarana) of God, the meditative recalling of the attributes of the divine Person, often in His human incarnation— for instance, as the lovely shepherd-boy Krishna.
4. "Service at the feet" (pada-sevana) of the Lord; this is ceremonial worship. The feet are traditionally considered a terminal of magical and spiritual power (shakti) and grace. In the case of one's living teacher, self-surrender is frequently expressed by bowing at the guru's feet. Here service at the Lord's feet is understood metaphorically, as one's inner embrace of the Divine in all one's activities.
5. Ritual (arcana), the performance of the prescribed religious rites, especially those involving the daily ceremony at the home altar on which the image of one's deity is installed.
6. Prostration (vandana) before the image of the Divine.
7. "Slavish" devotion (dasya) to God, which is expressed in the devotee's intense yearning to be in the company of the Lord.

8. Feeling of friendship (sakhya) for the Divine, which is a more intimate form of associating with God.

9. "Self-offering" (atma-nivedana), or ecstatic self-transcendence through which the worshipper enters into the immortal body of the divine Person.[9]

These nine stages form part of a ladder of continuous ascent to ever more fervent devotion and thus union with the Divine. Supporting this process is the disposition of faith (shraddha), which is true of all traditional forms of Yoga. In Vyasa's Yoga-Bhashya (I.20), faith is said to be like a good, protective mother. Faith is different from belief. Whereas belief is of the nature of an opinion, faith is more a positive attitude, here a disposition of trust in the yogic process.

Remarkably, the Bhagavata-Purana (VII.1.30) acknowledges the liberating power of emotions other than love, such as fear, sexual desire, and even hatred—so long as their object is the Divine. The secret behind this is simple enough: In order to fear God, feel hatred for Him, or approach the Lord with burning sexual love (as did the shepherdesses of Vrindavana in the case of the God-man Krishna), a person must place his or her attention on the Divine. This creates a bridge across which the eternally given grace can enter and transform that person's life, even to the point of enlightenment provided the emotion is intense enough.

The devotee feels a growing passion (rati) for the Lord, and this helps him or her to break down one barrier after another between the human personality and the Divine Person. This increasing love culminates in the vision of the cosmos penetrated, saturated, and sustained by the Lord. This is the kind of vision that overwhelmed and awed Prince Arjuna, as described in the famous eleventh chapter of the Bhagavad-Gita. Witnessing the divine splendor of Krishna, Arjuna exclaimed:

O God, in your Body I behold the gods and all the various kinds of beings, the Lord Brahma seated on the lotus throne, and all the seers and divine serpents! (XI.15)

Everywhere I behold you [who are] of endless Form, with many arms, bellies, mouths, and eyes. I can see no end, middle, or beginning in you, O All-Lord, All-Form! (XI.16)

I behold you with diadem, mace, and discus—a mass of brilliance, flaming all-round. You are hard to see, for you are entirely a brilliant radiance of sun-fire, immeasurable. (XI.17)

Beholding that great Form of yours, with its many mouths and eyes, its many arms, thighs, feet, bellies, and formidable fangs, O strong-armed [Krishna], the worlds shudder, and so do I. (XI.23)

With flaming mouths, you lick up and devour all the worlds entirely. Filling the whole universe with your brilliance, your dread-inspiring rays blaze forth, O Vishnu. (XI.30)

Tell me who you of dread-inspiring Form are. Salutations be to you! O Foremost God, have mercy! I wish to know you [as you were] at first [in your human form], for I do not comprehend your Creativity (pravritti). (XI.31)

The final moment of realization, when the Divine and the devotee become one, is often described as supreme love (para-bhakti). Prior to that event, devotion requires that God is an Other who can be worshipped in song, ritual action, or meditation. After that moment, the Divine and the devotee are inseparably merged in love.

In his Bhakti-Sutra, Sage Narada distinguishes between a primary and a secondary type of devotion. The latter is tinged by personal objectives and ulterior motives, such as the desire to be protectively embraced by the Lord or to be aided by him in worldly affairs. It can express itself in many different ways. Depending on the predominance of one of the three qualities (guna) of Nature, the devotee's love for the Divine can be more or less self-centered and more or less active.[10] By contrast, primary devotion is total surrender to God, pure devotion free of selfish motivation. As Narada puts it in his Bhakti-Sutra (5), the true devotee "sees nothing but love, hears only about love, speaks only of love, and thinks of love alone." The modern Indian scholar Surendranath Dasgupta characterized this spiritual practitioner as follows:

> Such a person is so attached to God that there is nothing else for which he cares; without any effort on his part, other attachments and inclinations lose their hold over him. So great is his passion for God that it consumes all his earthly passion. . . .
>
> The bhakta who is filled with such a passion does not experience it merely as an undercurrent of joy which waters the depths of his heart in his own privacy, but as a torrent that overflows the caverns of his heart into all his senses. Through all his senses he realizes it as if it were a sensuous delight; with his heart and soul he feels it as a spiritual intoxication of joy. Such a person is beside himself with this love of God. He sings, laughs, dances and weeps. He is no longer a person of this world.[11]

Bhakti-Yoga has been called a dualistic teaching par excellence, but this is not true of all schools of this Yoga. Even though at the outset all devotees relate to the Divine as a Person who is a separate being, the final goal of some schools is to merge so completely with the Divine that there is completely forgetfulness of one's own being: The Lord becomes one's only reality.

The History of the Bhakti Ideal

The devotional approach in India has a fascinating history that we know only imperfectly. Apart from the few monotheistic hymns of the Vedas that imply or express an emotional relationship to the invoked deity, the early Vedic religion is curiously devoid of devotionalism. It is almost as if sacrificial ritualism and love were mutually exclusive. The Vedic priests can almost be characterized as bureaucrats of the spirit. The proper performance of the various rituals seemed more important to them than either personal devotion to the Divine or the expression of love in interpersonal relationships. They were motivated more by a sense of duty than by the spontaneity of a happy heart.

Bhakti-Yoga calls for the exact opposite of ritualistic fixation, namely emotional fluidity and expressiveness. In archaic India, this unique attitude was rarely cultivated as a spiritual discipline. Either the religious-minded sought meaning in the exacting performance of the daily rituals, or they joined one of the more marginal groups of ecstatics, like the Vratyas, that traveled from place to place.[12] Later, perhaps as early as 1000 B.C., spiritual seekers were given a third option: They could drop out without risking censure, by becoming forest eremites. As hermits they were free to explore the hidden, mystical significances of the rituals and experiment with yogalike meditation or ascetic practices.

Early on, however, the monotheistic Pancaratra tradition of Vishnu worshippers offered a further alternative. It attracted a growing number of those who found the Vedic pantheon of gods unconvincing or the impersonal Absolute (brahman) of the orthodox theologians too abstract and who longed for personal intimacy with the Divine. The Pancaratra tradition flourished at the margins of ancient Indian society and was certainly not looked upon favorably by the Vedic priesthood. But this school did inspire the creation of the Bhagavata sect within the Vedic orthodox fold. It is largely because of the success of this sect as a movement—epitomized in the immense popularity of the Bhagavata-Purana and the Bhagavad-Gita—that Hinduism is what it is today: a religious culture of temples, sacred imagery, devotional worship, and (not least) Yoga. The Pancaratra tradition was instrumental in the development of Yoga by introducing the concept and practice of bhakti into what is all too often a somewhat heady or dry approach to Self-realization.

Although the bhakti path was originally most intimately associated with the religious worship of God Vishnu, the word *bhakti* is first used in the technical sense in a scripture dedicated to God Shiva. This is the Shvetashvatara-Upanishad (VI.23), a powerfully monotheistic work belonging perhaps to the third or fourth century B.C.[13] This text introduces the idea of love for God and love for the spiritual teacher, who should be loved in the same manner as God since he is the embodiment of the Divine.

In order to appreciate the evolution of the bhakti path, we must understand that the monotheistic teachings were developed largely, though not exclusively, in two sectarian circles, namely Vaishnavism (arising out of the Pancaratra tradition) and Shaivism. The Vaishnavas celebrate God Vishnu as the divine Person, and the Shaivas dedicate their lives to Lord Shiva. A third significant strand of development is known as Shaktism, which centers on the worship of the Divine in its female or power (shakti) aspect. Here, too, bhakti played an important role in the ritual worship of the Goddess, whether it be Kali, Durga, Parvati, or any of the other female deities.

The Bhagavad-Gita, a Vaishnava scripture belonging to approximately the same period as the Shvetashvatara-Upanishad, uses the word *bhakti* extensively. It describes the proper relationship between the spiritual practitioner and the Divine in the form of Lord Krishna. However, it not only signifies the appropriate response to the divine Person but also the final goal: Bhakti is the very essence of the liberated condition.[14]

The bhakti ideal found enthusiastic reception especially in south India, which was the home of a sensitive culture that was of non-Vedic origin and that celebrated its poets and artists. There the path of devotion was developed by both the Shaiva and the Vaishnava sects. Thousands of works extolling the virtue of devotion in its various forms were created in the millennium between 200 B.C. and A.D. 800. We will further explore these developments in Chapter 10 ("The Nondual Approach to God").

Among the Vaishnava minority of south India, the bhakti ideal and the worship of God Vishnu were particularly promoted by the Alvars, a group of twelve bhaktas (including only one woman). They sang their songs of praise in the eighth century A.D. The northern branches of Vaishnavism and Shaivism likewise popularized the bhakti approach in their own distinct fashion.

The Alvars were followed by the so-called Acaryas ("Instructors"), who attempted to systematize the monotheistic theology of Vaishnavism. Foremost among them was Ramanuja (A.D. 1017–1137), a southern brahmin. He was the principal exponent of Vishishta-Advaita, or Qualified Nondualism. His contribution to Hinduism equals that of Shankara, for what Ramanuja did was to make the idea of a suprapersonal Divine Being logically consistent with the teaching of Vedantic nondualism. He succeeded in integrating the northern and southern traditions of Vaishnavism, thereby greatly strengthening the religious worship of Vishnu and paving the way for the medieval bhakti-marga, or "way of devotion."

Ramanuja formulated a Yoga that is radically different from Patanjali's system in that the cultivation of bhakti, not meditation, is given prominence. For Ramanuja, devotion was not only the means to liberation but the goal of all spiritual endeavor. In this school, therefore, there is no end to spiritual practice.

The history of the bhakti cult and subsequent movement is vastly complex, and modern scholarship has only scratched the surface. The traditions of southern India have been especially neglected. What is clear, however, is that India has not only had its share of world-denying mystics but can also take pride in its many generations of thousands of love-intoxicated seekers and realizers.

The teachers of this tradition hail bhakti as the easiest way to emancipation. Loving devotion to the Lord bears fruit readily when it is constant, unswerving, and purposeless. The shepherdesses (gopi) of the Krishna legends symbolize that attitude perfectly. In their ardor for the God-man Krishna, they forgot everything—their husbands, children, family, friends, and daily duties. They were simply intoxicated with love, and it was their love that brought them closer to the divine essence of the beautiful young shepherd boy who was really God incarnate.

KARMA-YOGA: FREEDOM IN ACTION

To exist is to act. Even an inanimate object such as a rock has movement. And the building blocks of matter, the atoms, are in fact not building blocks at all but incredibly complex patterns of energy in constant motion. Thus, the universe is a vast vibratory expanse. In the words of philosopher Alfred North Whitehead, the world is *process*. It is on this insight, commonplace as it may seem, that Karma-Yoga is founded.

The word *karma* (or *karman*), derived from the root *kri* ("to make, do"), has many meanings. It can signify "action," "work," "product," "effect," and so on. Thus Karma-Yoga is literally the Yoga of Action. But here the term *karma* stands for a specific kind of action. More precisely, it denotes a particular inner *attitude* toward action, which is itself a form of action. What this attitude consists in is spelled out in the Bhagavad-Gita, the earliest scripture to teach Karma-Yoga.

> Not by abstention from actions does a man enjoy action-transcendence, nor by renunciation alone does he approach perfection. (III.4)

> For, not even for a moment can anyone ever remain without performing action. Everyone is unwittingly made to act by the qualities (guna) issuing from Nature. (III.5)

> He who restrains his organs of action, but sits remembering in his mind the objects of the senses, is called a self-bewildered hypocrite. (III.6)

> So—more excellent is he, O Arjuna, who, controlling with his mind the senses, embarks unattached on Karma-Yoga with his organs of action. (III.7)

> You must do the allotted action, for action is superior to inaction; not even your body's processes (yatra) can be accomplished by inaction. (III.8)

> This world is action-bound, save when this action is [intended] as sacrifice. With that purpose, O son of Kunti, engage in action devoid of attachment. (III.9)

> Therefore always perform unattached the proper (karya) deed, for the man who performs action without attachment attains the Supreme. (III.19)

Then God Krishna, who communicates these teachings to his pupil Arjuna, points to himself as the archetypal model of the active person:

> For Me, O son of Pritha, there is nothing to be done in the three worlds, nothing ungained to be gained—and yet I engage in action. (III.22)

For, if I were not untiringly ever to abide in action, people would, O son of Pritha, follow everywhere My "track" [that is, My example]. (III.23)

If I were not to perform action, these worlds would perish, and I would be the author of chaos, destroying [all] creatures. (III.24)

Just as the unwise act attached to action, O son of Bharata, the wise should act unattached, desiring the world's welfare. (III.25)

By the qualities (guna) of Nature, actions are everywhere performed. [Yet, he whose] self is deluded by the ego (ahamkara) thinks: "I am the doer." (III.27)

But, O strong-armed one, the knower of Reality [who understands] the relationship between the qualities and action is unattached and thinks: "Qualities abide in qualities." (III.28)

Always performing all [allotted] actions and taking refuge in Me, he attains through My grace the eternal, immutable State. (XVIII.56)

Renouncing in thought all actions to Me, intent on Me, resorting to Buddhi-Yoga, be constantly "Me-minded." (XVIII.57)

What Krishna, the divine Lord, is saying here is that all activity arises spontaneously as part of the program of Nature (prakriti). The idea that "I do this or that" is an illusion, a fatal presumption that we habitually superimpose on what is actually occurring. Thus, even our thoughts are not really generated by us. Thoughts, like all processes of Nature, are simply arising. We decide to type into a computer, play the piano, ride a bicycle, or speak to a friend—but these activities, according to Krishna (and the spiritual authorities of Hinduism in general), are not effects of the ego-personality in relation to which they seem to be occurring. In fact, the "I" itself arises as one of the activities of Nature, presuming itself to be the actor of certain deeds.

The objective of Karma-Yoga is stated to be "action-freedom." The actual Sanskrit term is *naishkarmya,* which means, confusingly enough, "nonaction." This literal meaning is misleading; it is not inactivity that is meant to be expressed here. Rather, naishkarmya-karman corresponds to the Taoist notion of wu wei, or inaction in action. That is to say, Karma-Yoga is about freedom *in* action, or the transcendence of egoic motivations. When the illusion of the ego as acting subject is transcended, then actions are recognized to occur spontaneously. Without the interference of the ego, their spontaneity appears as a smooth flow. Hence, truly enlightened beings have an economy and elegance of movement about them that is generally absent in unenlightened individuals. Behind the action of the enlightened being there is no author; or we could say that Nature is the Author.

Since, by definition, life is action, even any apparent inaction must be understood as a form of action. The principle of Karma-Yoga applies universally. This means that even the renouncers in the tradition of samnyasa, who formally abstain from secular activity, are still bound *to* action and bound *by* their actions, unless their withdrawal from the world is done in the spirit of Karma-Yoga.

Through Karma-Yoga, whether one lives the life of a householder or of a renouncer, every action is turned into a sacrifice. What is sacrificed is, in the last analysis, the self or ego. So long as the ego (ahamkara) is the author behind actions or inactions, these actions or inactions have a binding power. They reinforce the ego and thereby obstruct the event of enlightenment.

Egoic action or inaction generates karma. The word *karma* has become part of the English language, and *Webster's* explains it as "the force generated by a person's actions held in Hinduism and Buddhism to perpetuate transmigration and in its ethical consequences to determine his destiny in his next existence." This definition is essentially correct. Karma is not only action but also its invisible result that shapes a person's destiny.

The underlying idea is that we are what we are because of what we do or, rather, how we do it. In our actions, we express who or what we are (or presume ourselves to be). In other words, we externalize our inner being, so that our actions are a reflection of ourselves. But they are not only reflections. There is a "feedback loop" between our actions and our being. Every action acts upon our self and contributes to the entire structure of the person we tend to be.

Thus, put simply, if someone tends to be a good-hearted, benign individual, his or her actions are apt to be what would be judged good or benign, and they reinforce that person's native good-heartedness and benignity. On the other hand, if someone tends to be mean and destructive, his or her actions are likely to be of the kind that would be judged mean and destructive, and they reinforce that individual's native meanness and destructiveness.

Actions and inactions have their immediate, visible results, which may or may not have been intended. But just as important is their invisible aftereffect on the quality of our being, about which we in the West are mostly ignorant. We may send in our monthly donation to our favorite charity and thereby help those in need as well as obtain various advantages such as a tax break—the visible results of our action. But we also set in motion invisible forces that shape and transform our being and thus our future destiny: We reap as we sow. That India's religious geniuses have understood this very clearly is evident from the karma doctrine.

The link between action and its feedback effects is thought to be an iron law, or what has been called the law of moral causation. It appears that the karmic law is the only immutable aspect of our world of constant change, the samsara. It governs the cosmos on all its countless levels, and only the transcendental Reality itself is free of this peculiar arrangement.

This teaching is closely associated with another widespread belief shared by all Hindu, Buddhist, and Jaina schools. This is the notion that the human being is a multidimensional structure or process, which does not come to an abrupt end with the death of the physical body. Different traditions have offered different explanations for this postmortem continuity, and the interpretations range from naive to rather sophisticated. According to some, the surviving consciousness is clothed in a nonmaterial body awaiting its renewed incarnation on the material plane in another physical body, or on one of the supramaterial (or "subtle") planes in a supraphysical body. According to others, the ego-consciousness does not survive the death of the body, so that there is, strictly speaking, no stable transmigrating entity but only a continuity of different karmic forces.

All schools are agreed that the mechanics of destiny on the physical plane and on any other level of existence are controlled by the quality of a person's action or, more accurately, his or her *intention*. Karma-Yoga is the art and science of "karmically" aware and responsible action and action-intention. Its immediate purpose is to prevent the accumulation of unfavorable karmic effects and to reverse the effects of existing karma.

Karma-Yoga implies a complete reversal of human nature, for it demands that every action be performed out of a disposition that is radically distinct from our everyday mood. Not only are we asked to assume responsibility for appropriate (karya) action but also to offer up our work and its fruit to the divine Person. Such offering (arpana), however, necessarily entails a self-offering, or the surrender of the ego. Karma-Yoga is thus considerably more than doing one's duty. It goes beyond conventional morality and involves a profound spiritual attitude. The "easy" discipline of Karma-Yoga, when adopted conscientiously, becomes a fiery practice of self-transcendence.

Action performed in the spirit of self-surrender has benign invisible effects. It improves the quality of our being and makes us a source of spiritual uplift for others. Lord Krishna, in the Bhagavad-Gita, speaks of the karma-yogin's working for the welfare of the world. The Sanskrit phrase he uses is *loka-samgraha,* which literally means "world-gathering." What it refers to is this: Our own personal wholeness, founded in self-surrender, actively transforms our social environment, contributing to its wholeness. But this is not the goal of the karma-yogin, only an inevitable side effect of his practice of inaction in action.

It should be noted here that the law of karma does not intrinsically encourage fatalism, even though some individuals and sects have taken this stance. On the contrary, it is a call to assume responsibility for one's destiny. This is made clear in all the psychospiritual traditions of India, which, as liberation teachings, insist on the freedom of will: We are free to turn toward the transcendental Reality, or toward conditional existence under the thrall of karma.

The fulcrum of Karma-Yoga is that we can transcend all karmic necessity *in our consciousness.* We still have to endure certain karmic results (such as illness, misfortune, and of course death), but these need not determine our being. In our essence we are free, and the yogin who has realized the Self is abundantly aware of this truth. Action can improve the quality of our being and destiny, and this is the intent behind conventional religiosity: A person does good deeds because he or she wants to be spared the terrible blows of bad karma and instead enter one of the delightful realms after dropping the physical body.

Karma-Yoga, however, aims at the transcendence of all possible destinies in the conditional realms of the multilevel cosmos. The karma-yogin, and indeed all authentic spiritual practitioners of any tradition, aspire to the Unconditional beyond good and evil, pain and pleasure, beyond karmic necessity and embodiment. For when the Self is realized there is only bliss, and from this position the machine of Nature cannot touch our true being. A Self-realized yogin may suffer all kinds of adversities — the late Ramana Maharshi, one of modern India's great sages, died of cancer — but he knows himself to be infinitely above the arising qualities of conditional existence. The Self-realized adept *is* the transcendental essence of all qualities — seemingly desirable or undesirable — that impinge upon the physical body or the personality associated with it. Herein lies his triumph over the body, the mind, and all other finite aspects of human nature.

Historically, Karma-Yoga can be seen as the countering response of the conservative forces in ancient India to the growing social movement of world renunciation. Spiritually, however, it is much more than a compromise solution between conventional life (whether religious or secular) and the life of a forest-dwelling ascetic or wandering mendicant. It is an integral teaching that transcends both worldliness and otherworldliness. The Bhagavad-Gita, therefore, represents a genuine innovation.[15] Its teachings have exerted a lasting influence on many other Hindu traditions.

Another noteworthy work that must be mentioned in the present context is the Yoga-Vasishtha, composed well over a thousand years after the dialogue between Krishna and Arjuna. Although it espouses a form of nondualism that is so radical as to regard the world as entirely illusory, it nevertheless favors an even more positive affirmation of mundane existence than does the Bhagavad-Gita. In the Yoga-Vasishtha, the yogin is invited to fully participate in the activities of his family and society. Wisdom (jnana) and action (karma) are compared to the two wings of a bird; it needs both to fly. Emancipation is said to be achieved by the harmonious development of both means.

A similar teaching is found in the Tri-Shikhi-Brahmana-Upanishad, a late medieval work:

> Yoga is deemed twofold: Jnana-Yoga and Karma-Yoga. Now then, O best of brahmins, listen to the Yoga of action (kriya-yoga). The binding of the undistracted consciousness (citta) to an object, O best among the twice-born [i.e., brahmins], is union (samyoga). It is attained in two ways: The constant binding of the mind (manas) to prescribed action — since action is to be performed — is called Karma-Yoga. The continual binding of consciousness to the supreme Object should be known as Jnana-Yoga, which is auspicious and yields all accomplishments. He whose mind is immutable, even though the twofold Yoga characterized here [is followed], goes to the supreme Good, which is of the nature of liberation. (II.23–28)

Karma-Yoga is the most grounded of all yogic approaches. Its great ideal of inaction in action (naishkarmya-karma) applies to all other spiritual disciplines and is as relevant today as it was when the Indian sages first formulated it well over 2000 years ago.

MANTRA-YOGA: SOUND AS A VEHICLE OF TRANSCENDENCE

Sound is a form of vibration, and it was known as such to the yogins of ancient and medieval India. According to the dominant theory of the science of sacred sound (known as mantra-vidya or mantra-shastra), the universe is in a constant state of vibration (spanda or spandana). The discovery that sound, particularly repetitive sound, affects consciousness was made a very long time ago, possibly in the Stone Age. We may safely assume that some form of simple chanting and drumming, possibly with animal bones as drumsticks, was associated with paleolithic rituals. It is not surprising, therefore, that by the time the Vedic religious community was flowering in north India, sound (both as speech or chanting and as music) had become a rather sophisticated ritual means.

The Vedic hymns are known as mantras. There is no adequate English equivalent for the word *mantra*, which derives from the root *man* ("to think, be intent"), as found in the term *manas* ("mind"). A mantra is sacred utterance, numinous sound, or sound that is charged with psychospiritual power. A mantra is sound that empowers the mind or that is empowered by the mind. It is a vehicle of meditative transformation of the human body-mind and is thought to have magical potency.

The Sanskrit hymns of the Vedas, envisioned by the seers, were composed in fifteen different meters that called for punctilious recitation in ritual contexts and required carefully regulated breathing to ensure the necessary accuracy. It is here that we may find the origins of the later yogic technique of breath control (pranayama). One of the four Vedic hymnodies, the Sama-Veda, contains a large number of hymns that were sung by special priests during the great sacrificial rites; the songs sounded rather like the medieval plain-chants.

Four types of priests were involved in the formal ceremonies. The hotri recited the hymns, the ugatri and his helpers accompanied the rituals with songs (chandas) and music, the adhvaryu performed the manual rites while pronouncing the various sacrificial formulas, and the brahmana or brahmin acted as overseer, protecting the ceremony through his intense attention to liturgical details. As the German Yoga researcher J. W. Hauer has shown, the melodies (saman) of these songs were not of Vedic origin but belonged to the Vratya brotherhoods, which were connected with the early development of Yoga. The Vedic priests simply adopted them for their own hymns.

It is a well known fact that prolonged and concentrated chanting leads to changes in consciousness. Combined with the intoxicating effects of the liquid used in the daily soma sacrifice, it is easy to imagine that the priests were experts on altered states of consciousness. It is not absolutely clear from which plant the soma juice was pressed; some think it was the fly agaric mushroom.[16] The soma juice was not merely poured into the sacrificial fire—the Vedic people drank it for its hallucinogenic effects.

The most remarkable speculation about sound is found in a hymn of the

Rig-Veda (I.164), the most important of the four Vedic collections of hymns. That hymn speaks of Vac (related to the Latin *vox,* "speech"), a feminine deity, the "mother" of the Vedas. She is said to have four "feet" (pada), or aspects. Three of these are beyond the ken of mortals; only one is known, belonging to human speech. Only the seers (rishi) know how to track down Vac in her hidden dimension. Another hymn (X.71.4) expresses regret at those who see and hear without seeing and hearing Vac.

In other hymns, Vac is related to the sacred cows (vacas) who are called "auspiciously voiced." Could the mooing of cows have been associated with the sacred syllable *om,* which is the primal sound of the cosmos? At any rate, in these archaic hymns we have the foundations of the later Mantra-Yoga.

The single most important sound in Vedic ritual chanting was *om,* and it is to this day the most widely recognized and venerated sacred phoneme of Hinduism. It is even found in Buddhist Tantrism (e.g., in the Tibetan mantric formula *om mani padme hum,* "Om, hail to the jewel in the lotus"). The syllable *om,* which "contains a whole philosophy which many volumes would not suffice to state,"[17] is held to be or to express the pulse of the cosmos itself. It was through meditative practice rather than speculation that the seers and sages of the Vedas arrived at the idea of a universal sound, eternally resounding in the universe, which they saw as the very origin of the created cosmos. The Vedic seers "heard" that sound in their moments of deepest meditation when they had successfully blocked out all external sounds.

Agehananda Bharati (1965), a Western Swami and professor of anthropology, made the useful observation that a mantra is a mantra only when it has been imparted by a teacher to a disciple during an initiatory ritual. Thus, the sacred syllable *om* is not a mantra to the uninitiated. It acquires its mantric power only through initiation. The Mantra-Yoga-Samhita, a work possibly of the eighteenth century A.D., acknowledges this fact when it states: "Initiation (diksha) is the root of all recitation (japa);[18] initiation is likewise the root of asceticism; initiation by a true teacher accomplishes all things" (I.5).

Mantras, which may consist of single sounds or a whole string of sounds, can be employed for many different purposes. Originally, mantras were undoubtedly used to ward off undesirable powers or events and to attract those that were deemed desirable, and this is still their predominant application. In other words, mantras are used as magical tools. But they are also employed in spiritual contexts as instruments of empowerment, where they aid the aspirant's search for identification with the transcendental Reality. Thus, a

The sacred syllable om, most famous of all the mantras of Hinduism

mantra like aham brahma-asmi, "I am the Absolute," is a potent affirmation of our fundamental identity as the Self (atman), which is the Ground of the world.

The beginnings of Mantra-Yoga, as we have seen, date back to the ancient Vedas. But Mantra-Yoga proper is a product of the same philosophical and cultural forces that gave rise to Tantrism in medieval India. In fact, Mantra-Yoga is Tantric in nature and is treated in numerous works belonging to that movement. Hence its metaphysical or esoteric basis is discussed in Chapter 13, "The Esotericism of Medieval Tantra Yoga."

There are also a number of scriptures that specifically expound Mantra-Yoga, notably the encyclopedic Mantra-Mahodadhi ("Ocean of Mantras"), which was composed by Mahidhara in the fifteenth century A.D.[19] This work has recently been translated into English, as has the Mantra-Yoga-Samhita. To these must be added several dictionaries that try to explain the esoteric meaning of mantras—a rather doubtful enterprise, which is borne out by the fact that these reference works frequently contradict each other.

According to the above-mentioned Samhita, Mantra-Yoga has sixteen limbs:

1. Devotion (bhakti), which is threefold: (a) prescribed devotion (vaidhi-bhakti), which consists in ceremonial worship; (b) devotion involving attachment (raga-atmika-bhakti)—that is, which is tainted by egoic motives; and (c) supreme devotion (para-bhakti), which yields superlative bliss.

2. Purification (shuddhi), which is distinguishable by the following four factors: body, mind, direction, and location. This practice involves (a) cleansing the body, (b) purifying the mind (through faith, study, and various virtues), (c) facing in the right direction during recitation, and (d) using an especially consecrated location for practice.

3. Posture (asana), which is meant to stabilize the body during meditation; it is said here to comprise two principal forms, svastika-asana and the lotus posture (padma-asana), which are both depicted in Chapter 13 ("Yoga as Spiritual Alchemy").

4. Serving the five limbs (panca-anga-sevana), the daily ritual practice of reading the Bhagavad-Gita and the Sahasra-Nama ("Thousand Names") of the Divine, and reciting songs of praise (stava), of protection (kavaca), and heart-opening (hridaya). These five are thought of as the "limbs" of the Divine; their practice is understood as a powerful means of granting attention and energy to God and thereby becoming assimilated into him.

5. Conduct (acara), which is of three kinds: divine (divya), or that which is beyond worldly activity and renunciation; left-handed (vama), which involves worldly activity; and right-handed (dakshina), which involves renunciation.

6. Concentration (dharana), which may have an external or an internal object.
7. "Serving the divine space" (divya-deva-sevana), which has sixteen constituent practices that convert a given place into consecrated space.
8. "Breath ritual" (prana-kriya), which is singular but accompanied by a variety of practices, such as the various types of "placing" (nyasa) the life-force into different parts of the body.
9. Gesture or "seal" (mudra), which has numerous forms; these hand gestures are used to focus inwardly. They are described in more detail in Chapter 13 ("Yoga as Spiritual Alchemy").
10. Satisfaction (tarpana), the practice of offering libations of water to the deities, delighting them and thereby making them favorably disposed toward the yogin.
11. Invocation (havana), the calling upon the deity by means of mantras.
12. Offering (bali), which consists in making gifts of fruit, etc., to the deity; the best offering is said to be the gift of oneself.
13. Sacrifice (yaga),[20] which can be either external or internal; the inner sacrifice is praised as superior.
14. Recitation (japa), which is of three kinds: mental (manasa), quiet (upamshu), and voiced (vacika).
15. Meditation (dhyana), which is manifold, because of the great variety of possible objects of contemplation.
16. Ecstasy (samadhi), which is also known as the "great state" (maha-bhava), in which the mind dissolves into God or the chosen deity as a manifestation of the Godhead.

As is evident from this outline of the sixteenfold path of Mantra-Yoga, this school has a pronounced ritualistic flavor. This reflects well the overall bias of Tantrism. Today, when mantras are widely sold and published, it is perhaps good to remember that they originated in a sacred setting. Mantra-Yoga has through the ages been touted as the easiest of all approaches to God; what could possibly be easier than to recite a mantra? However, it is obvious that this Yoga is, in the final analysis, as demanding as any other. The mindless repetition of mantras, especially by the uninitiated, can hardly lead to enlightenment or bliss. Paradoxically, we must be intensely attentive in order to transcend the game of attention and realize the Being-Consciousness-Bliss in which the ego and its attentive states arise of their own accord.

LAYA-YOGA: DISSOLVING THE UNIVERSE

Laya-Yoga makes meditative absorption (laya) its focus. The laya-yogin seeks to transcend all memory traces and sensory experiences by dissolving the microcosm, the mind, in the transcendental Self-Consciousness. His goal is to gradually dismantle his inner universe by way of intense contemplation, until only the one transcendental Reality remains. Laya-Yoga is a frontal attack on the illusion of individuality.

The spiritual work of the laya-yogin appears to have already been misunderstood in medieval times. This is evident from the following stanza found in the Hatha-Yoga-Pradipika, one of the standard manuals of Hatha-Yoga:

They exclaim "absorption, absorption," but what is the character of absorption? Absorption is the nonremembering of objects as a result of the nonemergence of previously [acquired] impressions (vasana). (IV.34)

The "nonremembering of objects" is not a temporary lapse of memory but the condition of objectless ecstasy, or what in Vedanta is called nirvikalpa-samadhi. In yogic circles, memory is explained as a network of subliminal impressions (vasana). These are rather like the scent lingering in our noses after we have smelled a fragrant flower. But they are dynamic and hence also known as activators (samskara), since they give rise to mental activity.

The laya-yogin is concerned with transcending these karmic patterns to the point where his inner cosmos becomes dissolved. In this endeavor he borrows many practices and concepts from Tantrism and Hatha-Yoga, especially the Tantric model of the subtle body with its psychic centers (cakra) and life-currents (nadi). Central to Laya-Yoga is the notion of the kundalini-shakti, the serpent power, which represents the universal life-force as manifested in the human body. The arousal and manipulation of this tremendous force is also the concern of the hatha-yogin. In fact, Laya-Yoga can be understood as the higher, meditative phase of Hatha-Yoga.

As the awakened kundalini ascends from the energy center at the base of the spine to the crown of the head, it absorbs a portion of the life-energy in the limbs and trunk. The body temperature drops measurably in those parts, whereas the crown feels as if on fire and is very warm to the touch. The physiology of this process is still little understood. Subjectively, however, the yogin experiences a progressive dissolution of his ordinary state of being, until he recovers the ever-present Self-Identity that knows no bodily or other limits.

The significance of this fundamental process of Laya-Yoga will become clearer in my subsequent treatment of Tantrism and Hatha-Yoga in Chapters 12 ("The Esotericism of Medieval Tantra Yoga") and 13 ("Yoga as Spiritual Alchemy").

योग त्रानन्दकल्पनः

chapter 3
Yoga and Other Hindu Traditions

A BIRD'S-EYE VIEW OF THE
CULTURAL HISTORY OF HINDUISM

The Indian subcontinent is the home of thousands of local animistic and polytheistic cults, paralleling the richness of the shamanic cultures of the African continent. But India has also spawned four major spiritual traditions that rank among the world religions—Hinduism, Buddhism, Jainism, and Sikhism. Thus, India's contribution to world spirituality is second to none. More than any other people, the Indians have demonstrated an incredible versatility in spiritual matters, which has inspired many other nations and which in our century has led to a much-needed enrichment of our spiritually ailing Western civilization.

The dominant tradition of the Indian subcontinent has for centuries been Hinduism, which today has more than 660 million adherents around the world. The term "Hinduism" is ambiguous. Sometimes it is used to refer to the total culture of all the inhabitants of the Indian peninsula apart from those who belong to such clearly defined religions as Buddhism, Sikhism, and Christianity. More specifically, the word applies to the numerous traditions that are historically more immediately connected with the ancient Vedic culture of 3000 years ago and that assumed their characteristic form at the beginning of the first millennium A.D. In this volume, the term is understood in the broader sense.

Hinduism is more than a religious school of thought. Like the other world religions, it is an entire culture or lifestyle, which includes a distinct social structure: the caste system. From roughly the middle of the first millennium B.C. on, Hindu society has been organized into four estates (varna), which are often wrongly referred to as "castes": the priestly class, the brahmanas or brahmins; the warrior class, kshatriyas; the merchant class, vaishas; and the servile class, shudras, who are also considered outcastes. Each estate has its own subdivisions, which are properly called castes. This social hierarchy is governed by elaborate conventions that forbid intermarriage between castes and carefully regulate behavior and activities (such as occupations and communal meals) between castes.

This vast structure has frequently been challenged by visionaries; Gautama, the founder of Buddhism, was among the first to reject it. Yet it continued to persist over the centuries and to exert a compelling influence on all other traditions of the Indian subcontinent. Social innovators who rejected the caste system generally also had to reject the Vedic revelation that sanctioned it. For the pious Hindu, the caste system with its social inequality is as natural as democracy is to us. Just as we justify democratic principles by pointing to the worth of the individual, the caste system is justified by invoking the law of karma: Each person has his or her station in life because of former volitions and deeds. A brahmin is a brahmin because of his virtuous and spiritual pursuits in previous lifetimes. An outcaste is an outcaste perhaps because of his past lack of motivation toward a higher life, or because of serious misdeeds. The caste system may offend our modern Western sensibilities, but not too long ago our ancestors held opinions and values similar to those of the traditional Hindus. It was only with the emergence of individualism in the Renaissance that the ancient social order, which was pointedly hierarchical, came to be questioned, challenged, and finally abolished.

The rigidity of the caste system has been balanced by a strong tendency toward ideological flexibility. Thus, Hinduism has proved to have an amazing capacity for assimilating even the most extreme opposites within itself. For instance, at one end of the spectrum we find the radical nondualist school of Shankara (A.D. 788–820), and at the other end the strict dualistic and atheistic school of Classical Samkhya, which even denies the Vedic revelation while still being regarded as orthodox. Another example of such widely contrasting philosophical positions is the cool, contemplative approach of Jnana-Yoga on the one side and the fervent emotionalism of some schools of Bhakti-Yoga on the other. Moreover, the spongelike absorptive power of Hinduism is such that even a distinctly autonomous religious tradition like Christianity fell under its spell and, in the sixteenth and seventeenth centuries, had to be rescued by Jesuit missionaries from complete Hinduization.

Hinduism is best understood as a complex process that has unfolded in the dynamics between continuity and discontinuity, or the persistence of ancient forms and the assimilation of new expressions of cultural and religious life. Thus, from one point of view, Hinduism can be said to have commenced with the Vedic culture (1800–1000 B.C.) of the Indo-European invaders, or even earlier, with the native Indus valley civilization (2500–1800 B.C.), many of whose artifacts are amazingly "Hindu" in form and style. From another point of view, there are real and important differences between the Vedic culture or the indigenous Indus valley civilization and Hinduism as we know it today. The historical development of Hindu-dominated India can conveniently be organized into nine periods, expressing distinguishable cultural styles.

Pre-Vedic Period (2500–1800 B.C.)

Prior to the conquest of the peninsula by the Indo-European nomads from Russia, who called themselves aryas ("noble folk"), ancient India was under the influence of the Indus valley civilization, whose origins and final end are as yet obscure. This great civilization, however, was probably not as significant to the evolution of the Vedic culture into later Hinduism as were the many rural or folk cultures of India, which may or may not have had much contact with the Indus civilization and its direct descendants.

It is these rural cultures that proved decisive in the gradual emergence of Hinduism, particularly in the formation of the powerful sectarian movements of Vaishnavism, Shaivism, and (not least) Shaktism, which revolve around the worship of God Vishnu, Shiva, and the feminine cosmic power called Shakti respectively. Indeed, the creative stimulus of these rural cultures was such that scholars speak of the Indianization of the many traditions imported into India at different periods, beginning with the settlement of the Aryan peoples and continuing with the Moslem invasions. The contribution of the Indus civilization will be discussed in more detail in Chapter 4 ("Yoga in Ancient Times").

Vedic Period (1800–1000 B.C.)

Probably around 2000 B.C., the first family groups of Indo-European nomads, whose original home was somewhere in the steppes of what is now central Russia, started to cross the Hindukush Mountains of Iran and enter the Indus River basin. More massive waves of immigration occurred several hundred years later and may have coincided with the disappearance of the native Indus civilization around 1800 B.C.

What we know of these Sanskrit-speaking invaders stems almost entirely from the Rig-Veda, which is a collection of hymns that give us glimpses of the psychology, beliefs, and daily life of the early Vedic settlers. Because of the prominence given to the Rig-Veda and the other Vedic hymnodies (Sama-Veda, Yajur-Veda, and the somewhat later and unorthodox Atharva-Veda), the "this-worldly" but still sacred culture of the period between 1800 and 1000 B.C. is known as the Vedic Age. We will further investigate this era and its contribution to the evolution of Yoga in Chapter 4.

Brahmanical Period (1000–800 B.C.)

The Indo-European nomads gradually expanded their territory from the Indus River in the west to the Ganges, which runs all the way to the northeastern boundary of the peninsula. As they settled and grew in numbers, their social system became more complex. One result was that a priestly elite, the so-called brahmanas (or brahmins), emerged, which soon dominated the Vedic religion. Their theological-mythological speculations and preoccupations with sacrificial rites are captured in the Brahmana literature, after which this period is generally named. More will be said about this phase in the development of Hinduism and its relationship to the creation of Yoga in Chapter 4.

Upanishadic Period (800–500 B.C.)

The period of Brahmanism came to its conclusion with the appearance of the earliest Upanishads, the first full-fledged mystical treatises on Indian soil of which we have knowledge. In these anonymously composed teachings we can see the beginnings of India's psychospiritual technology. The Upanishadic sages "internalized" the ritual technology of the Brahmanas; they invented the path of meditation as the "inner sacrifice." The old prose and metric Upanishads were originally spoken and remembered, and only much later written down.

Even though Upanishads were composed as recently as our own century, subsequent to the sixth or fifth century B.C. the religious life in India had become so diversified that the Upanishads were no longer the innovation they once represented. This fourth period could also be designated as the Period of the Early Heresies, since it saw the emergence of both Jainism and Buddhism. The Upanishads themselves were a quasi-heretical development within the Vedic religion, which was ritualistic rather than mystical. In their lofty metaphysical idealism and their focus on ecstatic self-transcendence, the Upanishads can be compared to the Kabbalah within Judaism, or the Gospel of John within biblical Christianity. The connection between the principal Upanishads and the Yoga tradition will be examined in some detail in Chapter 5 ("The Whispered Wisdom of the Early Upanishads").

Epic Period (500 B.C.–A.D. 200)

During the fifth period in the present scheme, Indian metaphysical and ethical thought was in considerable ferment. It had reached a degree of sophistication that led to a fertile confrontation between the different religio-philosophical schools of thought of India. Here we witness the emergence of the immense diversity for which Hinduism is renowned. At the same time, this era is marked by a healthy inclination to integrate the immense multiformity of psychospiritual paths, notably the two great orientations of world renunciation on the one side and the acceptance of social obligations on the other. This syncretistic spirit is best typified in the Mahabharata epic, in which the earliest complete Yoga work, the Bhagavad-Gita, is embedded. It was in the period from 500 B.C. to A.D. 200 that the massive bulk of the Mahabharata as we know it was created and enjoyed increasing popularity. The Epic Period, an important phase in the evolution of Yoga, will be investigated in Chapter 8 ("The Flowering of Yoga").

Classical Period (A.D. 200–800)

The cultural and religious synthesis epitomized in the teachings of the Mahabharata continued in the post-Christian centuries. It was largely borne by the sectarian cults centered on the gods Vishnu and Shiva. This was also the age in which the six classical schools of Hindu thought, now carefully defined, intensified their long-drawn struggle for supremacy. During this period the Yoga-Sutra of Patanjali was composed. This standard work on the formal philosophical system of Yoga will be examined in Chapter 9 ("Yoga as Philosophy and Religion").

Tantric Period (A.D. 800–1500)

Around the time of the adept Shankara (A.D. 788–820), who for the first time formulated the philosophy of nondualism (Advaita Vedanta) in a more rigorous way, we witness the beginnings of the great cultural revolution of Tantrism. This tradition, whose extraordinary psychotechnology will be discussed in Chapter 12 ("The Esotericism of Medieval Tantra Yoga"), represents a grand synthesis between the highest philosophical ideas and ideals and popular religious beliefs and practices. Tantrism understood itself as the gospel of the new "dark age" (kali-yuga). By the turn of the first post-Christian millennium, Tantric teachings had swept across the entire Indian subcontinent, transforming the spiritual life of Hindus, Buddhists, and Jainas alike.

On the one hand, Tantrism simply continued the millennia-long process of amalgamation and synthesis; on the other hand, it represented a genuine innovation. Although it added little to India's philosophical repertoire, Tantrism was of the utmost significance in the matter of spiritual practice. It promoted a spiritual lifestyle that was in contrast to most of what had hitherto been considered legitimate within the fold of Hinduism, Buddhism, and Jainism. In particular, Tantrism lent philosophical respectability to the feminine psychocosmic principle (known as shakti), which had long been acknowledged in more local cults.

This period could also be referred to as the Puranic Age, because during this era the great encyclopedic (and mostly sectarian) compilations known as the Puranas were created. At their core they are sacred histories, around which a web of philosophical, mythological, and ritual knowledge has been woven.

Many of these works show the influence of Tantrism, and many contain valuable information about Yoga during that period.

Sectarian Period (A.D. 1500–1700)

The Tantric rediscovery of the feminine principle for philosophy and yogic practice set the stage for the next phase in India's cultural history: the bhakti movement. This movement of religious devotionalism was the culmination of the monotheistic aspirations of the great sects of the Vishnu and Shiva worshippers; hence the title Sectarian Period.

By including the emotional dimension in the psychospiritual process, the bhakti movement—or bhakti-marga—completed the pan-Indian synthesis that had been initiated during the Epic Period. The path of devotionalism will be treated at length in Chapter 10 ("The Nondual Approach to God").

Modern Period (A.D. 1700–)

The ferment created by the sectarian bhakti movement was followed by the modern period, beginning with the collapse of the Mogul empire in the first part of the eighteenth century and leading to the establishment of British rule in India. From then on, we witness the gradual but steady impact of Western secular civilization upon the age-old religious cultures of India, leading to their progressive undermining through industrialization and the importation of the kind of secular values that seem to ride tandem with modern technology.

The Indian genius has not passively suffered these developments. There has been a promising spiritual renaissance, which, among other things, has created for the first time in history a missionary sense among Hindus: Ever since the appearance of the imposing figure of Swami Vivekananda at the Chicago World Conference of Religions in 1893, there has been a steady flow of Hindu wisdom, especially Yoga and Vedanta, to the Euro-American countries. Much could be said about this revival of the Hindu tradition abroad, but this subject lies beyond the scope of the present work.

The above attempt at periodization is only an approximation, and the dates given are flexible. Indian chronology is notoriously conjectural until we come to the modern period. The Hindu historiographers have seldom been concerned with recording actual dates and tended to freely mingle historical fact with mythology, symbolism, and uninspected ideology. Western scholars have therefore often remarked on the "timelessness" of the Hindu consciousness and culture. The reader should obviously bear this in mind when studying the materials in the extensive treatment of the history of Yoga in Part Two of this book.

In addition to the division into religious traditions and chronological periods, a useful distinction can also be made between the fundamental orientations of asceticism (tapas), renunciation (samnyasa), and mysticism (yoga) in the broadest sense of the term. These cut across all the religious traditions of India. The differences and similarities between these major approaches will be made clear in the following sections of this chapter.

THE GLOW OF PSYCHIC POWER: YOGA AND ASCETICISM (TAPAS)

Long before the word *yoga* acquired its customary meaning of "spirituality" or "spiritual discipline," the Indians had developed a body of knowledge and techniques aimed at the transformation of ordinary consciousness. This stock of ideas and practices formed the matrix out of which grew the complex historical phenomenon that later came to be called Yoga. In a certain sense, Yoga may be looked upon as internalized asceticism. Where the earlier ascetic stood stock-still under the burning sun in order to win the favor of one deity or another, the yogin's work occurs primarily in the laboratory of his own consciousness.

A typical example of the ascetic is the royal sage Bhagiratha, whose exploits are told in the Mahabharata. In ancient times, during a long spell of drought, he took it upon himself to stand on one foot for a thousand years and, for another thousand, to hold his arms up high. In this manner he compelled the gods to grant his request that the heavenly river Ganges should release its waters to flood and regenerate the parched earth. The downpour from the celestial river was so great that God Shiva had to slow its speed by catching the water with his head. The water ran through his tangled hair, forming the riverine basin of the Ganges of northern India.

The earliest term for yogalike endeavors in India is *tapas*. This ancient Sanskrit word means literally "heat." It is derived from the verbal root *tap* meaning "to burn" or "to glow." The term is often used in the Rig-Veda to describe the quality and work of the solar orb (or its corresponding deity, God Surya), or of fire (or its corresponding deity, God Agni). In these contexts it is frequently implied that the heat of sun and fire is painful and distressing in its burning intensity. We can see in this the root of the subsequent metaphoric usage of *tapas* as psychic heat in the form of anger and aggression, and also as fervor, zeal, or painstaking self-application.

Thus the word *tapas* came to be applied to the religious or spiritual struggle in the form of voluntary self-disciplining through the practice of austerities. The term is hence frequently rendered as "asceticism." The earlier portions of the Rig-Veda still refer to *tapas* in its naturalistic or psychological connotations. But the tenth book of this hymnody, which belongs to a more recent era, contains many references to its spiritual significance.

In one of the most exquisite hymns of the Rig-Veda (X.129), which is an early philosophical treatment of the theme of creation, the manifest worlds are said to have been produced by virtue of the excessive self-heating (tapas) of the primordial Being.[1] This self-exertion and self-sacrifice by the incommensurate Being that abides prior to space and time is the great archetype for spiritual practice in general. That the Vedic seers and sages were aware of this is borne out by this and many other hymns.

The Rig-Veda documents the emergence of tapas as a religious means of creating inner heat or the kind of creative tension that yields ecstatic states, visions of the gods, perhaps even transcendence of object-consciousness itself, and not least magical powers (siddhi). The Vedic sacrificial ritual (yajna) involved great concentration, for success depended on the correct pronunciation and intonation of the prayers and on the correct performance of the ceremony. It is easy to see how the Vedic ritual should have given rise not only to a whole sacrificial mysticism but also to ascetic practices that were intended to prepare the sacrificer for the actual ritual.

However, the typical ascetic (tapasvin) in the Vedic period is not the householder-sacrificer or even the seer (rishi), but the muni. The muni is an ecstatic for whom silence (mauna) is an important part of his penance. He belongs to what one might call the Vedic counterculture, composed of religious individuals and groups who pursued their sacred aspirations at the margins of Vedic society. The muni has frequently been regarded as the prototype of the later yogin. In his ecstatic oblivion he resembles a madman. Indeed, many elements in his lifestyle anticipate the unconventional behavior of the later crazy adept (avadhuta) as celebrated in the Avadhuta-Gita and other medieval works.

Tapas continued as an independent tradition alongside Yoga. This parallel development is documented, for instance, in the Mahabharata epic, which relates many stories of such celebrated tapasvins (or tapasas) as Vyasa, Vishvamitra, Vashishtha, Ahalya, Cyavana, Bharadvaja, and Uttanka. Indeed, in many parts of the epic, the tradition of tapas is given preeminence over Yoga, which is an indication of the relative age of those passages.

Tapas is generally pursued through the observance of chastity (brahmacarya) and the subjugation of the senses (indriya-jaya). The frustration of the body-mind's natural inclinations is held to generate psychophysical effulgence (tejas), radiance (jyotis), great strength (bala) or vitality (virya). Another term closely associated with asceticism since Vedic times is *ojas* (apparently related to the Latin *augustus,* "majestic"). It stands for a particular kind of numinous energy that charges the entire body-mind. Ojas is generated especially through the practice of chastity, as a result of the sublimation of sexual energy. According to the Atharva-Veda (XI.5–19), the deities themselves acquired their state of immortality through the practice of chastity and austerities.

Tapas is typically associated with the acquisition of psychic powers (siddhi), which often proved the downfall of unwise ascetics who abused these capabilities. The tradition of tapas, both in the Vedic Age and the Epic Age, unfolded against the backdrop of a magical world-view according to which the cosmos is filled with personalized sources of psychic power. Thus, the tapasvins are frequently depicted as combating evil spirits or as pitting themselves against different deities to win a boon from them. More often than not the ascetics emerge as victors, and only pride or sexual profligacy are held to diminish their formidable puissance. To this day, the practitioners of tapas are thought of by the villagers of India as magicians able to accomplish any feat—from reading people's minds, to predicting the future, to stopping the sun in its course.

Yoga spiritualized the orientation of the earlier tradition of tapas by emphasizing self-transcendence over the acquisition of magical powers. At the same time, the yogins adopted and adapted many of the techniques and practices of the tapasvins. Chastity remained central to its practice, as is clear from the eight-limbed path outlined in the Yoga-Sutra. In this work, Patanjali states (II.38) that the yogin who is grounded in chastity gains vigor (virya). He also mentions (II.32) tapas as one of the five observances or disciplines (niyama) and declares (II.43) that through asceticism the body and its senses are perfected. Manifestly, tapas is here relegated to the status of a preparatory practice. The real concern of Yoga is meditation and its intensified form, ecstatic transcendence (samadhi).

The tradition of tapas existed alongside the schools of Yoga for centuries, and this is no different today. The remarkable story of a modern tapasvin and saint, who reputedly lived for 185 years, is told in the hagiography *Maharaj*.[2] The hero of the story, known as Tapasviji Maharaj, was born around 1820 into a princely family but left everything behind in his late fifties and girded himself with a loincloth. During his lifetime he was widely hailed as a mighty ascetic and miracle worker. He performed startling feats of endurance, conquering both pain and boredom. For three years he stood on one leg with one arm stretched upward; for another twenty-four years he never lay down, while walking many miles every day. In the 1960s this saint attracted much attention in the United States because of his extreme longevity, which he claimed was the result of undergoing on three different occasions the kaya-kalpa, a rejuvenating treatment known to native Indian medicine. The success of this treatment depends largely on the disposition of the individual, who must be able to endure long periods of almost complete isolation. Only a skilled meditator of the stature of Tapasviji Maharaj could possibly cope with the ordeal of self-denial involved. Clearly, Western medicine has much to learn from the tapasvins of ancient and modern India.

DELIGHT IN NOTHING: YOGA AND THE WAY OF RENUNCIATION (SAMNYASA)

Tapas, as we have seen, represents a more magical-shamanic type of spirituality. Unlike Yoga, which is primarily concerned with the achievement of contemplative states and self-transcendence, the technology of tapas focuses on the attainment of inner strength, visionary experiences, and magical powers.

The cultivation of willpower is central to this approach. By contrast, Yoga embodies a more refined orientation to psychospiritual growth. It recognizes, among other things, the need for the transcendence of the will, which is a manifestation of the egoic personality.

Many facets of tapas have been integrated into the practice of Yoga, and the popular image of the yogin is that of a thaumaturgist, or miracle-working ascetic. Yet Yoga is closer in spirit to another tradition, that of the renunciation (samnyasa) of worldly life, which first appeared in the Upanishadic Age. It was around 800 B.C. that the ideal of world renunciation entered the sphere of Hinduism, perhaps from older indigenous sources. Suddenly, or so it appears, a growing number of householders left the villages and cities to live out the rest of their days in the wilderness, often on their own but occasionally with their spouses.

These renouncers are known as samnyasins, practitioners of samnyasa. The word *samnyasa* is composed of the prefixes *sam* (expressing the idea of union, similar to the Greek *syn-*) and *ni* ("down"), as well as the verbal root *as* ("to cast, throw"). Thus, it signifies one's "casting down" or "laying aside" of all worldly concerns and attachments.

Although renunciation can be identified as a lifestyle, it cannot be performed as one might perform austerities or meditation. It is, rather, a fundamental *attitude* to life. Hence the tradition of renunciation can be said to be counter-technological: It aims at leaving everything behind, including, if it is pursued rigorously enough, all methods of seeking. The German indologist Joachim Friedrich Sprockhoff has rightly described renunciation as "a phenomenon at the margin of life"[3] and compared it to other borderline experiences, such as fatal illness and old age.

Renunciation is a response to the insight that human existence, and cosmic existence in general, is ultimately unfulfilling, if not altogether illusory. In either case, the renouncer seeks to realize a higher state of being, which is equated with Reality itself. Depending on whether the world is regarded as illusory or merely morally unworthy (but rooted in the Divine), renunciation can be expressed in at least two principal ways. On the one side is literal renunciation, on the other is symbolic renunciation. The former position understands renunciation, pure and simple, as the abandonment of ordinary life: The renouncer leaves everything behind—wife, children, property, work, social respectability, worldly ambitions, and any concern for the future. The latter position perceives renunciation in metaphorical terms, as primarily an inner act: the voluntary letting-go of all attachments and, in the final analysis, of the ego itself.

Both orientations have had their advocates throughout the long history of Indian spirituality. In the Bhagavad-Gita, we find the earliest record of an attempt to reconcile the two approaches. Thus, the God-man Krishna teaches Prince Arjuna the distinction between mere abandonment and inner renunciation, clearly favoring the latter. In response to Arjuna, who was confused about the difference between renunciation of actions and the Yoga of Action, Krishna explained:

Of yore I proclaimed a twofold way of life in this world, O sinless [Arjuna]—the Yoga of Wisdom (jnana-yoga) for the [followers of] Samkhya, and the Yoga of Action (karma-yoga) for the yogins. (III.3)

Not by abstention from actions does a man enjoy action-transcendence (naishkarmya), nor by renunciation (samnyasa) alone does he approach perfection (siddhi). (III.4)

Renunciation (samnyasa) and the Yoga of Action (karma-yoga)—both lead to the highest. But of the two, the Yoga of Action is more excellent than [mere] renunciation of action. (V.2)

He who does not hate or desire is forever to be known as a renouncer. (V.3a)

But renunciation, O strong-armed [Arjuna], is difficult to attain without Yoga. The sage (muni) yoked in Yoga approaches the Absolute without delay. (V.6)

Yoked in Yoga, with the self purified, with the self subdued, and the senses conquered, whose self has become the Self of all beings—even though active, he is not defiled. (V.7)

"I do nothing whatsoever"—thus reflects the yoked one, the knower of Reality, [even as he is] seeing, hearing, touching, smelling, eating, walking, sleeping, breathing, talking, excreting, grasping, opening and closing [his eyes], and thinking "the senses move among their [appropriate] sense objects." (V.8, 9)[4]

He who acts, assigning [all] actions to the Absolute, and having abandoned attachment (sanga), is not defiled by sin (papa), just as a lotus leaf [is not stained] by the water. (V.10)

The symbolic interpretation of renunciation was, understandably, favored by the orthodox powers within ancient Hindu society, which were greatly concerned about the growing mood of resignation and spreading pessimism. If it had been only the older generation that found the eremitic existence in forests or caves attractive, the Hindu establishment would have had little cause to worry. But the ideal of flight from the world also held considerable appeal among the middle-aged population and even young men (and, more rarely, women). Their renunciation of worldly life led to abandoned families and fields as well as kingdoms. The sociocultural reasons for this trend are ill understood; some scholars have blamed the hot, dry climate of many parts of the peninsula.

In the Maitry-Upanishad, a work belonging to the centuries just before the beginning of the Christian era, King Brihadratha is portrayed as suffering from excessive existential ennui. He articulated a sentiment that, at one time or another, overwhelmed thousands of others when he said:

In this ill-smelling, pithless body, which is a conglomerate of bone, skin, muscle, marrow, flesh, semen, blood, mucus, tears, rheum, feces, urine, wind, bile, and phlegm—what good is the enjoyment of desires? In this body, which is afflicted with lust, anger, greed, delusion, fear, despondency, jealousy, separation from what is loved, union with what is unloved, hunger, thirst, senility, death, illness, grief, and the like—what good is the enjoyment of desires?

We see that all this is perishable, like these gnats, mosquitoes, and so on, like the grass and the trees that grow and decay. Indeed, what of these? There are the great ones, mighty warriors, some rulers of empires like Sudyumna, Bhuridyumna . . . and kings like Marutta, Bharata, and others, who, before the eyes of their whole family, surrendered their great wealth and passed on from this world to that. . . . (I.2ff.)

Radical relinquishment of conventional existence clearly threatened the social fabric and established order. Consequently, the Hindu policymakers discouraged what they considered premature renunciation and instead proposed the alternative social ideal of the stages of life (ashrama)—studentship, householder stage, forest-dweller existence, and finally total renunciation. In this new hierarchical framework, renunciation was fully sanctioned but only after a person had fulfilled his or her obligations as a householder (grihastha).

Two levels of renunciation came to be distinguished. The first, known as vana-prasthya ("forest-dwelling"), is the stage of the hermit, who practices a kind of esoteric ritualism in the seclusion of the forest. The second, known as samnyasa, consists in leaving behind even the forest-dweller's sedentary existence and sacrificial ritualism, taking up a life of constant wandering. These two lifestyles anticipated the modern Western custom of retirement, though by turning the evening of an individual's life into a sacred opportunity, the Hindu orthodoxy granted older people—at least in theory—a dignity that they are denied by our own society.

The tradition of renunciation has been as persistent a feature of Indian spirituality as has been the tradition of asceticism. Often the two overlapped. Although the word *samnyasa* is first mentioned in the Mundaka-Upanishad (III.2.6), which belongs to the third or second century B.C., the idea and ideal are much older. Thus, the Brihad-Aranyaka-Upanishad (IV.4.22), which is reckoned as the oldest work of the Upanishadic genre, speaks of the pravrajin, the person who has "gone forth"—that is, left house and home and is wholly intent on Self-realization. In another memorable passage, Yajnavalkya, the grand old man of Upanishadic wisdom, instructs a disciple as follows:

That which is beyond hunger and thirst, sorrow and delusion, old age and death [is the transcendental Reality]. The brahmanas who know that as the very Self overcome the desire for sons, the desire for wealth, the desire for the worlds, and lead a mendicant's life. The desire for sons is the desire for wealth, and the desire for wealth is the desire for the worlds; thus both these are merely desires. Therefore let a brahmana despair of scholarship and desire to live [in innocence] as a child. When he has despaired both of scholarship and childlikeness, then he becomes a sage (muni). When he despairs both of sagehood (mauna) and nonsagehood (amauna), then he becomes a [true] brahmana. (III.5.1)

Thus, Yajnavalkya characterizes renunciation as the transcendence of attachment to every desire, including the desire for renunciation itself. Elsewhere (III.8.10) he expressed his doubts about the usefulness of asceticism (tapas), saying that even a millennium of austerities will be of no avail unless the Absolute is intuited first.

Even though the Hindu orthodoxy made provisions for those who felt an irresistible urge to "drop out," renunciation was at best condoned, never actively encouraged. And in some quarters renunciation was viewed as unlawful. In the Mahabharata (XII.10.17ff.), for instance, is the story of Yudhishthira, who, fatigued from the brutalities of the great Bharata war, felt moved to embrace the life of a forest eremite. His teacher Bhishma reminded him, as Krishna had reminded Arjuna, that renunciation was inappropriate for a warrior. Bhishma also aired the cynical opinion (no doubt based in part on reality) that only those assailed by misfortune adopt such a lifestyle.

This ambivalence toward renunciation explains, among other things, why the Upanishads specifically dedicated to the ideal of renunciation never quite achieved the status of being part of the Vedic revelation (shruti). Their teachings embody a tradition that has thrived for hundreds of years at the margins of Hindu society.

That renouncers were not all of the same ilk becomes readily apparent when one delves into the various Sanskrit scriptures dealing with renunciation, notably the so-called Samnyasa Upanishads. The Jabala-Upanishad, dating back to around 300 B.C. and thus one of the oldest works of this genre, differentiates between renouncers who maintain the sacred fire and those who do not—that is, between those who in their retirement continue to engage the Vedic sacrificial ritualism and those God-seekers who simply leave it all behind. This work celebrates the parama-hamsa ("great swan"), who drifts through life unconcerned by any of its problems, as the foremost of all renouncers. Some 600 years later, the Vaikhanasa-Smarta-Sutra (VIII) furnishes a more detailed picture. It mentions four types of forest anchorites and four types of wandering renouncers. The forest-dwelling ascetics can be married, whereas the wandering renouncers live on their own, seeking Self-realization.

An almost identical list is found in the Ashrama-Upanishad (c. A.D. 300). This scripture mentions four types of forest anchorite:

1. Vaikhanasas, who perform the traditional fire ritual (agni-hotra) and live on wild grain and vegetables available in their forest environment. The appellation *vaikhanasa* is derived from the prefix *vi* ("dis-") and the word *khana* ("food"). It hints at these eremites' discipline relative to their nourishment.

2. Audumbaras, who sustain themselves by eating wild grain and fruit, especially figs (udumbara).
3. Valakhilyas, who get their name from wearing their hair (vala) in a tuft (khilya). Their diet is as meager as that of the other anchorites; they gather food for eight months of the year and basically fast during the remaining months. This ascetic practice is known as catur-masya ("the four months").
4. Phenapas, whose name means literally "froth-drinkers." Perhaps this curious designation stems from their practice of drinking the morning dew from leaves. Their diet is stark, consisting chiefly of certain kinds of fruit. Unlike the other eremites, the phenapas have no fixed abode.

The wandering renouncers (parivrajaka) comprise the following categories:

1. Kuticakas: The name refers to the wearing of a tuft but has other connotations as well. The word *kuti* can mean both "house/home" and "sexual intercourse," whereas the stem *caka* means "to tremble." Hence the kuticaka is one who trembles when he ponders the lure of sexual attachment; that is, he practices chastity. He wanders from place to place, wearing a loincloth and carrying a renouncer's staff and water vessel. He practices meditation by means of sacred syllables or chants (mantra).
2. Bahudakas: Their lifestyle is as simple as that of the kuticakas. They subsist on eight morsels a day, which they gather from different places "like a bee." The appellation means literally "abundant water" and refers to the fact that renouncers of this type tend to frequent sacred places along rivers.
3. Hamsas: These itinerant ascetics are so named because they live like "swans" (strictly speaking, the word refers to Indian geese), like migratory birds, leaving no tracks in the sky. They do not even beg their food but live from the products of cows, including urine and dung.
4. Parama-hamsas, "great swans": Their way of life is still more spartan. They are described as smearing their bodies with ashes as a sign of total renunciation of conventional existence. Different scriptures prescribe different rituals for them, such as the wearing of a single loincloth or the carrying of a bamboo staff. But the important fact about the parama-hamsas is that they are considered to be fully Self-realized beings. According to some texts, such as the Vaikhanasa-Smarta-Sutra, the parama-hamsas wander about in the nude and frequent graveyards. This strange custom foreshadowed the later left-hand rituals of Tantrism, which will be introduced in Chapter 12 ("The Esotericism of Medieval Tantra Yoga").

The Narada-Parivrajaka-Upanishad (c. A.D. 1200) adds two more classes to the above schema—the Turiyatitas and the Avadhutas. Both are Self-realized adepts. The former, whose name means "transcending the Fourth," live on the little food that is placed directly in their mouths—a practice that is called "cow-face" (go-mukha). The latter depend equally on the charity of others. The most telling distinction between the two is that the Avadhutas walk about naked, thus demonstrating their ecstatic obliviousness to all differences: There is only the One Reality, which is sexless. All else has, as the name *avadhuta* suggests, been "cast off."

As can be seen, the term "renunciation" covers a wide range of possible lifestyles—from the householder who simply performs an inner or symbolic renunciation to the forest-dweller who continues to observe certain ritual obligations, to the naked wanderer whose way of life can be described as a form of sacred anarchy. Some practiced one or another form of Yoga, while some simply contemplated the mystery of the Self without any external aids. All these different types have, over the millennia, contributed to the rich tapestry of Indian spirituality.

YOGA AND HINDU PHILOSOPHY

In Hinduism the distinction between philosophy and religion is not as clear-cut as it is in our contemporary Western civilization. Sanskrit, the sacred language of Hinduism, does not have straightforward equivalents for either the term "philosophy" or "religion."[5]

For the Hindu, philosophy is not a matter of pure abstract knowledge, but metaphysics that has moral implications. In other words, whatever one's theoretical conclusions about reality are, these must be applied in daily life. Thus, philosophy is always regarded as a way of life and is not merely pursued as an inconsequential exercise in logical thinking. More than that, Hindu philosophy (and Indian philosophy as a whole) has a spiritual orientation. With the exception of the materialist school (known as Lokayata or Carvaka), which was not without influence in ancient India, all Hindu philosophical schools recognized that there is a transcendental reality and that a person's spiritual well-being depends on how he or she relates to that reality. Hindu philosophy is therefore closer to the spirit of ancient Greek philosophy (the "love of wisdom") than to the contemporary academic discipline of conceptual analysis.

Hindu philosophy comprises the same areas of rational inquiry that have preoccupied the philosophers of the West since the times of Socrates, Plato, and Aristotle—namely, ontology (which deals with the nature of being), epistemology (which is concerned with the processes of knowledge by which we come to know what there is "in reality"), logic, and ethics. But, in contrast to Western philosophy, the Indian genius has not included aesthetics in its philosophical program, nor did it develop a philosophy of history. However, Hindu philosophy, like Christian philosophy, is greatly concerned with the ultimate spiritual destiny of humankind. Hence it often describes itself as atma-vidya, the "science of the Self."

The earliest philosophical speculations or intuitions of Hinduism are found in the ancient Rig-Veda, though the first proper philosophical schools developed in a much later era, after the emergence of Buddhism in the sixth century B.C. Traditionally six systems are distinguished, which are referred to as "viewpoints" (darshana). This phrase hints at two significant things about Hindu philosophy: Each system is not merely the product of rational thinking but also of visionary-intuitive processes; and each system is a particular perspective from which the *same* truth is viewed, which suggests a position of tolerance (at least in theory, if not in practice). And that identical Truth is what has been handed down by word of mouth (and by esoteric initiation) as the ultimate or transcendental Reality, whether it is called "God" (ish, isha, ishvara), the "Self" (atman, purusha), or the "Absolute" (brahman).

Tradition is a key element in Hindu philosophy, and tradition means the Vedic revelation, particularly the Rig-Veda. In order to establish their schools within the orthodox fold, the Hindu philosophers had to pay allegiance, or at least lip service, to the ancient Vedic heritage. The six schools recognized by

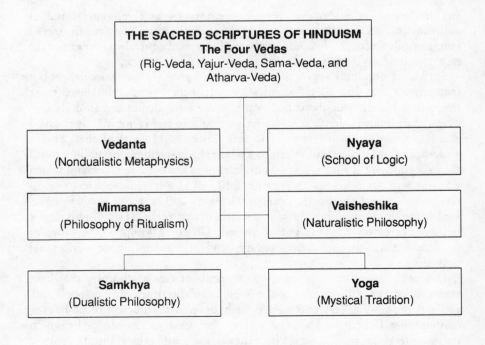

The Vedic revelation and the six orthodox traditions of Hinduism.

the Hindu orthodoxy as representing valid points of view within the context of the Vedic revelation are the following: Purva-Mimamsa (which puts forward a philosophy of sacrificial ritualism), Uttara-Mimamsa or Vedanta (which is the nondualist metaphysics espoused especially in the Upanishads), Samkhya (whose principal contribution concerns the evolution of Nature), Yoga (which here refers specifically to the philosophical school of Patanjali, the author of the Yoga-Sutra), Vaisheshika (which, similar to the Samkhya school, is an attempt to philosophize about Nature), and Nyaya (which is primarily a theory of logic and argument). I will briefly describe each school and highlight its relationship to the Yoga tradition.

Purva-Mimamsa

The school of Purva-Mimamsa ("earlier discussion") is so called because it interprets the "earlier" two portions of the Vedic revelation, the Vedic hymnodies themselves and the Brahmana texts that explain and develop their sacrificial rituals. It is contrasted to the Uttara-Mimamsa or "later discussion," represented by the nondualist teachings of the Upanishads. The Purva-Mimamsa school originated with the Mimamsa-Sutra of Jaimini (c. 200 B.C.). It expounds the art and science of moral action in keeping with Vedic ritualism. Its focal point is the concept of dharma, or virtue, insofar as it affects the religious or spiritual destiny of the individual. The secular, social applications of dharma are left to the authorities of ethics (dharma-shastra) to define and explain.

The Mimamsa thinkers regard ethical action as an invisible, extraordinary force that determines the appearance of the world: The human being is intrinsically active, and action determines the quality of human existence both in the present incarnation and in future incarnations. Good actions (actions in keeping with the Vedic moral code) bring about positive life circumstances, whereas bad actions (actions contradicting the Vedic moral code) lead to negative life circumstances.

The purpose of living a morally sound life is to improve the qualities of one's existence in the present, in the hereafter, and in subsequent embodiments. Because the individual has free will, he or she can accumulate positive results, and even annul existing negative results, through good actions. Free will is guaranteed by the fact that the essential Self, or soul, of the person is transcendental and eternal. In contrast to Vedanta, the Mimamsa school postulates many such Selves (atman). These are deemed intrinsincally unconscious and come to consciousness only in conjunction with a body-mind. Consciousness is, therefore, always I-consciousness for the Mimamsakas, the adherents of Mimamsa. There is no God over and above those many eternal and omnipresent Selves, although from the fifteenth century on, some representatives of this school started to believe in a Creator God.

Since the Self is held to possess neither consciousness nor bliss, the earlier

Mimamsakas naturally found the ideal of liberation pursued by other schools quite undesirable. This orientation was rejected by the eighth-century philosopher Kumarila and his pupil and later rival Prabhakara. They both taught that abstention from prohibited and merely optional actions, and the dutiful performance of prescribed actions, automatically lead to the dissociation of the Self from the body-mind—that is, liberation. They looked upon the Self as consciousness, though they failed to develop a viable metaphysics.

The practice of yogic techniques has no place in this school, which extols the ideal of duty for duty's sake. As Sarvepalli Radhakrishnan, a former president of India, remarked about this school of thought, "as a philosophical view of the universe it is strikingly incomplete. . . . There is little in such a religion to touch the heart and make it glow."[6] However, Purva-Mimamsa was one of the cultural forces encountered by the Yoga tradition, and therefore it needs to be taken into account here.

By Western standards, this system of thought would hardly be called philosophical, though Purva-Mimamsa was instrumental in developing logic and dialectics. Apart from Jaimini, Kumarila, and Prabhakara, the most outstanding thinker of this school, which has produced a rather comprehensive literature, is Mandana Mishra (ninth century A.D.), who later became converted to Shankara's nondualist Vedanta and assumed the name Sureshvara.

The story of the electrifying encounter between the adept Shankara and the philosopher Mandana Mishra is told in the Shankara-Dig-Vijaya, a spurious medieval biography of Shankara. According to this legend, the young Shankara, who had adopted the life of a renunciate, visited Mandana Mishra's stately mansion just as the great scholar of Vedic ritualism was about to embark on one of his ceremonies. He was at once annoyed with Shankara, who wore neither the traditional hair tuft nor the sacred thread. After a barrage of insulting remarks, which Shankara took calmly and not without amusement, Mandana Mishra, rather proud of his learning, challenged the visitor to a debate. They agreed that, as was customary in those days, whoever lost the debate was to assume the lifestyle of the winner.

This combat of knowledge and wit lasted over several days and drew large crowds of scholars. Mandana Mishra's wife, Ubhaya Bharati (who was really Sarasvati, the Goddess of Learning, in disguise), was appointed umpire. Before long she announced the defeat of her husband but then promptly argued that Shankara had defeated only one half; for his victory to be real, he would also have to defeat her. Slyly, she challenged the young renunciate to a discussion on sexuality.

Without losing his composure, Shankara asked for an adjournment so that he could acquaint himself with this area of knowledge. It so happened that the ruler of a neighboring kingdom had just died, and Shankara, wasting no time, used his yogic powers to enter the corpse and reanimate it. Under the joyous exclamations of the king's relatives, he returned to the palace. In the spirit of Tantrism, Shankara explored the delights of sexual love among the dead king's wives and courtesans. In fact, he got so absorbed in this newfound life that his disciples had to steal into the palace and remind him of his former life as a renunciate.

Restored to his true identity, Shankara dropped the king's body and resumed the debate with Mandana Mishra's wife. Of course, he won. Mandana Mishra declared himself a pupil of Shankara, and his wife revealed herself as the Goddess Sarasvati. Shankara's victory is generally seen as a victory of his superior nondualist metaphysics over the less sophisticated philosophy of the Mimamsakas. This may be so, but it was also a triumph of Yoga over intellectualism.

Uttara-Mimamsa

The many-branched school or tradition of Uttara-Mimamsa ("later discussion"), also known as Vedanta ("Veda's end"), gets its name from the fact that it evolved around the consideration of the "later" two portions of the Vedic revelation: the Aranyakas, forest treatises composed by hermits, and the Upanishads, esoteric gnostic scriptures composed by sages. Both the Aranyakas and the Upanishads represent a metaphoric reinterpretation of the ancient Vedic heritage: They preached the "internalization" of the archaic sacrificial ritual in the form of meditation. Especially the Upanishadic teachings gave rise to the whole consciousness technology associated with the Vedanta tradition. The literature of Uttara-Mimamsa, or Vedanta, comprises the Upanishads (of which there are over 200), the Bhagavad-Gita (which is regarded as an Upanishad), and the Vedanta- or Brahma-Sutra of Badarayana (c. A.D. 200), which systematizes the often contradictory teachings of the "revealed" Upanishads and the Bhagavad-Gita.

Vedanta is metaphysics par excellence. Its different subschools all teach some form of nondualism, according to which Reality is a single, indivisible whole. The fundamental idea of Vedantic nondualism is articulated in the following stanzas from the first chapter of the Naishkarmya-Siddhi authored by Sureshvara (the former Mandana Mishra):

Nonrecognition of the singular Selfhood [of all things] is [spiritual] ignorance (avidya). The mainstay of [that ignorance] is the experience of one's own self. It is the seed of the world-of-change. The destruction of that [spiritual ignorance] is the liberation (mukti) of the self. (7)

The fire of right knowledge (jnana) arising from the brilliant Vedic utterances burns up the delusion of [there being an independent] self. Action does not [remove spiritual ignorance], because it is not incompatible [with that ignorance]. (80)

Because action arises from [spiritual] ignorance, it does not do away with delusion. Right knowledge [alone can remove ignorance], since it is its opposite, rather like the sun is [the opposite of] darkness. (35)

Upon mistaking a tree stump for a thief, one becomes frightened and runs away.

> Similarly, one who is deluded superimposes the Self upon the buddhi [i.e., the higher mind] and the other [aspects of the human personality], and then acts [on the basis of that mistaken view]. (60)

Advaita Vedanta stood the earlier Vedic ritualism on its head. It is a gospel of gnosis: not intellectual or factual knowledge but the liberating intuition of the transcendental Reality.

The two greatest exponents of Vedanta were Shankara (c. A.D. 788–820) and Ramanuja (A.D. 1017–1137). The former succeeded in constructing a coherent philosophical system out of the Upanishadic teachings, and has done more for the survival of Hinduism and the displacement of Buddhism from India than any other single individual. Ramanuja, on the other hand, came to the rescue of the Advaita Vedanta tradition when it was threatened with losing itself in dry scholasticism. His notion of the Divine as entailing rather than transcending all qualities encouraged the popular thrust toward a more devotional expression within Hindu spirituality.

Both Shankara and Ramanuja, as well as many other Vedanta teachers, have had strong links with the Yoga tradition. This is explored in Chapter 10 ("The Nondual Approach to God").

Samkhya

The tradition of Samkhya ("number"), which comprises many different schools, is primarily concerned with enumerating and describing the principal categories of existence. This approach would be called "ontology," or the "science of being," in Western philosophy. In their metaphysical ideas, Samkhya and Yoga are closely akin and in fact once formed a single Pre-Classical tradition. But whereas the followers of Samkhya use discrimination and renunciation as their principal means of salvation, the yogins proceed chiefly through the practice of meditation and renunciation. Samkhya is often characterized as the theoretical aspect of Yoga praxis, but this is inaccurate. Both traditions have their own distinct theories and practical approaches. Because of its emphasis on discriminative knowledge rather than meditation, Samkhya in later times has tended toward intellectualism, whereas Yoga has always been exposed to the danger of deviating into mere psychotechnology with magical goals.

Next to Vedanta, the Samkhya philosophy has been the single most influential system of thought within the fold of Hinduism, and Shankara regarded it as his main opponent. Samkhya is said to have been founded by the Sage Kapila, who is credited with the authorship of the Samkhya-Sutra. Kapila is more fiction than reality, although a teacher by that name is likely to have lived in ancient times, perhaps as early as the sixth century B.C. At any rate, the Samkhya-Sutra appears to be the creation of a much later age.

In the framework of the six orthodox Hindu schools of thought, the

Samkhya referred to is the school of Ishvara Krishna (c. A.D. 350), author of the Samkhya-Karika. In striking contrast to Vedanta and the earlier Samkhya schools mentioned in the Mahabharata epic, Ishvara Krishna taught that Reality is not singular but plural. On the one side are the countless mutable and unconscious forms of Nature (prakriti), and on the other side are the innumerable transcendental Selves (purusha), which are pure Consciousness, omnipresent and eternal. Looked at more closely, this pluralism is illogical; if countless Selves are all omnipresent, they must also be infinitely intersecting each other, so that logically they should be considered as one. This problem has been tackled again and again by different philosophers, and while Shankara's monism is intellectually the most elegant, Ramanuja's qualified nondualism perhaps best satisfies both reason and intuition.

Ishvara Krishna further taught that Nature (prakriti) is a vast composite created by the interplay of three primary forces, the dynamic qualities (guna). The word *guna* means literally "strand" but has a wide range of connotations. In the context of Yoga and Samkhya metaphysics, the term denotes the irreducible ultimate "reals" of the cosmos. These gunas can be said to resemble the energy quanta of modern physics. They underlie all material as well as psychomental phenomena. In the Samkhya-Karika, their respective characters are described as follows:

> The gunas are of the nature of joy, joylessness, and dejection and have the purpose of illuminating, activating, and restricting. They overbear each other, are interdependent, productive, and co-operative in their activities. (12)

> Sattva is regarded as buoyant and illuminating. Rajas is stimulating and mobile. Tamas is inert and concealing. The activity [of the gunas] is purposive like a lamp [made up of various parts that together produce the single phenomenon of light]. (13)

The gunas *are* Nature, just as the atoms *are* matter-energy. Together they are responsible for the variety of natural forms on all levels of existence other than that of the transcendental Selves, which are unqualified Consciousness. The German Sanskritist Max Müller observed about the gunas:

> We can best explain them by the general idea of two opposites and the middle term between them, or as Hegel's thesis, antithesis and synthesis, these being manifested in nature by light, darkness, and mist; in morals by good, bad, and indifferent, with many applications and modifications.[7]

According to the Samkhya-Karika, the gunas are in a state of balance in the transcendental aspect of Nature, known as prakriti-pradhana ("Nature's foundation"). The first product to appear in the evolution from this transcendental matrix to the multiplicity of space-time forms is mahat ("great one [principle]"). It has the appearance of luminosity, intelligence, or consciousness, and is therefore also known as buddhi ("intuition, cognition"), or what I call the "wisdom-faculty." But, in reality, mahat is in itself quite unconscious and only a particularly refined form of matter-energy. It depends on the transcendental Self-Consciousness for its "light" of intelligence.

Out of the mahat, or buddhi, emerges the ahamkara (lit., "I-maker"), the principle of individuation, which gives rise to the distinction between subject and object. This category, in turn, causes the appearance of the mind (manas), the five cognitive senses (sight, smell, taste, touch, and hearing), and the five

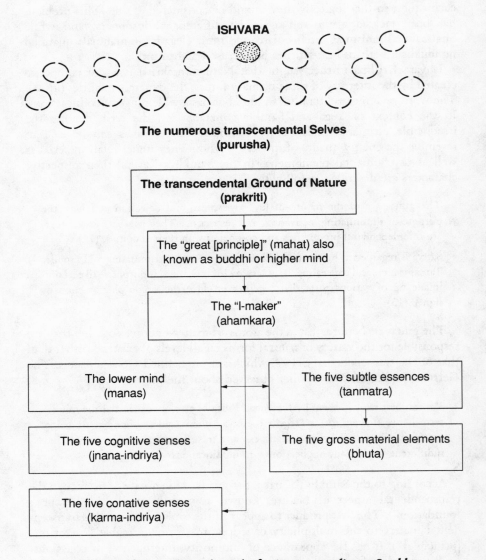

The twenty-four categories (tattva) of existence according to Samkhya

conative senses (speech, prehension, movement, excretion, and reproduction). The ahamkara principle further gives rise to the five subtle essences (tanmatra) underlying the sensory capacities. They in turn produce the five gross material elements (bhuta), namely earth, water, fire, air, and ether.

Thus, Classical Samkhya recognizes twenty-four categories of "material" existence in all. Beyond the guna triad and its products are the countless Self-monads, which are untouched by the ramifications of Nature.

The whole evolutionary process is triggered by the proximity of the transcendental Selves to the transcendental matrix of Nature. Moreover, the entire process is for the sake of the liberation of those Selves that, mysteriously and wrongly, identify themselves with a particular body-mind rather than the condition of pure Consciousness.

The psychocosmological evolutionism of the Samkhya tradition is not meant so much to explain the world as to help transcend it. It is a practical framework for those who desire Self-realization and who encounter the different levels or categories of existence in their practice of meditation.

Yoga

In the context of the six schools of Hindu philosophy, Yoga ("union") refers specifically to the school of Patanjali, the author of the Yoga-Sutra. This school, frequently referred to as Classical Yoga, is considered a cousin of the Samkhya school of Ishvara Krishna. Both are dualistic philosophies, which teach that the transcendental Selves (purusha) are radically separate from Nature (prakriti), and that the former are eternally unchanging whereas the latter is forever undergoing transformation and is therefore not conducive to lasting happiness. We need not go into further detail here, because Patanjali's school will be presented at length in Chapter 9 ("Yoga as Philosophy and Religion").

Vaisheshika

Vaisheshika ("distinctionism") is concerned with the differences (vishesha) between things. It teaches that liberation is attained through a thorough understanding of the six primary categories of existence:

1. Substance (dravya), which is ninefold: earth, water, fire, air, ether, time, space, mind (manas), and Self (atman)
2. Quality (guna), of which there are twenty-three types, such as color, sensory perceptions, magnitude, etc.
3. Action (karma)
4. The universal (samanya or jati)
5. The particular (vishesha)

6. Inherence (samavaya), which refers to the necessary relationship between wholes and parts or substances and their qualities, and so on

The Vaisheshika school was founded by Kanada, the legendary author of the Vaisheshika-Sutra, who lived around 500 or 600 B.C. The name Kanada appears to be a nickname, meaning literally "particle eater." Presumably it refers to the kind of philosophy elaborated by him, though some Sanskrit authorities suggest that the name immortalizes the fact that the mighty ascetic lived on particles (kana) of grain. Perhaps both interpretations are right.

The origins of Kanada's school of thought are quite obscure. Some scholars regard it as an offshoot of the older Mimamsa school, others see in it a development of the materialist tradition, and yet others have proposed that it has its earliest roots in a schismatic branch of Jainism. In its general orientation as well as its metaphysics, the Vaisheshika school is close to the Nyaya system, with which it is traditionally grouped. Both these schools come closest to what we in the West understand by philosophy. They made a lasting contribution to Indian thought, but neither school has retained a prominent position. Vaisheshika is virtually extinct, and Nyaya has only a few representatives, mostly in Bengal.

Nyaya

The Nyaya ("rule, precedent") school of thought was founded by a certain Gautama (c. 500 B.C.), who lived in an age of great controversy between Vedic ritualism and such heterodox developments as Buddhism and Jainism—an age in which thinking and debating were, as in ancient Greece, a newfound passion. His was one of the earliest attempts to formulate valid rules for logic and the art of rhetorics.

Gautama proceeded from the insight that in order to live rightly and to pursue meaningful goals, we must first determine what constitutes right knowledge. True to the Indian flair for classification, he elaborated sixteen categories important for anyone desiring to know the truth. These range from the means by which valid knowledge (pramana) can be acquired, to the nature of doubt, to the difference between debate and mere wrangling. This is not the place to examine these categories more closely. What is of interest is the metaphysics of the Nyaya school.

According to the followers of Nyaya, there are numerous transcendental Subjects, or Selves (atman). Each infinite Self is the ultimate agent behind human consciousness, and the Self also enjoys and suffers the fruits of its actions. God is considered a special atman, as in Classical Yoga, and alone is Conscious. Notwithstanding that the human Selves are all deemed unconscious, as in the Mimamsa school, the Nyaya philosophers proposed the pursuit of liberation as the noblest goal in life. Of course, their opponents did not fail to point out the undesirability of a liberation that would lead to a rocklike, insentient existence. How little the adherents of Nyaya were convinced by their own metaphysics is evident from the fact that they looked for spiritual refuge in the religious teachings of Shaivism.

There are several points of contact between Nyaya and Yoga. Yoga is mentioned in the Nyaya-Sutra (IV) as that condition in which the mind is in contact with the Self alone, as a result of which there is mental equilibrium and insensitivity to bodily pain. In discussing various forms of perception, the Sutra's composer Vatsyayana further notes that the yogins are able to perceive remote and even future events, a skill that he felt could be cultivated by the regular practice of meditative concentration. Liberation is called apavarga, a term also found in the Yoga-Sutra.

A further curiosity is that both Nyaya and Classical Yoga subscribe to the obscure doctrine of sphota, which concerns the eternal relationship between a word and its sound. The idea here is that, for instance, the letters *y, o, g,* and *a,* or even the entire word *yoga,* cannot explain the knowledge we have of the thing called "Yoga." Over and above these letters or sounds is an eternal concept, the essence of a thing. When we hear a sequence of sounds, this eternal essence "bursts forth" (sphuta) or reveals itself spontaneously in our mind, leading to comprehension of the thing thus denoted. Finally, the followers of Nyaya are also known as yauga, "those who have to do with Yoga." It is not clear just what is hidden in this designation.

The division of Hindu philosophy into six schools is somewhat artificial. There are many other schools — notably those associated with certain sectarian movements — that at one time or another played an important role in the evolution of Hindu thought. We will encounter some of them in later chapters. What should be remembered is that Yoga influenced most of these approaches and traditions, though it did so more as a loose body of ideas, beliefs, and practices than as the philosophical system (darshana) articulated by Patanjali.

YOGA, AYUR-VEDA, AND SIDDHA MEDICINE

Ayur-Veda (lit., "science of life") is the name given to the native Indian system of medicine. Ayur-Veda is essentially naturopathic medicine, emphasizing prevention but also having an extensive curative repertoire. It is practiced in India alongside modern medicine and is put forward as a way of life for those wishing to enjoy longevity and good health. Although Ayur-Veda cannot be regarded as a philosophical tradition, it is founded in Hindu metaphysics. Ayur-Veda is traditionally considered to be a supplement to the ancient Atharva-Veda, in which we find the earliest recorded speculations on anatomy and on curative as well as preventive medicine. Because of its cultural importance, Ayur-Veda has sometimes been regarded as a fifth branch, or "collection," of the Vedic heritage.

The Ayur-Vedic body of knowledge is said to have originally amounted to 100,000 stanzas distributed over 1000 chapters. While medicine was undoubtedly practiced in the early Vedic era, no work of such comprehensiveness has survived into our time. The earliest extant medical works of encyclopedic scope are the Sushruta-Samhita ("Collection of Sushruta") and the Caraka-Samhita ("Collection of Caraka"). The former dates back in its oldest portions to pre-Buddhist times but was completed in its present form only in the early post-Christian era. The latter collection, which was also frequently revised, belongs in its present shape to the period around A.D. 800. However, its reputed author, Caraka, probably lived many centuries earlier, since he is said to have been the court physician of King Kanishka (A.D. 78–120).

Like Classical Yoga, the Ayur-Vedic system of medicine is divided into eight branches: (1) surgery, (2) treatment of diseases of the head, (3) treatment of other physical diseases, (4) treatment of childhood diseases, (5) processes for counteracting baneful occult influences, (6) antidotes to poisons, (7) processes for rejuvenating the body, known as *rasayana,* and (8) techniques for sexual revitalization. This formal similarity between Ayur-Veda and Patanjali's Yoga, though remarked on by the native authorities, is purely coincidental.

Ayur-Veda and Yoga do have a number of concepts and techniques in common. Most significantly, the authors and editors of the above-mentioned medical reference works have availed themselves of the spiritual philosophy of the Yoga-Samkhya tradition. Thus, at one point, the Sushruta-Samhita was revised in light of Ishvara Krishna's dualistic system of thought, as propounded in his Samkhya-Karika around A.D. 350. The Caraka-Samhita, on the other hand, contains echoes of epic Samkhya-Yoga metaphysics. Here it should also be mentioned that some of the ancient Sanskrit commentators believed that the same Patanjali who composed the Yoga-Sutra also wrote a famous treatise on grammar and on medicine.

Both Ayur-Veda and Yoga insist on the interactive unity of body and mind. Physical diseases can affect the mind adversely, and mental imbalance can lead to illnesses of all kinds. Ayur-Veda's notion of a healthy life includes that it must be both happy (sukha) and morally good (hita). A happy life, by Ayur-Vedic definition, is one that is physically and mentally hale and vigorous but also moral and wise. The intimate relationship between ethical conduct and happiness is often noted in the Yoga literature as well.

The authorities of Ayur-Veda recommend the cultivation of tranquility, self-knowledge, and prudence. Today we might say that the Hindu physicians incorporated self-actualization (in Abraham Maslow's sense[8]) into their medical theory and practice. We can readily appreciate that such a life would form a sound basis for the pursuit of the spiritual value of Self-realization (atma-jnana).

A strong connecting point between Ayur-Veda and Yoga is the theory of the different life-currents (vayu) in the body, which originated at the time of the Atharva-Veda, around 1000 B.C. The medical authorities generally list thirteen conduits (nadi) along or in which the different types of life-force are thought to travel, whereas Hatha-Yoga scriptures usually mention fourteen such principal pathways.

In Hatha-Yoga, the importance of commencing the practice of breath control in the right season is recognized. The medical basis for this custom is furnished by Ayur-Veda, according to which the bodily humors (dosha) undergo changes in the different seasons. The concept of the doshas is also referred to in different Hatha-Yoga works. Three principal humors are distinguished: wind (vata), bile (pitta), and phlegm (kapha). Health is a matter of the right balance between these bodily constituents.[9]

Furthermore, Hatha-Yoga and Ayur-Veda share certain purificatory techniques, notably the practice of self-induced vomiting (vamana) and physical cleansing (dhauti). These techniques have, among other things, a salutary effect on the body's metabolism. Ayur-Veda, furthermore, knows of thirteen kinds of internal heat (agni), of which the digestive heat (jathara-agni) is often mentioned by the authorities of Hatha-Yoga.

Physical well-being (arogya) is definitely one of the prerequisites and intermediate goals of Hatha-Yoga. Even Patanjali, in his Yoga-Sutra (III.46), mentions "adamant robustness" of the body as one of the aspects of bodily perfection (kaya-sampad). Elsewhere in his work (II.43), Patanjali speaks of the perfection of the body and the senses as a result of the dwindling of impurities by virtue of asceticism. Moreover, he states in one aphorism (II.38) that vitality (virya) is gained through chastity. In aphorism I.30, again, Patanjali lists sickness (vyadhi) as one of the distractions (vikshepa) of the mind that prevent progress in Yoga. The Sanskrit commentators explain that "sickness" means an imbalance of the bodily constituents (dhatu)—that is, the humors wind, bile, and phlegm. (These three elements are also sometimes viewed as doshas, "defects.")

In the Shiva-Svarodaya, a yogic work that is several hundred years old, breath control is hailed as the foremost means of achieving or maintaining well-being and for gaining occult knowledge and powers, wisdom, and even liberation. In one verse (314), the technique of svarodaya—from *svara*, "sound [of the breath]," and *udaya*, "rising"—is stated to be a science promulgated by the siddha-yogins.

In the Sat-Karma-Samgraha ("Compendium of Right Acts"), a Yoga text authored by Cidghanananda, a disciple of Gaganananda of the Natha sect, a whole range of purificatory practices is outlined. These are intended to stave off or cure all kinds of illnesses resulting from sheer misfortune or from carelessness in observing the prescribed dietary and other rules, such as those relative to the proper location and time. Cidghanananda advises the yogin first to use postures (asana) and occult medications to heal himself. When these fail, he should proceed with the techniques disclosed in the text.

The close connection between Ayur-Veda, Yoga, and also alchemy (rasayana) is particularly apparent in the medieval Siddha tradition of northern India. The adherents of this important tradition, which will be treated in Chapter 12 ("The Esotericism of Medieval Tantra Yoga"), sought bodily immortality through a sophisticated psychophysiological technology known as kaya-sadhana, "body cultivation." Out of this grew the different schools of Hatha-Yoga—which, on one level, can almost be looked upon as the preventive branch of Hindu medicine. Interestingly, one book on medicine, by a certain Vrinda, has the title Siddha-Yoga. Another medical treatise, ascribed to Nagarjuna, bears the title "Century [of Verses] on Yoga," or Yoga-Shataka. The link between Yoga and Ayur-Veda is, moreover, clearly acknowledged in the sixteenth-century work by Yogananda Natha, entitled Ayur-Veda-Sutra, in which the author specifically makes use of Patanjali's Yoga-Sutra.

South India has produced a second independent medical system that is the equivalent of Ayur-Veda. This system is associated with the Siddha tradition as it has developed in the Tamil-speaking south of the peninsula. Even more than Ayur-Veda, it has a strong connection to alchemy, and employs a large number of remedies derived from vegetables and chemicals. Its three principal diagnostic and therapeutic tools are astrology, mantras, and drugs, known in Tamil respectively as mani, mantiram, and maruntu. It also makes use of postures (asana) and breathing practices.

This rival system of medicine, which has scarcely been researched, was founded by the legendary Akattiyar (Sanskrit: Agastya), to whom over 200 works are attributed. He is the first of the eighteen siddhas, or accomplished adepts, venerated in the south. I will say more about the southern and northern branches of the Siddha tradition in Part Two.

The recognition by native Indian physicians that the human mind plays an instrumental role in the health of the body proved a significant bridge between medical care and the psychospiritual technology of Yoga. This relationship between Yoga and Indian naturopathic medicine deserves closer study. It might lead to insights that could be useful to modern medicine, which is beginning to rediscover the role of the human mind and psyche in illness and health.

PART TWO

FIVE THOUSAND YEARS OF GLORIOUS HISTORY

Yoga has been called a living fossil. It belongs to the earliest heritage of India's humanity. Thanks to the missionary efforts of Hindu swamis, it has entered a new phase of flowering in our century, both in India and in other parts of the world. Today hundreds of thousands of Westerners are actively practicing some form of Yoga, yet they do not always have a clear understanding of its traditional goals and purposes. To a large extent this is because they are generally uninformed about its richly textured history. Therefore, Part Two of this book is dedicated to outlining the essential developments in the long and complex evolution of Yoga.

History provides a vital context for our understanding of the world, especially human culture. More than that, history tells us about ourselves, because our beliefs and attitudes are largely shaped by the culture to which we belong. We are what we are, not only because of our own personal history but also because of the collective history of human civilization. As the German philosopher and psychiatrist Karl Jaspers commented:

> No reality is more essential to our self-awareness than history. It shows us the broadest horizon of mankind, brings us the contents of tradition upon which our life is built, shows us standards by which to measure the present, frees us from unconscious bondage to our own age, teaches us to see man in his highest potentials and his imperishable creations. . . . We can get a better understanding of our present experience if we see it in the mirror of history.[1]

Without adequate understanding of the historical unfoldment of Yoga, it is hard to imagine that we could arrive at a genuine appreciation of its spiritual treasures, or could practice it meaningfully and with ultimate effectiveness. A study of the history of Yoga gives us a broader picture than we can glean from most of the popular literature on the subject.

To learn about the historical evolution of Yoga is more than an academic exercise; it actually furthers our self-understanding and hence our efforts to

93

swim free of the boundaries of the ego. The following chapters will reveal some of the glory of the Yoga tradition, which has generated such immense wealth of insight into the human condition. It is, of course, impossible to capture even in a few hundred pages everything that scholarship has brought to light. Indeed, no one has so far attempted to integrate all the available data, which would require mastery of several languages (especially Sanskrit and Tamil) and a truly encyclopedic knowledge. Therefore, what I will attempt in this volume is the more modest goal of erecting a preliminary framework for our understanding of Yoga.

In Part One, we have seen how the history of Hinduism can conveniently be arranged into nine periods, extending from the pre-Vedic age to our present-day era—a span of well over 5000 years. In reading the following chapters, it will be helpful to bear that schema in mind. Since yogic ideas and practices are not unique to Hinduism but are also found, for instance, in Buddhism and Jainism, it is possible to write quite different histories. However, given the superlative position of Hinduism in the historical development of India's civilization, this would only add needless complication. In the following, therefore, the development of Yoga is presented from the point of view of Hinduism, though I have included short chapters on Buddhism and Jainism. These two traditions are treated in their relative chronological sequence: Jainism appears after the earliest Upanishads and is followed by Buddhism, which is a slightly younger heretical offshoot from archaic Hinduism (known as Brahmanism).

I begin my panoramic treatment of the history of Yoga with a tradition far older than Hinduism, Jainism, or Buddhism—the hoary magical tradition of Shamanism.

योग आनन्दकल्पनः

chapter 4
Yoga in Ancient Times

FROM SHAMANISM TO YOGA

Shamanism is the sacred art of changing one's awareness, or consciousness, in order to enter nonordinary realms of reality, which are experienced to be populated by spirits. The shaman (the word is of Siberian origin) is a seasoned traveler in those realms. By listening to the monotonous sound of a drum, click stick, or other percussion instrument, or by means of psychotropic substances (such as the fly agaric mushroom), the shaman achieves a radical shift in his perceptual field. He does so in order to communicate with the spirit world. His purpose is not idle curiosity; he hopes to retrieve power and information that are vital to the psychological and bodily welfare of his community.

Some scholars suggest that shamanism gave birth to Yoga, but this is true only in the broadest possible sense. According to Michael Harner, an American expert on shamanism, the transition from shamanism to Yoga occurred at the time of the rise of the city-states in the Near East, when shamans were suppressed by the representatives of the official religion.[1] In order to avoid detection, they had to cease drumming loudly and instead elaborated quiet methods of altering consciousness. Out of this, in Harner's reconstruction of history, grew the tradition of Yoga.

While Harner's hypothesis is ostensibly plausible, the waning of the shamanic tradition was probably more connected with the rise of the city-states coinciding with the collapse of tribal communities that the shamans served. This collapse, in turn, is best understood as a shift in consciousness toward a more individuated self-awareness.[2]

Whereas the shaman was a privileged sacred technician who acted on behalf of his community, the yogin is a sacred technician who seeks his own salvation. He does not, as a rule, endeavor to make any social contribution. Yet, of course, the yogins and holy folk of India have always been great religious and spiritual models for the people.[3]

While the hypothesis that derives Yoga from shamanism is thus problematical, clearly many aspects and motifs of shamanism have survived in Yoga. Mircea Eliade, who has pioneered research on both Yoga and shamanism, furnished the following characteristics for shamanism:

> Among the elements that constitute and are peculiar to shamanism, we must count as of primary importance: (1) an initiation comprising the candidate's symbolical dismemberment, death, and resurrection, which, among other things, implies his descent into hell and ascent to heaven; (2) the shaman's ability to make ecstatic journeys in his role of healer and psychopompos (he goes in search of the sick man's soul, stolen by demons, captures it, and restores it to the body; he conducts the dead man's soul to hell, etc.); (3) "mastery of fire" (the shaman touches red-hot iron, walks over burning coals, etc., without being hurt); (4) the shaman's ability to assume animal forms (he flies like the birds, etc.) and to make himself invisible.[4]

Yoga, as we have seen, is an initiatory tradition. Its entire course is governed by the idea of the progressive transcendence ("dismemberment") of the human ego-personality. Later we will encounter the Kshurika ("Dagger")-Upanishad, a work that explains the yogic process in terms of a step-by-step dismantling of our ordinary consciousness. The yogin's ecstatic introversion and mystical ascent is the equivalent of the shaman's ecstatic flight, and the yogin's teaching function corresponds to the shaman's role as a guide of souls. Furthermore, many of the shamanic powers are also recognized in Yoga, where they are known as siddhis ("accomplishments"), including the ability to become invisible. Finally, the shaman's "mastery of fire," an external feat, is paralleled by the yogic "inner fire," especially the psychophysiological heat generated during the awakening of the life-force in Kundalini-Yoga.

We have already spoken of the tradition of asceticism (tapas), the precursor of Yoga. Here too we can see a striking parallel to shamanism: Where the shaman demonstrates his mastery of fire by touching red-hot objects, the tapasvin excels in "self-heating"—that is, in disciplining himself to the point where he sweats from all pores. Whether through prolonged retention of the breath or through transmutation of the sexual drive into a higher energy (called ojas), the yogin similarly frustrates the "natural" tendencies of the body-mind and thereby creates an inner pressure that translates into physiological heat. He feels as if he were burning up. Then, at the peak of this experience, a radical breakthrough occurs where his whole being is flooded with light. He discovers that he *is* that light, which has no apparent source but is the Source of everything.

The condition of illumination, or enlightenment, is to the yogin what the magical journey into other realms is to the shaman. Both events represent a radical departure from conventional reality and consciousness. Both have a profoundly transformational power. Yet only the yogin who journeys inward discovers the ultimate futility of all journeying, because he realizes that he is never traveling outside the Self that was the goal of his spiritual odyssey. He goes beyond the subtle dimensions explored by the shaman, to the transcendental Being that is transdimensional and unqualified, and which he knows to be his most authentic identity.

YOGA AND THE ENIGMATIC INDUS CIVILIZATION

Yoga as we know it today is the product of several millennia. The earliest beginnings are lost in the obscurity of ancient Indian prehistory. The Bhagavad-Gita (IV.3), which was composed around the middle of the first millennium B.C., speaks of Yoga as being already archaic (puratana). Western scholars have generally underestimated the antiquity of Yoga, whereas Indian pundits have tended to exaggerate in the other direction. Studies by Jakob Wilhelm Hauer and Maryla Falk have supplied ample proof that Yoga was not the creation of the Upanishadic sages in the sixth or seventh century B.C., as earlier generations of Indologists had assumed.[5] They have convincingly shown that Yoga, as a loose structure of ideas and practices, dates back at least to the time of the Rig-Veda—about 1500 B.C.—the earliest literary signpost of the Indo-European tribes.

More significantly, according to most contemporary scholars, traces of an early form of Yoga can even be detected in the Indus civilization that flourished in the second and third millennia B.C. According to this view, Yoga thus antedates the invasion of the Sanskrit-speaking tribes from the steppes of southern Russia, who called themselves Aryans ("noble folk") who had long been thought to have given birth to the tradition of Yoga.

The gigantic Indus civilization was discovered in the early 1920s just after the world had come to the comforting belief that, with the surprise discovery of the Hittite empire, the last of the great civilizations of antiquity had been found. The discovery of the Indus civilization was made during the Archaeological Survey conducted by Sir John Marshall over six decades ago. The survey found a number of soapstone seals that clearly did not belong to any of the known cultures of the ancient world.

The extent of the Indus civilization, whose origins are indefinite, outstripped the keenest imagination of modern scholarship. So far, some sixty sites have been excavated over an area of 1000 miles, from the Arabian Sea upwards to the foothills of the Himalayas. These sites appear to be grouped around two major cities, Mohenjo-Daro in the south and Harappa 350 miles farther north, with the Indus River serving as the main artery of communication. More recent evidence obliged archaeologists to revise their estimate about the size of this ancient civilization, which appears to have extended another 600 miles south of Mohenjo-Daro.

Mohenjo-Daro, the larger of the two metropolises excavated in the Indus valley, covered an area of about one square mile—enough living space to accommodate at least 35,000 people. The cities show meticulous planning and

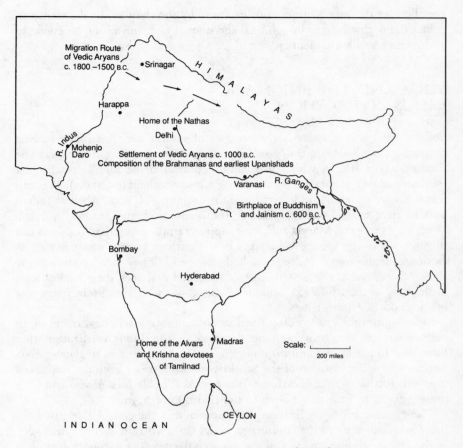

Map of India showing important traditional sites.

a high degree of standardization, suggesting a sophisticated sociopolitical organization. These two cosmopolitan cities, which incidentally have a common ground plan, survived for about 1000 years, during which time there was astonishingly little change in technology, written language, or artistic creativity. This stability prompted the British archaeologist Stuart Piggott to remark:

> There is a terrible efficiency about the Harappa civilization which recalls all the worst of Rome, but with this elaborately contrived system goes an isolation and a stagnation hard to parallel in any known civilization of the Old World.[6]

The excavations revealed elaborate drainage systems, including rubbish shutes, which are unique for pre-Roman times. They also showed an abundance of bathrooms, and this suggests the kind of ritual ablution that is typical of modern Hinduism. The mostly windowless buildings, including three-story houses, were made from kiln-burnt bricks, one of the finest known building materials. The nucleus of each big city is a huge citadel, some 400 by 200 yards in extent, built on an artificial mound.

In the case of Mohenjo-Daro, this central structure includes a large sacred bath, assembly halls, a large structure that was presumably a college for priests, and a great granary (grain storage was a government function). The urban layout points to a centralized authority, undoubtedly of a priestly nature. Although no temples have so far been definitely identified, it is assumed that religion played an important role in the lives of these early people. This assumption is mainly borne out by finds that show a striking resemblance to the religious motifs of later Hinduism.

Of special interest are the numerous soapstone (steatite) seals used by merchants, which depict animals, plants, and mythological figures reminiscent of later Hinduism. A number of the over 2000 terra-cotta seals that were found show horned deities seated in the manner of the yogins. One seal in particular, the so-called pashu-pati seal, has attracted attention and excited the imagination of archaeologists and historians. It portrays a divinity enthroned on a low seat and surrounded by an elephant, a tiger, a rhinoceros, and a buffalo. Beneath the seat is a pair of antelope-like creatures. This figure has been identified with God Shiva, the arch-yogin and lord of the beasts (pashu-pati). Though widely accepted, this interpretation has not remained unchallenged, and it is best to suspend judgment until further evidence is forthcoming once the highly developed pictographic script has been deciphered. Certainly the imagery is striking and suggestive.

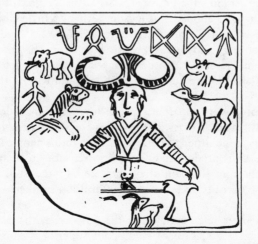

The famous "pashupati" seal, thought to be the earliest depiction of God Shiva as "Lord of the beast."

What we know about the religion of the Indus valley people is largely conjectural. However, the remarkable continuity in symbolism and design of certain cultural artifacts, such as ornaments, between the Indus civilization and modern India allows us to make informed guesses. There is good evidence for the existence of a goddess cult in the Indus civilization. One seal depicts a female from whose womb a plant grows, which suggests fertility beliefs and rituals, as one would expect of an early agricultural society. Associated with this are objects reminiscent of the later Tantric phallus (linga) and female organ (yoni). In fact, in the Rig-Veda of the invading Sanskrit-speakers, the native people are deprecatingly called "phallus-worshippers." Seals depicting the fig tree, which to this day is considered sacred in India, furthermore suggest the existence of a tree cult. As Stuart Piggott observed:

> The links between the Harappa [Indus] religion and contemporary Hinduism are of course of immense interest, providing as they do some explanation of those many features that cannot be derived from the Aryan traditions brought into India after, or concurrently with, the fall of the Harappa civilization. The old faiths die hard: it is even possible that early historic Hindu society owed more to Harappa than it did to the Sanskrit-speaking invaders.[7]

Piggott's closing suggestion is more than likely correct. Although the Vedic tribes were vital and spirited like all frontier people, they were by far outnumbered by the native population. But who were those invading "Aryans"?

Archaeological finds point to military violence in the latter days of Mohenjo-Daro. The cities had been in a state of cultural decline for a long time, and their final death is usually connected with the invasion of the Indo-European or Aryan tribes, creators of the Rig-Vedic culture, who started to enter northern India about 1500 B.C. or perhaps a little earlier. Numerous passages in the Rig-Veda speak of the destruction of fortified cities (pur), of massacres and looting, and of the breaking of dams that had regulated the waters of the Indus river for centuries. It was the latter act that forced the townspeople to abandon their cities and take refuge in the surrounding forests.

The Indus people were apparently peace-loving, well-to-do urbanites who had few weapons. In some cases, the towns were under siege for a year before they fell. Scholars are inclined to believe that the Indus people spoke an archaic form of Dravidian, the predominant language of south India, and that after the destruction of their civilization they migrated to the southern tip of the peninsula. Today there are an estimated 100 million speakers of the Dravidian languages.

Judging from their self-portrayal in the Rig-Veda, the Sanskrit-speaking invaders were aggressors, sure of their own superiority, proud, and rather merciless. They feared only the enemy's magical spells, suggesting that the Indus people must have had competent priests or magicians. Nevertheless, as so often happens in the history of conquests, the invaders were ultimately absorbed by the land and the native cultures, though not without modifying their social patterns and ideology.

Various hypotheses have been advanced to explain the apparent continuity between the culture of the Indus civilization and post-Vedic India, yet none of the explanations proffered is entirely satisfactory.[8] Whatever the historical truth may be, it is fairly certain that the death of this giant civilization did not imply the extinction of its cultural heritage. Undoubtedly, many of the beliefs, practices, and much of the acquired knowledge survived in one form or another in the rural communities.

It is clear from the Rig-Veda that, after the fall of the great cities, the Vedic tribes gradually assimilated many of the notions and customs of the non-Vedic native population. This is reflected already in the language of the Rig-Vedic hymns, which contain many non-Sanskrit words. At any rate, the presumption common among earlier scholars that Yoga is entirely a creation of the Indo-European invaders has been demonstrated to be incorrect in light of modern archaeological finds. Yoga is a tree with many roots, and its taproot is undoubtedly to be found in the Indus civilization.

SACRIFICE AND MEDITATION: THE RITUAL YOGA OF THE RIG-VEDA

The iconographic evidence for the presence of Yoga-like practices in the Indus civilization is fascinating. Yet it is not sufficient to prove definitely the existence of Yoga as a full-fledged tradition in that early period. More palpable evidence is found in the Rig-Veda and the Atharva-Veda. The former body of hymns, consisting mostly of prayers, invocations, and metaphysical speculations, was probably composed shortly after the invading Indo-European tribes had settled in the area of the modern Punjab. The latter hymnody, filled with magical spells and incantations, points to the geographical area of Bihar in the eastern corner of the Indian peninsula, where some of the tribes migrated in the course of time. Fifteen hundred years later, the Bihar region was part of the cradle of the great syncretistic movement of Tantrism, in which, among other things, magic and metaphysics entered a new marriage.

The Vedic tribes, who hailed from the steppes of southern Russia, had traveled through Persia, entering the Indian peninsula through the Khyber pass—the same pass in the Hindukush Mountains through which Afghan refugees have fled to Pakistan in recent years. The reason for their centuries-long migration is not known; they may have been forced to abandon their homeland because of severe drought or overpopulation. The early Vedic people were fair-skinned, blue-eyed, and light-haired, which distinguished them from the dark-complexioned natives whom they (rather unkindly) called snub-nosed serfs. The Vedic invaders were semisedentary cattle breeders who, with their horse-drawn chariots and bronze weapons, were militarily superior to the native population of India. They settled in villages in the Indus valley, where they applied not only their military but also their agricultural skills—undoubtedly they had much to learn in this regard from the Indus people.

Soon the Vedic invaders spread into the fertile basin of the Ganges all the way across northern India. Their conquest was seldom peaceful, and the invading tribes, in their hunger for land, cattle, and political supremacy, did not fail to go to war against one another. Thus, the fight between the Kurus (or Bharatas) and the Pancala tribe is recorded in the Mahabharata, the longest poem in the world. This feud is generally believed to have actually occurred, probably between 1000 and 900 B.C. According to the Mahabharata, the God-man Krishna served as the charioteer of Prince Arjuna, who had married into the royal house of the Pancala tribe. Other mythological accounts of those pioneering days are found in the Puranas, the great Sanskrit encyclopedias— which were, however, composed many hundreds of years after the event.

That warlike behavior and religious aspirations are not necessarily incompatible is apparent from the history of Christianity and Islam. Indeed, war is a crisis situation that confronts us with our mortality, impelling us to think about metaphysical matters. The greatest book on Yoga, the Bhagavad-Gita, was delivered by Lord Krishna on the eve of one of the fiercest battles fought on Indian soil.

But the hills and valleys of northern India did not resound only with battle cries and the sound of conches. The Vedic people were fond of singing and dancing, and counted among themselves many splendid poets and accomplished musicians—drummers, flutists, and lute players. Even though the Vedic settlers knew how to celebrate life, they also had a penchant for deep thought, solitary concentration, and penance.

Yoga in the Vedas

The Vedic evidence for an early form of Yoga can be arranged into two broad categories. The first consists of yogic practices and ideas found in the religious world of the Vedas themselves. The second comprises yogic elements that do not properly pertain to Vedic religion but are referred to or hinted at in the Vedas. In the former case, one may speak of the proto-Yoga as an early form of sacrificial mysticism, since the Vedic religion consisted essentially in the performance of sacrificial rites.

The central role played by ritual sacrifice (yajna) in Vedic society must be appreciated. Every household had its own daily sacrificial ceremony to perform. In addition, the village or tribe came together on special occasions to participate in large-scale sacrifices, such as the famous fire sacrifice (agnishtoma) and the horse sacrifice (ashva-medha), which was performed especially to ensure the continued reign of a successful king.

The daily sacrifice (homa), performed by both husband and wife, was quite simple. It involved the ritual pressing of the soma plant, which has been identified by some as the fly agaric mushroom. Mixed with milk, a portion of the soma liquid was poured into the carefully tended fire. The rest of this intoxicating libation was imbibed by the participants. Food offerings were also made. All this ritual activity was accompanied by invocations to Indra (the god of lightning and war), Agni (the fire god), and other deities of the Vedic pantheon.[9] The purpose of the sacrifice was to win the favor of a particular deity. Most of the gods were male; the few goddesses (notably Aditi and Sarasvati) that were recognized occupied a rather subordinate position in the Vedic religion, reflecting the strong patriarchal order of that tribal society.

There were also periodic large-scale complex sacrifices that required the participation of many priests as well as expensive offerings of gold and herds. Such ceremonies could stretch over several days, even weeks. They demanded the highest degree of concentration from the priests and their numerous helpers.

The Vedic settlers had neither temples nor idols, and the priests, though respected, did not have the stifling authority of the brahmins of later periods. Their religious aspirations were down-to-earth; in their prayers they petitioned for a long, healthy, and prosperous but also righteous life. The hereafter was imagined to be rather similar to a happy earthly existence for those who were free of sin or guilt, whereas sinners could look forward to eternal damnation. There was yet no sign of a belief in rebirth, which gained prominence in subsequent eras.

Examining the Rig-Veda from the point of view of spiritual practice, the British vedicist Jeanine Miller has concluded that the practice of meditation (dhyana) as the fulcrum of Yoga goes back to the Rig-Vedic period. She observes:

> The Vedic bards were *seers* who *saw* the *Veda* and sang what they saw. With them vision and sound, seership and singing are intimately connected and this linking of the two sense functions forms the basis of Vedic prayer.[10]

Miller's exacting and sensitive studies have revealed unsuspected depths of spiritual practice among the Vedic settlers, and a spectacular world of symbols and ideas that evince a people who were as fond of introspection and contemplation as they were of earthly delights.

The Vedic hymns were expressions of their deep spirituality. To compose a hymn meant to envision it in a state of contemplation. The envisioner was known as a rishi, or "seer," by virtue of his vision. By means of the performance of the prescribed sacrifices, the rishi "sent forth" his vision (dhi) to the Divine. The proto-Yoga of the rishis contains many elements characteristic of later Yoga: concentration, watchfulness, austerities, regulation of the breath in connection with the recitation of sacred hymns during the ritual, painstakingly accurate recitation (foreshadowing the later Mantra-Yoga), visionary experience, the idea of self-sacrifice (or surrender of the ego), and the encounter with a Reality larger than the ego-personality.

Sri Aurobindo, modern India's finest seer-poet, championed a spiritual interpretation of the Vedic hymns. He wrote:

> The Veda possesses the high spiritual substance of the Upanishads, but lacks their phraseology; it is an inspired knowledge as yet insufficiently equipped with intellectual and philosophical terms. We find a language of poets and illuminates to whom all experience is real, vivid, sensible, even concrete, not yet of thinkers and systematisers to whom the realities of the mind and soul have become abstractions. . . . Here we have the ancient psychological science and the art of spiritual living of which the Upanishads are the philosophical outcome.[11]

The Vedic Sanskrit language had two words for prayerful meditation—*brahman* and *dhi.* The former is derived from the verbal root *brih,* meaning "to grow, expand," whereas the latter stands for intensive thought, inspired reflection, or meditative vision. Miller describes the brahmic meditation as follows:

> This is the essence of the Vedic *brahman*—the Vedic magic: an invocation and an evocation, an active participation, by means of mental energy and spiritual insight, in the divine process, rather than a mere passive reception of external influences; a deliberate drawing forth out of a probing deep within the *psyche,* and the appropriate formulation thereof; the words themselves into which the orison [prayer], now mentally conceived, is finally couched, being but the form in which is clothed the *inspiration—vision—action.*[12]

Vedic Meditation

According to Jeanine Miller, the meditative practice in Vedic times displays three distinct but overlapping aspects, which she calls mantric meditation, visual meditation, and absorption in mind and heart. By mantric meditation she means mental absorption via the vehicle of sound, or sacred utterance (mantra). Visual meditation is epitomized in the concept of dhi (the later dhyana), in which a particular deity is envisioned. Absorption in mind and heart is the highest meditative stage, in which the seer, on the basis of what Miller calls a seed-thought, explores the great psychic and cosmic mysteries that led to the composition of the remarkable cosmogonic hymns, such as the above-mentioned hymn of creation.

Meditation, when successful, leads to illumination, the discovery of the "immortal light." Thus in one hymn (V.40.6) the ancient sage Atri is said to have "found the sun hidden by darkness" in the course of the fourth stage of prayer, which can be equated with ecstatic transcendence (samadhi). Miller sees in this the "culmination of the Vedic quest for truth."[13]

In view of the this-worldly, or earthly, nature of many of the Vedic hymns, which Aurobindo reinterpreted as cryptic symbolism, some scholars have concluded that the whole ascetic and contemplative tradition was merely borrowed from the aboriginal cultures. But there is no reason to deny the Vedic Aryans the religious impulse, or even enthusiasm for metaphysical thinking. The religion they brought with them from their homeland around the Caspian Sea had strong shamanic features. The Vedic figure of the muni or silent sage can be looked upon as a shaman.

In the Keshi-Sukta, the long-haired muni is said to ride the winds and to benefit his fellow beings, which are both typical shamanic motifs. The muni points to a more primitive religious world than the Vedic rishi, though the world of the muni was still very much alive when the rishis were composing their inspired hymns. While the rishis represent the Vedic orthodoxy, the munis, who are "mad with silence," appear to stand for a different stream of Aryan culture: those who stood midway between the sacrificial mysticism of the Vedic orthodoxy and the esoteric traditions of non-Vedic peoples. And we may well see in them forerunners of the later yogins in their more eccentric appearance, as avadhutas or crazy adepts.

Among the 1028 hymns of the Rig-Veda, five are of special relevance to the student of Yoga.

The first is the nasadiya-sukta, often called the hymn of creation (X.129). This cosmogonic hymn foreshadows the later metaphysical speculations of the Samkhya school of thought, which was so closely allied with Yoga.[14] Cosmogony (from Greek kosmos and gonia, "birth") concerns itself with the origins of the universe. The ancient cultures have proffered ingenious theories about the beginnings of the world, and this hymn of creation is one of the most remarkable.

The second noteworthy hymn is X.72. This is another cosmogonic speculation, addressing the riddle of how the universe came into existence. The third and fourth verses mention the term *uttanapad,* "one whose feet are turned upward," which is one name of the goddess Aditi ("Boundless"), who gave birth to the world. This peculiar expression is reminiscent of the uttana-carana posture referred to in verse III.198 of Yajnavalkya's Smriti ("Memory"), a text on ethics and jurisprudence composed in the early post-Christian centuries. This posture is executed by raising the legs above the ground, as in the shoulderstand.

The third example is the purusha-sukta, "hymn of man" (X.90). Of the various cosmogonic hymns, which are important for a study of Yoga inasmuch as they describe not only the evolution of the cosmos but also the genesis of the human psyche, the hymn of man is one of the most striking. In the first verse the primeval male (purusha) is said to have covered the entire creation and extended ten digits beyond it. This is meant to suggest that the Creator transcends his creation, that the manifest world emanates from the transcendental Reality but does not define it. A more elaborate version of this hymn is found in the Atharva-Veda (XIX.6).

The fourth hymn is I.164 (=Atharva-Veda IX.9–10). This composition is a collection of profound mystical riddles. The sixth verse, for instance, asks about the nature of the One that is unborn and is yet the cause of the manifested universe. Verses 20–22 speak of two birds that occupy the same tree; one is said to eat of its fruit while the other merely looks on.

The tree can be read as a symbol of the world. The unenlightened being devours the tree's fruit, impelled by egoic desires. The enlightened being, or the sage, abstains and merely looks on dispassionately. The tree can also be seen as a symbol of the tree of knowledge, of whose fruit the sage partakes but not the uninitiated. A more strictly vedantic interpretation is the following: The onlooking bird is the uninvolved Self beyond the realm of nature; the other bird is the embodied being enmeshed in conditioned existence.

In verse 46, we find the oft-quoted utterance that the nameless one Being is called differently by the sages.[15] The author, or envisioner, of this particular Rig-Vedic hymn is known by name—Dirghatamas ("Long Darkness"), who was undoubtedly one of the deepest thinkers of that early period. The Indian scholar Vasudeva A. Agrawala, who has written a detailed study of this asya-vamiya-sukta, remarked:

> Dirghatamas is the type of all men of philosophy and science who have cast their eyes of comprehension on the visible world. Their vision is focussed on the invisible source, the First Cause which was Mystery of yore and a Mystery now. Dirghatamas stands at the apex of them all asking: "Where is the Teacher, knowing the solution? Where is the pupil, coming to the Teacher for revelation? . . . He takes quick snaps of the Cosmos itself, pointing to many symbols that carry the tale of its secret. The Seer seems to take the confident view that the imprisoned divine splendour, although a veritable Mystery, is present in every manifest form and is open to understanding.[16]

The fifth and final hymn (X.136), which is especially important, is known as the keshi-sukta, "hymn of the long-haired one." Here a special type of non-Vedic ascetic, the keshin, is eulogized, in whom some scholars have seen a forerunner of the later yogin.

Even though this hymn does not belong to the earliest portions of the Rig-Veda, it gives us a precious glimpse into a very archaic type of religious specialist, the shamanic ecstatic. The keshin—who, as the name indicates, wears long hair—is said to exult in his seeing of and participation in truths that are concealed from the ordinary mortal. He is as compassionate as he is mindlessly god-intoxicated or "god-impelled" (deva-ishita).

There are several obscure phrases and statements in this hymn. In interpreting them, I have largely followed Jeanine Miller's lead, though in a few instances I am putting forward my own divergent views and intuitions. The "tawny dust" with which the keshin clothes himself could refer to the Hindu practice of smearing sandalwood paste on certain parts of the body, especially the forehead.

The phrase "wind-girt" has generally been interpreted to mean "nude."

But this could also have deeper symbolic significance. As is clear from other verses of this hymn, the keshin is closely associated with Vayu, god of the wind or life-force. If we read this hymn from a yogic point of view, we could easily wrest from this phrase a different meaning: that the keshin armed himself with the breath—that is, practiced breath control. This would explain the first-person exclamation "upon the winds we have ascended." In that case, it is through the regulation of the breath that the keshin enters a different state of consciousness (and its corresponding reality).

> The long-hair [endures] fire; the long-hair [endures] poison; the long-hair endures the world (rodasi) [both physical and psychic]; the long-hair gazes fully on heaven; the long-hair is said to be that [transcendental] Light. (1)
>
> The wind-girt sages (muni) have donned the tawny dust. Along the wind's course they glide when the gods have penetrated [them]. (2)
>
> Exulted by our silence (mauna), upon the winds we have ascended. Of us, you mortals, you behold only our bodies. (3)
>
> Through the mid-region (antariksha) flies the sage shining down upon all forms; for his goodness, he is deemed the friend of every god. (4)
>
> The wind's steed, [God] Vayu's friend, is the god-intoxicated sage; within both oceans he dwells, the upper and the lower. (5)
>
> In the paths of apsaras [female spirits], gandharvas [male spirits], and beasts wanders the long-hair, knower of [the most hidden] thoughts, a gentle friend, most exhilarating. (6)
>
> For him has [God] Vayu churned and pounded the unbendable (kunamnama), when the long-hair drank with [God] Rudra ("Howler") from the poison cup. (7)

God Rudra was apparently intimately connected with the ecstatic munis. He later became assimilated into the powerful figure of Shiva. It is not clear what is meant by the "unbendable" (kunamnama) in the concluding stanza. Miller speculates that it may be the gross aspect of the human body-mind—that is, the material vehicle that resists psychospiritual transformation. Lord Vayu, the master of the life-force (prana), is said to have "churned" and "pounded" the kunamnama for the keshin. Here perhaps we see an early reference to the dormant psychospiritual power of the human body, which later came to be known as the kundalini-shakti.

Neither is the reference to the poison cup altogether clear. Some scholars think that the "poison" (visha) was a concoction similar to the soma, which produced hallucinations. Jeanine Miller prefers a symbolic interpretation: The poison is the poison of the world, which the spiritual practitioner can absorb with impunity because of his inner purity. These interpretations are not mutually exclusive, however, and given the widespread ritual employment of soma in Vedic times, the existence and use of other similar intoxicants is probable. Similarly, in later Tantrism the ritual use of wine is sanctioned in left-hand schools. It is said to lead to spiritual degradation in those who consume it casually, for purely egoic reasons, but it can be a gateway to the Divine for the spiritual aspirant. In other words, what is poison for the worldling is ambrosia for the initiate.

What we find, then, in the Vedic era is a fairly developed body of lofty ideas and practices centering on meditation and the contemplation of the divine Mystery. These notions and techniques, notably the soma ritual, were associated with a vital sacrificial cult. We also find in the Vedic hymns evidence for a more ecstatic approach to spirituality, as embodied in the figure of the wild, long-haired ascetic. Clearly, the religious environment of the Vedic tribes was one of the taproots of later Yoga.

SPELLS OR TRANSCENDENCE: THE MAGICAL YOGA OF THE ATHARVA-VEDA

As the creeper has completely embraced the tree, so may you embrace me. May you love me. May you not withdraw from me.

As the eagle, flying forth, beats its wings toward the earth, so do I beat down your mind. May you love me. May you not withdraw from me.

As the sun travels swiftly in [the space between] heaven and earth here, so do I go about your mind. May you love me. May you not withdraw from me. (VI.8.1–3)

*　　*　　*

Having harnessed the chariot [of my mind], here has come forth the thousand-eyed curse, seeking after my curser, as a wolf [seeks out] the dwelling of a shepherd.

O curse, avoid us like a burning fire [avoids] a pool. Strike our curser here, as the [lightning-]bolt from heaven [strikes] a tree.

Whoever shall curse us not cursing, and whoever shall curse us cursing, him [who is] whithered I cast unto death, as a bone [is cast to] a dog. (VI.37.1–3)

*　　*　　*

Night after night, we bring to You, o Agni, [our offerings] without mixture, as fodder to a standing horse. Let us, Your neighbors, not experience harm, [but] enjoy abundance of wealth and food.

Whatever arrow [of destiny] of You who are good is in the air, that is Yours. With it, be gracious to us. Let us, Your neighbors, not experience harm, [but] enjoy abundance of wealth and food.

Evening after evening, Agni [the God of Fire] is our household's lord. Morning after morning, He is the giver of good intentions. May You be for us the giver of good of every kind. May we adorn ourselves by kindling You.

Morning after morning, Agni is our household's lord. Evening after evening, He is the giver of good intentions. May You be for us the giver of good of every kind. May we thrive a hundred winters by kindling You.

May I not fall short of food. To the food-eating Lord of Food, to Agni [who is Rudra] be homage. (XIX.55.1–5)[17]

The first of the above hymns from the Atharva-Veda is a love charm, the second is a spell against curses, and the third is an incantation addressed to Agni for prosperity. These prayers and spells give some indication of the range of concerns expressed in this "fourth" Veda.

Like the other Vedic hymnodies, the Atharva-Veda contains sacred knowledge (veda). It was collected by the magician and fire-priest Atharvan, who may have been a native of what is now Bihar. As a collection, the Atharva-Veda is several centuries younger than the Rig-Veda, but much of its content is at least as old as the oldest hymns of the Rig-Veda.

The Atharva-Veda consists of about 6000 verses and 1000 lines in prose, most of which deal with magical spells and charms designed to promote peace, health, and material and spiritual prosperity or to call down disaster on an enemy. Even though the Atharva-Veda was undoubtedly used widely, for a long time it was not counted as part of the sacred Vedic canon (consisting of Rig-Veda, Yajur-Veda, and Sama-Veda). Even after its incorporation it was never granted the same elevated position as the other three Vedas by the orthodox priesthood. The reason for this is the marginal social status of the followers of Atharvan. While they were undoubtedly consulted by the Vedic villagers for their skill in the "black arts," they were also feared. Moreover, they kept themselves apart and carefully guarded their arcane learning.[18]

Of the many mystical passages in the Atharva-Veda, most of which defy full comprehension, the following selection of hymns appears to imply some esoteric knowledge that could feasibly be linked with primeval Yoga and the related Samkhya tradition.

1. II.1: This hymn speaks of the seer Vena. It is said that he saw the highest secret, "where everything becomes of one form."
2. IV.1: Another enigmatic hymn, this tells of Vena's mystic Realization. Vena is said to have uncovered the womb (yoni) of being and nonbeing.
3. V.1: This hymn is purposely obscure and probably grammatically corrupt in many parts. However, judging from the sophisticated concepts expressed, its composer was evidently aware of a deep mystical tradition.
4. VII.5: This hymn teaches of the inner sacrifice, which became the

main theme of the early Upanishads. It starts with the enigmatic line, "By sacrifice the gods sacrificed to the sacrifice." That is, the deities themselves performed sacrifices, and their sacrifices had no other purpose than the action of sacrifice, which is the giving of oneself. The sacrifice is described as being the overlord of the gods who extended—that is, taught the sacrifice to human beings.

5. VIII.9: This cosmogonic hymn poses a number of esoteric riddles and extols Viraj, the female (in other hymns also male) creative principle that, the anonymous author declares, can be seen by some and not seen by others. "Breathless, she goes by the breath of breathing ones."

6. VIII.10: The subject of this hymn is again Viraj, who is said to ascend and descend into the householder's fire. The householder who knows this secret is said to be "house-sacrificing" (griha-medhin).

7. IX.1: This cosmogonic hymn intimates the secret of the "honeyed whip" (madhumati-kasha). This mysterious substance is said to have sprung from the elements generated by the gods, upon which the sages contemplate. From what we can gather from the difficult passages, the honeyed whip corresponds to the later idea, found in Tantrism and Hatha-Yoga, of the internal ambrosia, the nectar of immortality, thought to drip from a secret place near the palate. The Vedic mystic aspired to win the honey, to experience the transcendental splendor within his own body-mind. The honey doctrine (madhu-vidya) can be encountered in the ancient Brihad-Aranyaka-Upanishad, where we find this significant passage:

The Self (atman) is honey for all things, and all things are honey for this Self. This shining, immortal Person who is in this Self, and, with reference to oneself, this shining, immortal Person who exists as the Self—he is just this Self, this Immortal, this Absolute, this All. (II.5.14)

8. X.7: This mystical hymn discloses the secret doctrine of the world-pillar (skambha) that sustains the entire creation and is known by those who know the transcendental Reality, or brahman, within their own hearts. In verse 15, the nadis (currents of the life-force) are mentioned, which shows the age of such speculations about the subtle or energic body.

9. X.8: This hymn hints at the author's occult understanding about the origin of the cosmos and expresses wonder at the complexity of creation. Particularly revealing is verse 43:

The lotus-flower of nine doors [i.e., the body and its nine orifices], covered with the three strands (guna) [i.e., skin, nails and hair?]—whatever mighty being (yaksha) is within it, that the knowers of the Absolute (brahman) know.

10. XI.4: This hymn extols the life-force (prana), which is said to clothe man as a father would clothe his dear son (verse 11).
11. XI.5: Here the Vedic novice (brahmacarin) is spoken of, and the symbolism of his initiation and subsequent spiritual practice are briefly discussed.
12. XV: This is the famous vratya-khanda (book of the Vratyas), which will be discussed in the next section.

Whether we talk about the mainstream (orthodox) Vedic society, guided by the brahmins who were masters of sacrificial ritualism, or whether we consider such marginal cultural groups as the magician-priests of the Atharva-Veda or the ecstatic mystics (keshin), they all were possessors of esoteric knowledge. We can only speculate about the origins of those early traditions and deploy our historical imagination to reconstruct, in faint outlines, a picture of their most ancient roots—in the mysterious religion of the Indus civilization and the shamanic religion of the Indo-European tribes prior to their emigration from Russia to India. What we see is a constant concern with states of consciousness that are far removed from our ordinary awareness. It is here that we have the cradle of Yoga.

THE MYSTERIOUS VRATYA BROTHERHOODS

Ancient India holds many riddles for the modern historian. The spiritual brotherhood of the Vratyas is perhaps the most intriguing enigma. Their importance for the present survey lies in the fact that they were connected with the earliest evolution of Yoga and probably invented the practice of breath control (pranayama). The Vratyas were instrumental in the transmission of Yoga-like knowledge and in all probability were the first among the Indo-European immigrants to assimilate the cultural—and in particular the religious—wisdom of the conquered Indus civilization.

Who exactly were these Vratyas? The statements about the Vratyas in Indian literature are confusing and often contradictory, and the only authentic text is the vratya-khanda (book XV) of the Atharva-Veda.[19] Unfortunately, many of its hymns are scarcely intelligible. Nevertheless, there are a number of well-established points that, when viewed together, result in at least a rough picture of these people.

The Vratyas were one of the many communities that did not belong to the orthodox kernel of Vedic society but had their own set of customs.[20] They roamed the country, mostly the northeast of India, in groups (vrata) bound together by vow (also vrata). Some of them apparently traveled on their own and were known as eka-vratya, the word *eka* meaning "one" or "solitary." They spoke the same language as the Vedic settlers and hence have been regarded as an earlier wave of the Indo-European-speaking immigrants from Eurasia.

In the eyes of their orthodox cousins who upheld the Vedic sacrificial religion, the Vratyas were despicable outcasts who spoke the same tongue by accident and who were fit to become victims in human sacrifice (purusha-medha), which was apparently enacted literally at this early period. Nonetheless, the Vratyas must have been numerous and influential, for later on the orthodox priesthood, the brahmanas (brahmins in English), introduced special rites by which a Vratya could be purified and accepted into the mainstream of Vedic society. After their conversion most seem to have settled down and taken up a trade.

The Vratyas frequented especially the country of Magadha (modern Bihar) in northeastern India—the country of the two great heresies Buddhism and Jainism, and later also of Tantrism. They also appear to have had a vital relationship with the kshatriya, or warrior, estate that played a substantial role in the formation of early Upanishadic thought. Thus, according to one hymn of the Atharva-Veda (XV.8), the eka-vratya, or solitary Vratya, was the originator of the warrior (rajanya) estate. Kings like Ajatashatru and the incredibly wealthy Janaka were among the first to promote the teaching of nondualism that is associated with the Vedanta of the Upanishads, and it would not be too farfetched to surmise that in many cases they may have been inspired directly by the Vratyas. Noteworthy is the case of the mighty King Prithu, who, according to the Jaiminiya-Upanishad-Brahmana, received instruction about the sacred syllable *om* from the seer Vena, the "divine Vratya."

The Vratyas apparently traveled in groups of thirty-three, and each group had its own head. Members were distinguished on the principle of seniority. Some are said to have "quietened the penis"—that is, mastered their sexual drive. The ancient Sanskrit phrase for this accomplishment is *shamanica medhra,* which reminds one of the yogic state of urdhva-retas, the upward conduction of semen in those who are adepts in celibacy. Interestingly enough, the phrase *urdhva-retas* is also employed in conjunction with God Rudra, whom the Vratyas worshipped together with Vayu, the God of Wind and ecstatic flight.

The Vratyas wore simple garments tied to their loins, with red or black borders, and a red turbanlike headdress. They used silver ornaments for neck or breast, wore sandals, and carried a whip and a small bow but no arrows. This and other evidence point to the fact that the Vratyas were sacred brotherhoods, most likely of a military nature originally. They traveled in primitive carts drawn by a horse and a mule; during their religious ceremonies the carts served as sacrificial altars. Each group was accompanied by a professional bard, known as magadha or suta, and a female called pumshcali ("man-mover"). Bard and sacred prostitute performed the sexual rite in the midsummer ceremony called maha-vrata ("great vow"), which also involved railing and obscene dialogues. Without question, the bard and the sacred prostitute enacted the creative play between god and goddess. Anticipating the bipolar metaphysics of later Tantrism, the Vratyas pictured God Rudra ("Howler" or "Roarer") as being accompanied by a drum-beating female deity reminiscent of the Kali of Hinduism.

This important agricultural fertility ritual also included the use of a swing, which was regarded as a "ship bound for heaven." The chief priest swung on this apparatus while muttering prayers, which included references to the three types of life-force that were thought to animate the body—prana, apana, and vyana.

The Vratyas were experts in magical matters, and some of their magical lore has survived in the hymns of the Atharva-Veda. In view of the unorthodox nature of the Vratya beliefs and practices, the Vedic priests did everything to obscure or obliterate as much of the sacred lore of the Vratyas as possible, and it is something of a miracle that the vratya-khanda has survived at all.[21]

From the yogic point of view, the most interesting feature of Vratya lore is their apparent practice of pranayama and other similar austerities. It is in such practices that we can detect one of the roots of later Yoga and Tantrism. Thus, the Atharva-Veda (XV.15.2) mentions the Vratyas' knowledge of seven pranas, seven apanas, and seven vyanas. These are the various functions of the life-force circulating in the body and are related to the breath as it is inhaled, exhaled, and retained. The three sets of seven are analogically linked with a variety of different things.[22] This practice of giving far-flung psychocosmic associations for the breath evinces the archaic mentality preserved in the Vedas.

The following extract from the Atharva-Veda (XV.1) is another typical example of this style of magical thinking:

[Once] there was a Vratya roaming about. He stirred up the Lord-of-Creatures. (1)

He, the Lord-of-Creatures beheld gold within himself. He brought it forth. (2)

That [gold] became the One; that became the Forehead-sign-bearer (lalama); that became the Great (mahat); that became the Foremost (jyeshtha); that became the brahman; that became the creative-power (tapas); that became Truth (satya); by this He brought [himself] forth. (3)

He grew; he became the Great (mahan); he became the Great God. (4)

He surrounded [? pari + ait] the supremacy of the gods; he became [their] ruler. (5)

He became the One Vratya; he took a bow; that was Indra's bow. (6)

Its belly was blue; red the back. (7)

With the blue [side of the bow] he encompasses hostile clans; with the red [side] he pierces the hateful [enemy]. Thus say the teachers-of-brahman. (8)

It is impossible to make strict rational sense of the above hymn. Its composer moved in a different frame of reality, that of mythopoeic thought rather than abstract reasoning. He delighted in mystical equations and analogies, and he was obviously aware of esoteric meanings that we can only dimly intuit.

To return to the historical picture: The Vratyas appear to have had some kind of relationship to Jainism, which is one of the two prominent rival traditions to Hinduism, the other being Buddhism. Unlike Buddhism, however, which was the creation of a member of the warrior estate within late Vedic society, Jainism claims a much longer history reaching back into pre-Vedic times. The first "ford-maker" (tirthankara), or adept-teacher of the Jainas, was Rishabha. The name means "bull," which is also Rishabha's emblem, and it is the bull that figured prominently in Indus art. If we can believe the line of succession of teachers given in the Jaina canon, Rishabha's date was around 1200 B.C., which puts him close—by three centuries—to the final days of the Indus civilization.

Some scholars have suggested that the Jainas, with their pronounced emphasis on nonharming (ahimsa) and renunciation, represent more faithfully than any other known tradition the mood of that vanquished civilization. It is certainly interesting to note that in the Acara-Anga-Sutra, which must be reckoned among the oldest extant works of the Jaina canon, the accomplished traveler on the spiritual path is commonly referred to as a muni. This affords a direct connecting point with the culture of the Atharva-Veda, where, as we have seen, the muni is a celebrated ecstatic.

The following hypothesis suggests itself: The origins of Jainism may be found in the native rural communities that were the principal carriers of the heritage of the Indus civilization after the destruction of the big cities. The sacred Vratya brotherhoods assimilated much of that rural tradition without, however, forsaking their Indo-European roots. If Jainism made withdrawal from the world into an art form, the Vratyas combined a disposition of renunciation with a more virile attitude of magical mastery of the body and nature. The Jainas may have been the prototypes of the later Hindu tradition of renunciation (samnyasa), but the Vratyas laid the foundations of Yoga and Samkhya.

योग आनन्दकल्पनः

chapter 5
The Whispered Wisdom of the Early Upanishads

OVERVIEW

Some historians regard the period from 1500 B.C., marking the collapse of the Indus civilization and the arrival of the Vedic tribes, to the time of the Buddha a thousand years later as the Dark Ages of India. This designation is as inappropriate here as it is in the European context, for those days were far from decadent or sinister. Rather, they were a time of great cultural adventure in which the Vedic tribal society and the native cultures of India encountered each other and, after centuries of hostilities, gradually became integrated.

More than anything, the expression "Dark Ages" betrays our lack of detailed and accurate historical knowledge of that period. Of course, it is just as inappropriate to speak of it as the Golden Age, as have some historians who idealized the spiritual status of the early Indians. The period was marked by war and death and the disappearance of old ways of life, as well as reconstruction and the emergence of new patterns of living and thinking.

The absence of precise historical knowledge also hampers our study of the early Yoga movement. We have seen in the previous chapter that proto-yogic ideas and practices were present in both the sacrificial ritualism of the orthodox Vedic priesthood and in the religious world of the nonbrahmanical circles at the fringe of Vedic society, particularly the mysterious Vratya brotherhoods. As the Vedic people grew increasingly dissatisfied with the highly formalized ritualism requiring the constant services of their hereditary priesthood, the Vratyas and other "heretics" gained steadily in importance. It was among these marginal religious folk that early Yoga was fashioned.

There is no evidence of Yoga in the Brahmanas (c. 1000–800 B.C.), Sanskrit works expounding and systematizing the Vedic sacrificial ritual, composed by the Vedic priests. The only possible exception is the late Shata-Patha-

Brahmana. This scripture, which dates back to perhaps 800 B.C., bridges the gap between the strictly ritualistic world-view of the Brahmanas and the symbolic ritualism of the Upanishads. It contains speculations about the world-ground, life-force (prana), and rebirth, all woven into the fabric of Vedic sacrificial mysticism.

Although Yoga is not mentioned in the Brahmana scriptures, we can see in their sacrificial ritualism one of the contributing sources of the later Yoga tradition. Thus, their treatment of the ceremony of prana-agni-hotra, the "fire sacrifice of the breaths," which consists in the offering of food to the various kinds of breath, shows lines of thought that prepare the ground for the yogic theory and practice of breath control (pranayama). The prana-agni-hotra is a symbolic substitute for the earlier Vedic fire ritual (agni-hotra), the most popular of all rites. In the prana-agni-hotra, the life-force takes the place of the ritual fire and is identified with the transcendental Self, the atman.

However, this is not yet a full-fledged mental sacrifice as is yogic meditation or lifelong celibacy. The prana-agni-hotra was enacted bodily.[1] This important sacrifice was a decisive stepping-stone toward what historians of religion have called the interiorization of sacrifice—the conversion of external rites to inner or mental rites.

There is also no reference to Yoga in the Aranyakas, or "forest books." Similar in nature to the Brahmanas, these were meant as ritual texts for the orthodox brahmin who retired to the forest to live in solitude, dedicated to a life of quiet contemplation and mystical rituals. These forest-dwellers—vana-prasthas, as they were later called—are the first sign of the increasingly powerful trend in India toward world-renunciation. The Aranyakas can be looked upon as preparing the ground for the subsequent Yoga tradition in its ascetic mode.

The first real opponents to the formalized sacrificial cult of Vedic society, however, were not the forest anchorites of the Aranyaka period but the sages of the Upanishads. Who were these sages? They were a motley group: Some were brahmins, like the famous Yajnavalkya, who had broken away from the established sacerdotal tradition. Others were powerful kings, like Janaka, or popular local rulers like Ajatashatru, king of Kashi (modern Benares, or Varanasi). Others were forest-dwellers. What they had in common was a penchant for esoteric wisdom, or what in classical Greece was called gnosis, transcendental knowledge that would lift them beyond mundane life, even beyond Vedic ritualism and its promised heavens, to the realization of the unconditional Reality. That Reality they preferred to name brahman, the Absolute. The word brahman is derived from the verbal root brih, meaning "to grow." It denotes the vastness of the supreme Reality.

The oldest Upanishads, which grew out of the Aranyakas, were composed in the eighth and seventh centuries B.C. Although there is no mention of the word yoga in the technical sense in the most archaic works of this genre, it is evident that some important conceptions peculiar to later Yoga and its ally Samkhya had become widely adopted by the thinkers of that period. Probably the most significant fact is that the Upanishadic sages turned unanimously to meditative practice as the chief means of obtaining transcendental knowledge. In contrast to this, the meditation practiced by the orthodox priests was intimately bound up with sacrifice, which, as we have seen, was granted supreme status in the Vedic religion. Even the forest-dwelling ascetics continued to adhere to the sacrificial cult of mainstream Vedic society; they merely retired from the hustle and bustle of ordinary life.

The Upanishadic sages initiated what was to become an ideological revolution. They internalized the Vedic ritual in the form of intense contemplation, or meditation. This is best illustrated in the following passage from the Kaushitaki-Brahmana-Upanishad:

> Now next [follows the practice of] self-restraint according to Pratardana, or the inner fire sacrifice, as they call it. Verily, so long as a person (purusha) is speaking, he is unable to breathe. Then he is sacrificing the breath to speech. Verily, so long as a person is breathing, he is unable to speak. Then he is sacrificing the speech to breath. These are the two unending, immortal oblations. In sleeping and in waking, he sacrifices them continuously. Whatever other oblations there are, they are limited, for they consist in [ritual] actions. Understanding this, the ancestors did not offer the [external] fire sacrifice. (II.5)

The last line suggests that this symbolic fire sacrifice was practiced already by the predecessors of the composer of this Upanishad. He may well have received this tradition from his teacher, but we can be certain that it originated with the early Upanishadic sages.

The idea that behind the reality of multiple forms, our ever-changing universe, there abides an eternally unchanging single Being was communicated already in Vedic times. What was new was the Upanishadic discovery that this single Being is none other than the very core of one's own existence. Almost 3000 years ago, sage Yajnavalkya put it thus in the Brihad-Aranyaka ("Great Forest")-Upanishad:

> He who breathes with your inhalation (prana) is your Self (atman), which is in everything. He who breathes with your exhalation (apana) is your Self, which is in everything. He who breathes with your mid-breath (vyana) is your Self, which is in everything. He who breathes with your up-breath (udana) is your Self, which is in everything. He is your Self, which is in everything. (III.4.1)

When asked how that Self is to be conceived, Yajnavalkya continued:

> You cannot see the Seer of seeing. You cannot hear the Hearer of hearing. You cannot think the Thinker of thinking. You cannot understand the Understander of understanding. He is your Self, which is in everything. Everything other than Him is irrelevant. (III.4.2)

This passage epitomizes the essence of the Upanishadic mystery teachings that were passed on from Self-realized teacher to disciple by word of mouth: The transcendental Ground of the world is identical with the transcendental core of the human being; brahman equals atman. That supreme Reality cannot exhaustively be described or defined. It must simply be *realized*. Upon realization, the Self will be found to be infinite, eternal, utterly real and free, as well as immeasurably blissful (ananda).

How can the Self be realized? The Upanishadic sages emphasized the need for world-renunciation and intensive contemplation, but the earliests Upanishads contain few practical instructions about the art of meditation. This was apparently a matter to be settled between the teachers and their disciples. The spiritual path included extensive and wholehearted service to the teacher and constant discrimination between the real and the unreal—all sustained by a burning desire for Self-realization and a willingness to transcend the ego.

The Upanishads make much of the esoteric nature of this communication and enjoin the initiate to keep it concealed from undeserving ears. The word *upanishad* is composed of the verbal root *sad* ("to sit") prefixed with *upa* and *ni* (together meaning "near"). Thus the term conveys the idea of "sitting down near" the teacher, who quietly instructs the disciple. The esoteric wisdom of the Upanishads was whispered rather than proclaimed aloud. Today the most precious teachings are made available in paperback editions, and we tend to read the Upanishads as entertaining or, at best, inspired and inspiring literature, seldom approaching these ancient teachings with the respect and integrity they once commanded.

The Upanishads do not, however, speak only of the glory of the Self or the different avenues of approach to it. They contain a great mass of other teachings, not least the once hidden teaching of reincarnation (punar-janman) and moral causation (karma). It is generally believed that since these ideas are foreign to the Rig-Veda, they were adopted from the native peoples of the Indian peninsula. Only a handful of scholars assume that it was the Upanishadic sages themselves who discovered the cycle of births and deaths, governed by the iron law of karma. In any case, this notion became a prominent feature of Hinduism and the other religious traditions of India. Each tradition had its own interpretations of how reembodiment works and how the self-perpetuating mechanism of karma can be outwitted through spiritual practice. The escape from the round of successive births became a principal motive behind India's spirituality, and we will therefore encounter this idea again and again in the remaining portion of this book.

Over 200 Upanishads exist, and most have been translated into English. The earliest works date back to the eighth century B.C., whereas the youngest scriptures of this genre were composed as recently as our own century. Hindu traditionalists, following the list furnished in the 500-year-old Muktika-Upanishad, generally recognize 108 Upanishads, which are considered a continuation and conclusion of the Vedic revelation. Their teachings are known as Vedanta; the term means literally "Veda's end." All subsequent teachings are considered to be no longer shruti ("revelation") but smriti ("tradition").

The oldest principal Upanishads can be arranged in rough chronological order as follows: The first group (800–600 B.C.) comprises the Brihad-Aranyaka-, Chandogya-, Taittiriya-, Kaushitaki-, Aitareya-, and Kena-Upanishad. The second group (600–300 B.C.) includes the Katha-, Isha-, Shvetashvatara-, Mundaka-, Maha-Narayana-, Prashna-, Maitrayaniya-, and Mandukya-Upanishad.

The remaining Upanishads are generally divided into the following five groups: The first comprises the Upanishads that expound Vedanta in general. The second consists of the Samnyasa-Upanishads, which elaborate on the ideal of renunciation. The third group is made up of the Shakta-Upanishads, which disclose teachings related to shakti, the feminine aspect of the Divine. The fourth group comprises the so-called Sectarian Upanishads, which expound teachings related to specific religious cults dedicated to such deities as Skanda (God of War), Ganesha (elephant-headed remover of obstacles), Surya (Sun God), or even Allah (the Moslem Creator-God, who is reinterpreted in Vedantic terms), and so forth.

The final group comprises the Yoga-Upanishads, which explore different aspects of the yogic process, especially Hatha-Yoga. This category includes the Brahma-Vidya-, Amrita-Nada-, Amrita-Bindu-, Nada-Bindu-, Dhyana-Bindu-, Tejo-Bindu-, Advaya-Taraka-, Mandala-Brahmana-, Hamsa-, Mahavakya-, Pashupata-Brahma-, Kshurika-, Tri-Shikhi-Brahmana-, Darshana-, Yoga-Cudamany-, Yoga-Tattva-, Yoga-Shikha-, Yoga-Kundaly-, Shandilya-, and Varaha-Upanishad. These works will be described in Chapter 11 ("God, Visions, and Power").

It should be remembered that originally all these texts—the Vedas, Brahmanas, Aranyakas, and Upanishads—were not written down at all but memorized and transmitted from teacher to pupil by word of mouth. The Vedic corpus is what has been called a mnemonic literature. Given the bulk of this literature and its often complicated subject matter, it is astonishing how these works could have been memorized for centuries so accurately that in many cases only a few variants exist. Different lines of teaching, perhaps belonging to widely separated geographic regions, managed to preserve the original with remarkable faithfulness. To this day, there are some bards in India who can recite the entire Mahabharata or Ramayana from memory. The former comprises over 100,000 stanzas, the latter around 50,000 verses.

While memorization was not deemed a yogic feat in itself, it helped young students acquire a rare degree of concentration that proved useful in their later spiritual work. Besides, in learning the Vedic corpus by heart they were constantly exposed to the highest wisdom, which naturally opened their hearts to the spiritual path. Today, immersed as we are in a lopsided materialistic culture, it is sometimes difficult for us to find and maintain a spiritual perspective. Fortunately, the inspired creations of ancient and modern Hindu saints, yogins, and sages are readily available to us in book form. We need not abandon home and work to sit at the feet of the great adepts and benefit from their vision of humanity's potential and destiny. Modern technology brings their timeless wisdom and encouragement to our doorstep.[2]

THE BRIHAD-ARANYAKA-UPANISHAD

The oldest among the early Upanishads is the Brihad-Aranyaka- ("Great Forest") Upanishad, in which the meditative path is still closely connected with sacrificial concepts. It begins with a set of instructions about the horse sacrifice (ashva-medha) interpreted as a cosmological event. The horse sacrifice was a major ceremony performed in honor of a successful king to ensure the continued prosperity of his rule. The last-known performance took place in the eighteenth century at Jaipur in Rajasthan.

In the course of this sacrifice, the chief sacrificer's wife mimicked sexual intercourse with the dead horse just before it was dismembered and cooked. The parallel to the sexual symbolism of Tantrism is obvious: The horse does not loose its semen during this symbolic ritual, but the "copulating" woman partakes of the animal's vital energy. In later Hindu Tantrism, the yogic God Shiva is often depicted as a corpse and his spouse Shakti shown seated on him in a pose of sexual intercourse.

Early on, the horse came to signifiy the sun and, by further symbolic extension, the resplendent transcendental Self. The Self is the Source of all life and yet, because of its transcendental nature, is more appropriately understood as passive (like a corpse) rather than active. It is the Self's power, or shakti, aspect, in the form of the life-force animating the human personality and consciousness, that creates access to the Self. In the Great Forest treatise, these symbolic associations are vaguely hinted at.

For instance, we find speculations about the origin of the universe, which is said to spring from the One Being that split itself into two—male and female—thus creating the entire cosmos. Linked with this cosmological doctrine is a fundamental ethical conviction characteristic of the subsequent Vedantic technology of emancipation: Because there is essentially only the One, it is a heinous sin to cling to the multiple objects of the universe. This One Being is described as the true goal of humanity. Yajnavalkya, the most outstanding sage of the early Upanishadic period, is credited with these stanzas:

> As a tree, or lord of the forest,
> just so, truly, is man (purusha):
> his hairs are leaves,
> his skin the outer bark.
>
> Verily, from his skin flows blood,
> as sap from the bark.

Therefore, when the skin is torn,
blood issues from him,
as does sap from a wounded tree.

His flesh is the inner bark,
the tendons the inner layer, which is tough.
Beneath are the bones, as is the wood.
The marrow is comparable to the pith [of the tree].

If a tree, when felled, grows again
from its root into another,
from what root grows the mortal [person],
after he has been felled by death?

Do not claim, "From the seed":
that is generated in the living.
A tree grows indeed from seed.
After it has died, it springs forth [again].

If, however, the tree is destroyed with its roots,
it does not spring forth again.
From what root does the mortal grow
when he has been felled by death?

He is simply born [and then dies, you may argue].
No, [I say]. He is born *again*. Born by what?
The conscious, blissful Absolute (brahman),
the Principle of grace,
the refuge of him who knows and abides in It.
(III.9.28.1–7)

In this marvelous passage of the Brihad-Aranyaka is intimated the higher knowledge of the mystic and yogin, who knows the one indivisible Ground of Being and who, like Yajnavalkya, confidently declares: aham brahma-asmi, "I am the Absolute." The last stanza contains the key to the whole metaphor: The human "tree" is born again and again by force of his karma, as is made clear in other passages. It is this repeated drama of birth, life, and death that, to the sensitive psyche of the yogin, is but pain (duhkha). This cycle is imaged most potently in another passage:

Just as a leech, when it has reached the end of a blade of grass, draws itself together before making a further approach [to a different blade], so this Self, after having cast off the body and dispelled ignorance, draws itself together before making another approach [to a new body]. (IV.4.3)

Clearly, there is no solace in this cycle (samsara), and hence the Upanishadic sages taught the esoteric means by which the world of change and endless rebirth can be transcended. Elsewhere in the same scripture, Yajnavalkya proclaims:

> I have touched and found the narrow ancient path that stretches far afar. By it the wise, the knowers of the Absolute, go up to the heavenly world and are released. (IV.4.8)

> He who has found and awakened to the Self that has entered this perilous and inaccessible [body-mind], is the Creator of the world, for he is the Maker of all. The world is his. He is indeed the world. (IV.4.13)

> When one perceives directly the bright (deva) Self, the Ruler of what has become and what will be, then one does not recoil [from It anymore]. (IV.4.15)

> Those who know the Life (prana) of life, the Eye of the eye, the Ear of the ear, the Mind of the mind, have realized the ancient, primeval Absolute. (IV.4.18)

> It is to be seen by the mind alone. There is no difference in It whatsoever. He who sees difference in It, reaps death after death. (IV.4.19)

> It should be seen as single, immeasurable, perpetual. The Self is spotless, birthless, great, perpetual, and beyond [the subtle element of] the ether (akasha). (IV.4.20)

Emancipation, which is identical to immortality, is the realization of the Self in its immutable purity. This realization coincides with the transcendence of the limited mechanisms of the human body-mind and thus of conditional existence itself. What is more, Self-realization is the hidden program of the universe. Again it is Yajnavalkya who illustrates this point in a striking image in the Brihad-Aranyaka:

> As the ocean is the single locus of all waters, as the skin is the single locus of all touch, as the nostrils are the single locus of all smells, as the tongue is the single locus of all tastes, as the eye is the single locus of all forms, as the ear is the single locus of all sounds, as the mind is the single locus of all volitions (samkalpa), as the heart is the single locus of all knowledge, as the hands are the single locus of all acts, as the genitals are the single locus of all pleasure (ananda), as the feet are the single locus of all movement, as speech is the single locus of all the Vedas—so is this [Self].

> As a lump of salt, when thrown in water, dissolves in water, and no one can perceive it, because from wherever one takes it, it tastes salt—thus, my dear, this great, endless, transcendental Being is only a Mass of Consciousness (vijnana-ghana). (II.4.11–12)

Since the Self, or the Absolute, is all there is, It cannot be an object of knowledge. Therefore, Yajnavalkya argues that, ultimately, all descriptions of It are mere words. He responds to all positive characterizations of the Self by exclaiming "not thus, not thus" (neti neti). This famous procedure of negation is fundamental to Vedanta spirituality: The yogin of this tradition is asked to constantly remind himself of the fact that all the states and expressions of his body-mind are, in themselves, other than the transcendental Reality. No experience amounts to Self-realization. The body, as it is ordinarily experienced, is not the Self; nor are thoughts or feelings as they normally present themselves. The Self is nothing that could be pointed to in the finite world. This perpetual watchful discernment is called viveka, which literally means "separating out."

Through steady application to this practice of discernment, the yogin develops an inner sensitivity both to what is ephemeral in his nature and to the underlying eternal Ground of all his experiences. This awakens in him the will to renounce everything that he has identified as belonging to the world of change. Discernment and renunciation ultimately lead to the discovery of the universal Self, the atman, beyond all concepts and imagery.

THE CHANDOGYA-UPANISHAD

Another archaic Upanishad is the Chandogya, whose name derives from the words *chandas,* "hymn" (lit., "pleasure"), and *ga,* "going," here referring to those brahmins who sang the hymns of the Sama-Veda during the sacrificial ritual in Vedic times. Thus, the Chandogya-Upanishad consists of the esoteric teachings of the chandogas, the Vedic chanters.

It is therefore not surprising that this work commences with elaborate mystical speculations about the sacred syllable *om,* the most celebrated numinous sound, or mantra, of Hinduism. In his commentary on this Upanishad, Shankara, the great propounder of Vedantic nondualism, observes that this syllable is the most appropriate name of the Divine, or transcendental Reality.

The syllable *om* has a long history dating back to Vedic times. It can be considered the mother of all other mantras. It was used at the beginning and end of ritual pronouncements, just as Christians use the word *Amen.* Like all other words of the Vedas, *om* is regarded as divine revelation. The yogins of later periods have described how, in deep states of meditation, they could hear the sound *om* vibrating through the entire cosmos. This has a parallel in Pythagorean and Neoplatonic thought in the notion of the music of the spheres, the cosmic harmonic generated by the motion of the heavenly bodies.

In the third chapter, the sacred gayatri-mantra (to this day recited by all pious Hindus during the morning ritual) is introduced. The text of this ancient mantra, which dates back to the time of the Rig-Veda (III.62.10), runs as follows: om tat savitur varenyam bhargo devasya dhimahi dhiyo yo nah pracodayat—"Om. Let us contemplate that celestial splendor of God Savitri, so that He may inspire our visions." Savitri ("Stimulator") is the personification of the quickening aspect of the Vedic solar deity.

This chapter also contains a section (III.17) that speaks of Krishna, "son of Devaki," who is identified by some scholars as the Krishna of the Mahabharata war. Significantly, one passage (III.17.6) introduces Ghora, "son of Angiras" (after whom the Atharva-Veda was also named Angirasa-Samhita), as the teacher of Krishna. Here a teaching is mentioned according to which one should repeat, at the hour of death, three specific mantras from the Yajur-Veda, which contains the sacrificial formulas. The three mantras are: "You are the Undecaying! You are the Unchanging! You are the very essence of life!" This doctrine resembles the teaching in the Bhagavad-Gita (VIII.5–6) according to which a person's final thought should be of the Divine rather than any mundane concerns, for whatever one thinks, one becomes.

Here we also learn that, according to Ghora, austerity (tapas), charity (dana), rectitude (arjava), nonharming (ahimsa), and truthfulness (satya) are the sacrificial gift (dakshina). In other words, it is one's way of life that is the best recompense for what one has received from one's teachers. This notion is connected with the idea, expressed in a different passage (III.15.1), that a person—so long as he or she is a spiritual practitioner—is a sacrifice. In contemporary language, such a person is a self-transcender.

The disciplines mentioned by Ghora may be understood as components of the early Upanishadic proto-Yoga, and indeed some of them recur in the later Yoga-Upanishads as regular aspects of Yoga practice. Ghora affords a direct link between Krishna and the tradition of the Atharva-Veda, and this is further strengthened by the fact that in the Bhagavad-Gita (X.25), which is Krishna's song of instruction to Arjuna, the divine Lord exclaims: "Of the great seers I am Bhrigu." The fire priest Bhrigu was one of the leading lights of the Atharva tradition.

In another chapter of the Chandogya-Upanishad, the intriguing honey doctrine (madhu-vidya) is mentioned. This peculiar esoteric psycho-cosmology, alluded to already in the Rig-Veda and the Atharva-Veda, compares the world to a beehive.

> Verily, yonder sun is the honey of the gods. The sky is its cross-beam. The mid-region is the honeycomb. The particles of light are the brood. (III.1.1)

It is clear from the phrase "honey of the gods" that this passage should be understood metaphorically. Moreover, in another passage (III.5.1), where the "upward rays" of the world are spoken of, the Absolute (brahman) is said to be the flower from which the honey is gathered and which drips with nectar. As we read in another passage (III.6.3): "He who thus knows this nectar (amrita) . . . becomes content."

Honey (madhu), then, stands for the nectar of immortality, which in Tantric Yoga is thought to be secreted within the body itself. The Chandogya-Upanishad cryptically speaks of five kinds of nectar, which are obviously levels of realization. Ultimately, the scripture declares (III.11.1), the knower of the Absolute "neither rises nor sets but remains alone in the center."

The same chapter (III.13) includes an exposition of the different forms of the life-force (prana), which are called the "divine openings" (deva-sushi) of the heart, the "brahmic men," and the "door-keepers of the heavenly world." They are the gateway to the Absolute that is seated in the heart of all beings. This continues the speculations found in the Vedas and suggests a developing knowledge of the yogic practice of breath control (pranayama).

THE TAITTIRIYA-UPANISHAD

Third among the oldest Upanishads is the Taittiriya, which stands in the tradition of the Yajur-Veda, the Vedic hymnody containing the sacrificial formulas. The esoteric teachings of the Taittiriya go back to the teacher Tittiri, founder of the Taittiriya school, whose name means "partridge." The contents of this Upanishad are similar to that of the Chandogya. It emphasizes the mystical implications of the Vedic chants and sacrifice. Of its three chapters, the second and third are of particular interest to the student of Yoga history.

Probably the most peculiar teaching of the Taittiriya is the doctrine, received and transmitted by Bhrigu, that everything is to be looked upon as food (anna). This is an early "ecological" idea referring to the interlinkage of all things—the chain of life. In the words of the Upanishad:

From food, verily, creatures are produced—whatsoever [creatures] dwell on earth. Moreover, by food, in truth, they live, and into it they finally pass. (II.21)

This extends the notion, mentioned earlier, of the sacrificial nature of human existence to all forms of life. There is nothing dreadful about this, for, in the final analysis, life is blissful. This is a most important discovery: that the Absolute is not a dry, desertlike environment but conscious Bliss beyond description. The Taittiriya (II.8) teaches that there are degrees of bliss, extending from the simple joy of a prosperous human life to the delight on higher levels of existence (such as the realms of the gods and forefathers), up to the immeasurable Bliss of the Absolute itself—an idea that was later explored in Tantrism, with its Dionysian, world-positive orientation.

He who is here in man, and he who is there in the sun, is the One. He who knows this, on departing from this world, proceeds to the self consisting of food, proceeds to the self consisting of life-force, proceeds to the self consisting of mind, proceeds to the self consisting of consciousness, proceeds to the self consisting of bliss.

On this there is the following stanza:
He who knows wherefrom words recoil
together with the mind,
without attaining the Bliss of the Absolute,
fears nothing at all. (II.8–9)

This passage hints at a teaching of considerable importance in later Vedanta, the doctrine of the five sheaths (panca-kosha):

1. The anna-maya-kosha, or sheath composed of food; that is, of material elements: the physical body.
2. The prana-maya-kosha, or sheath composed of life-force: the etheric body in Western occult literature.
3. The mano-maya-kosha, or sheath composed of mind: The ancients considered the mind (manas) as an envelope surrounding the physical and the etheric body.
4. The vijnana-maya-kosha, or sheath composed of understanding: The mind simply coordinates the sensory input, but understanding (vijnana) is a higher cognitive function.
5. The ananda-maya-kosha, or sheath composed of bliss: This is that dimension of human existence through which we partake of the Absolute. In later Vedanta, however, the Absolute is thought to transcend all five sheaths.

Reaching the pinnacle of spiritual life, the sage realizes his essential oneness with the blissful transcendental Being. In his ecstasy he triumphantly proclaims:

Oh, wonderful! Oh, wonderful! Oh, wonderful!
I am Food! I am Food! I am Food!
I am the Food-Eater! I am the Food-Eater! I am the
Food-Eater!
I am the Maker of Poetry (shloka)![3] I am the Maker of
Poetry! I am the Maker of Poetry!
I am the first-born of the world-order (rita),
prior to the gods, [residing] in the hub of immortality!
He who gives Me [as food], he indeed has preserved Me!
I, who am Food, eat the Eater of Food!
I have overcome the whole world!
[My] effulgence is like the sun. (III.10.6–7)

The Taittiriya-Upanishad has preserved many archaic teachings that were part of the cultural background of those adepts who crafted the early yogic technology. It is in the Taittiriya (II.4.I) that we find the very first occurrence of the word *yoga* in the technical sense, probably standing for the sage's control of the fickle senses.[4] But it would take several more centuries for the Yoga tradition to emerge and to assume its place alongside the other paths of liberation within Hinduism.

OTHER ANCIENT UPANISHADS

The Aitareya-Upanishad

Of the three remaining Upanishads of the early period, the relatively short Aitareya is of interest because of its archaic cosmogonic material. This work, which is named after an ancient teacher, opens with a myth also found at the beginning of the Brihad-Aranyaka-Upanishad: "In the beginning"—that is, before the occurrence of space-time—the single Self (atman) decided to create, out of itself, the universe. First it created the material elements. Then the Self created various functions (called *deva,* "divinities"), such as hearing and sight, which joined with the human form. Next the Self created food for all creatures.

As the final act of the process of world creation, the Self enters the human body through the sagittal suture (siman), also known as the "cleft" (vidriti) and the "delighting" (nandana). According to later teachings, the yogin must consciously exit through that same opening at the crown of the head at the time of death. It is quite possible that this practice was known already in the pre-Buddhist era to which the Aitareya belongs.

The Kaushitaki-Upanishad

The Kaushitaki-Upanishad, titled after the old brahmin family in which this work was handed down, contains a valuable detailed exposition of the doctrine of rebirth and a description of the path to the "world of the Absolute," or brahma-loka. It also includes a long discourse on the life-force as being identical with the Absolute. One passage reads as follows:

> Life is prana, prana is life. So long as prana remains in this body, so long is there life. Through prana, one obtains, even in this world, immortality. (III.2)

In a subsequent section (III.3) prana is equated with consciousness (prajna). It is by means of consciousness that a person acquires true resolve (satya-samkalpa), the whole-body desire to transcend the finite world and thence achieve immortality. Thus, through the cultivation of the conscious life-force, the sage attains the universal prana, which is immortal and joyous.

In the fourth chapter of the Kaushitaki we encounter the widely traveled sage Gargya Balaki proudly instructing the famous king Ajatashatru in the mystery of the Vedas. However, Gargya Balaki's wisdom does not satisfy Ajatashatru, who promptly proceeds to initiate the mendicant in the secret of the universal prana or life, which is consciousness, and which can be known only by those who are pure in spirit. The Self, declared Ajatashatru, has entered the body from head to toes and is resident in it "like a razor lies concealed in its case." This is one of a number of instances in which a member of the warrior estate instructs a brahmin.

The Kena-Upanishad

Another archaic Upanishad is the Kena, which received its title from the opening phrase *kena,* meaning "by whom?" It starts with the question of who sent forth mind, speech, and sight, and so on, thus asking for the cause of our outer-directed consciousness. To be able to answer this question, one must apperceive, as the Upanishad insists, the underlying unitary substratum of all experience, which is the transcendental Self (atman). That which is responsible for our externalized awareness is the same Reality that is also responsible for the objects of that awareness. The transcendental Subject is the matrix of both the conditioned consciousness and the objective world.

The ancient Upanishadic sages were not alone in their mystical intuitions. The era they lived in was a time of great cultural ferment, in which the warrior estate had an important part. The Upanishadic sages simply gave expression, within the fold of post-Vedic society, to a widespread impetus for metaphysical thought and mystical experience. There were many other non-Vedic thinkers and visionaries, as well as mystics and seers who had broken away from mainstream Vedic society more severely than the Upanishadic sages. Among the latter were Vardhamana Mahavira and Gautama the Buddha. Both hailed from the warrior estate. Their "heretical" teachings are the substance of the next two chapters.

योग आनन्दकल्पनः

chapter 6

Jaina Yoga: The Teaching of the Victorious Ford-Makers

HISTORICAL OVERVIEW

The preceding chapters have outlined the gradual evolution of Hindu spirituality from the time of the Vedas about 1500 B.C. to the emergence of the secret teachings of the first Upanishads some 700 years later. With this chapter, we interrupt our historical survey of proto-yogic ideas and practices within the fold of Hinduism. Here we will briefly consider what from the Hindu point of view amounts to a rival teaching—the great religious tradition of Jainism.

Together with Hinduism and Buddhism, Jainism is one of the three major socioreligious movements to which the Indian spiritual genius has given birth. If we associate Hinduism with a breathtaking nondualist metaphysics and Buddhism with a stringent analytical approach to spiritual life, we find that Jainism excels in its rigorous observance of moral precepts, especially nonviolence (ahimsa). It was this lofty ideal, together with an extensive teaching about the moral force (karma) inherent in human behavior, that has exerted a lasting influence on the tradition of Yoga.

Jainism has preserved an archaic type of spirituality based on the practice of penance (tapas) combined with a strict code of ethics. However, the Jaina teachers of the post-Christian era adopted many ideas and practices from Hindu Yoga, particularly as formulated by Patanjali in the second century A.D. I will outline some of these borrowings shortly.

Jainism was founded by Vardhamana Mahavira, an older contemporary of Gautama the Buddha, who lived in the sixth century B.C., when Xenophanes, Parmenides, and Zeno taught in Greece. Vardhamana acknowledged his indebtedness to previous teachers, who are known as tirthankaras, or "ford-makers," and jinas, or spiritual "victors." In fact, Jainism celebrates Vardhamana as the twenty-fourth (and last) ford-maker, the first being the legendary Rishabha.[1]

129

Another legendary ford-maker, the twenty-second in line, is Arishtanemi or Neminatha, whom Jaina tradition makes a contemporary of Krishna, the disciple of Ghora Angirasa mentioned in the Chandogya-Upanishad. While this connection may be completely spurious, it suggests that the earliest beginnings of Jainism are to be found outside the Vedic ritualism in the culture of ascetics, known as shramanas. These renouncers were in all probability closely associated with the religion of the Indus valley civilization.

More readily believable is the historicity of the twenty-third ford-maker, Parshva, though the accounts of his life, too, are largely mythological. It is probable that he belonged, like Mahavira, to a well-to-do warrior family, perhaps resident in Varanasi, the modern city of Benares. It is certain that his teaching, about which we know very little, was immensely influential in the region of Magadha (modern Bihar) and beyond.

Vardhamana grew up under the influence of Parshva's religion but he did not know the man himself, who appears to have lived in the seventh century B.C. Mahavira gave Jainism its distinct shape, reforming the tradition of Parshva. He is said to have been born into a ruling family of the Licchavi tribe, which was probably of non-Aryan origin. His birthplace was a small town near Vaishali, the modern Besarh, to the north of Patna.

Most are agreed that he left his worldly life behind at the age of thirty to pursue a course of rigorous austerities, which included prolonged waterless fasting, as it is still practiced in the Jaina community today. He joined the order of Parshva but left after a few years because he found the monastic rules too lenient. Twelve years after setting out on his spiritual journey, he attained enlightenment. At once he started to preach the truth he had discovered for himself. He was a charismatic figure whose detachment and single-minded dedication to a self-transcending life inspired and awed many people. If his exemplary life and teaching did not make more of an impact both during his lifetime and subsequently, it is because Jainism demands a rare degree of renunciation and self-control. Vardhamana Mahavira died in 527 B.C. at the age of seventy-two, leaving behind a community of monks, nuns, and lay followers, numbering about 14,000 members. Today Jainism claims a membership of just over three million adherents.

Unlike Parshva, Mahavira is remembered to have walked about naked, thus declaring his uncompromising asceticism. We have encountered this practice already in connection with the long-haired ascetics (keshin) of the Vedas, who, as the Rig-Veda (X.136) has it, were "air-clad." The issue of nudity was in fact one of the principal reasons for the split of the Jaina community into two sects, which occurred about 300 B.C. Whereas the Digambaras ("Space-clothed") announce their renunciation of everything by going about naked, the Shvetambaras ("White-clothed") have opted for a more catholic and less literalist disposition. For them, the presence or absence of garments does not make a spiritual victor. But even the Digambaras do not permit their nuns to walk about in the nude. More than that, they assert that a woman cannot attain emancipation in this lifetime but has to be reborn in a male body first. By contrast, the Shvetambaras venerate a woman ford-maker, Malli, who was nineteenth in succession. There is one early sculpture of a nude female ascetic, which is generally held to be Malli.

When Alexander the Great invaded northern India in 327–326 B.C., his chroniclers reported the existence of gymnosophists, or naked philosophers. Some 1300 years later, the Moslem hegemonists put a stop to this practice, at least for a period of time. Naked ascetics, besmeared with ashes, can still be seen in India today. But it is not this curious custom for which Jainism should be noted. The lasting contribution of this minority religion lies rather in its minute examination of what constitutes a truly moral life.

The Anuvrata movement initiated by Acarya Tulasi in Rajasthan in 1949 is a sign that Jainism is by no means stagnant but continues to be an ethical force in the world. The movement's name, meaning "Small Vow," is meant to suggest that even the minor vows of Jainism can bring about big changes. The history of Jainism thus continues to be an important lesson in the efficacy of vows in a life that revolves around spiritual rather than material values.

THE PATH OF PURIFICATION

The Elimination of Karma through Morality and Meditation

Like Buddhism and Hinduism, the Jaina religion is essentially a path to emancipation, or what is called absolute knowledge (kevala-jnana). That superlative condition is defined in terms of freedom from the impact of the law of moral causation, (karma or karman). The doctrine of karma ("action") plays a vital role in Jainism, as it does in Hinduism and Buddhism. But the Jaina scholastics have elaborated this doctrine more than any other. The underlying idea of karma is that the law of cause and effect applies also to the psychic or moral realm, so that a person's actions or even violations determine his or her destiny, both in the present lifetime and future lifetimes.

Throughout the existence of a particular animate being (jiva), karma is produced and experienced through the application of the will, or intention. The Jainas conceive of karma as a kind of substance that can be generated, stored, and annihilated. The cycle of karma production and experience is regarded as an influx of karma into the body-mind, which needs to be stopped. As long as the inflow of karma continues, the being is bound to lifeless matter (ajiva-pudgala) and revolves continually in the wheel of repeated births and deaths.

In the enlightened condition, the human personality is utterly surpassed, and hence the law of moral causation is likewise transcended. The essence of the human individual is the Self (atman). The Jainas use the terms *atman* and *jiva* interchangeably, but whereas the former refers to the transcendental nature, the latter is the Self held in captivity by its own karmic actions.

As in the Samkhya school of thought, the Jainas believe in a plurality of ultimate or spiritual entities, the atmans. Like the Samkhya purushas or Self-monads, these are essentially infinite and pure Consciousness. But they become apparently confined to a certain form or body. Their self-limitation, which is regarded as a form of contraction of consciousness, results from the impact of karma. Only through the reduction of karmic influences, and ultimately the total obliteration of karma, can the jiva's consciousness be purified and transformed into the limitless transcendental Consciousness.

The spiritual process consists, first of all, in the warding off (samvara) of new karma. This is accomplished through proper moral conduct. The central virtue of the Jaina code of morals is ahimsa, nonharming. This entails the prohibition of killing animate beings for any purpose, be it for food or sacrifice, and even the mere intention of hurting another being. Jainism originally recruited its members primarily from the aristocratic families and warrior (kshatriya) estate. However, the strict regulations about nonharming have forced the Jaina laity into merchant careers. Ethics forms the foundation of Jaina Yoga, and it is stated that no amount of austerity or meditative practice can lead to emancipation unless they are accompanied by the careful observance of the moral rules.

Once the practitioner is grounded in a morally sound way of life, he or she seeks to exhaust the existing stock of karma through immersion into the highest form of ecstasy (samadhi), brought about by extreme penance. Such penance, especially the uncompromising practice of nonharming, not only stops the influx of karma into the body-mind but reverses all karmic effects. From this results, ultimately, the transcendental state of emancipation (moksha), or absolute knowledge.

In the ancient Acara-Anga-Sutra, Mahavira declares about this state of perfect freedom:

> All sounds recoil, where reason has no room, nor does the mind penetrate there. The liberated is not long or small, round or triangular; he is neither black nor white; he is disembodied, without contact [with matter] . . . not female, male, or neuter. Though he perceives and knows, there is no [fitting] analogy [to describe his perception or knowledge]. His being is formless. There is no condition of the Unconditioned. (330–332)

This doctrine is elaborated in the extensive exegetical literature of Jainism. For instance, in Kunda-Kunda's Niyama-Sara, a work of the fourth century A.D., we find the following reiteratively descriptive stanzas:

> The Self (atman) is free from punishment, without opposites, without me-sense (nirmama), impartite, without [objective] support, devoid of attachment, free from defects, free from delusion, and fearless. (43)

> The Self is free from contraction (nirgrantha), devoid of attachment, without

blemish, free from all defects, without desire, free from anger, free from pride, and without lust. (44)

Color, taste, smell, touch, male, female, male [or female] inclinations, etc., the [various kinds] of positions, and the [various types of] bodies—all these do not exist in the [transcendental] individual (jiva). (45)

Know the [transcendental] individual to be tasteless, formless, without scent, unmanifest [but] conscious, unqualified, soundless, not recognizable by [any external] sign, and without describable location. (46)

The Jaina Ladder to Liberation

At the heart of Jainism lies a carefully worked-out path that leads the faithful from the fetters of conditioned existence and suffering to absolute freedom, unexcellable joy, and incomparable energy. Although the recommended procedure for a prosperous spiritual life is to abandon everything and to dedicate oneself completely to a life of renunciation and penance, the Jaina authorities nevertheless think it possible in principle even for a householder to become emancipated. Indeed, it is thought that the reason for the persistence of Jainism in India is the high esteem in which it has held the laity since the earliest days. The displacement of Buddhism from Indian soil, on the other hand, is sometimes connected with the neglect of the laity by the monastic community.

According to a widely accepted model, the Jaina ladder to emancipation comprises fourteen stages, known as the levels of virtue (guna-sthana). This framework describes the course of a person's maturation from ordinary worldly life to spiritual liberation. It begins with the conventional state of unenlightenment, which is governed by false vision (mithya-drishti) involving the mistaken idea that one is identical with the finite body-mind. Gradually, a "taste" for right vision (samyag-drishti) appears. Now the practitioner understands that he or she transcends the skin-bound mortal frame. For a period thereafter, the person oscillates between truth and doubt, right vision and lack of self-discipline. Spiritual life proper can begin when self-control (virati) is cultivated. The importance of sound moral conduct is realized and the desire arises to renounce the world and become an ascetic. With this impulse ends the career of the householder.

From then on, the individual makes every effort to gain control over the mechanism of attention. Inattention is seen as a spiritual failure leading to such undesirable emotions as anger, pride, delusion, and greed. Through the disciplining of attention, the mind becomes purified and, as a side effect, sleep is overcome. Now the ascetic acquires the energy for intense concentration and meditative absorption. He or she discovers a joy far greater than any temporary pleasure, and step by step the sexual impulse is mastered. Finally, even the last trace of worldly interest is eradicated. This leads to the complete removal of the common delusion of being a separate physical entity, thus making room for the intuition of the universal Consciousness.

By dispelling the I-consciousness, all karmic hindrances are removed and absolute knowledge (kevala-jnana), or liberation, is attained. The "omniscient" ascetic can now resolve to propound his newly found wisdom to others, whereupon he becomes a ford-maker (tirthankara). This condition is known as active transcendence (sayogi-kevali). The ascetic who has won through to this sublime condition is known as a transcender (kevalin), a victor (jina), or a worthy one (arhat or arhant). The highest state, however, is inactive transcendence (ayogi-kevali). It is attained by a jina or arhat just prior to the death of the physical body. This stage corresponds to the "cloud of dharma ecstasy" (dharma-megha-samadhi) in Patanjali's Yoga. Beyond the fourteen stages of virtue lies liberation, the luminous condition of the perfected being (siddha), free from bodily existence and karma.

The main instruments governing the progression through these stages of spiritual attainment are the intricate ethical rules laid down in the Jaina canonical literature. As the following list of virtues will bear out, there is a great similarity between Jaina, Buddhist, and Hindu ethics. In Umasvati's famous Tattva-Artha-Sutra (IX.7), composed in the fifth century A.D., we find these qualifications of an ascetic, which are all considered forms of nonharming or ahimsa: forbearance (kshama), humility (mardava), uprightness (arjava), purity (shauca), truthfulness (satya), self-discipline (samyama), austerity (tapas), renunciation (tyaga), poverty (akinyana; lit., "having nothing"), and chastity (brahmacarya). For the layperson the following rules are binding: almsgiving (dana), virtuous conduct (shila), austerity (tapas), and spiritual disposition (bhava).

Jaina Yoga

In its higher aspects Jaina Yoga resembles its Hindu counterpart, and in fact the later Jaina writers, like Haribhadra (c. A.D. 750), made use of some of the codifications of Patanjali. Haribhadra was a philosopher, logician, and artist. He is reputed to have written no fewer than 1440 works, including several texts on Yoga, notably the Yoga-Bindu and the Yoga-Drishti-Samuccaya. In his Yoga-Bindu, Haribhadra praises Yoga as follows:

Yoga is the best wish-fulfilling tree (kalpa-taru). Yoga is the supreme wish-granting jewel (cinta-mani). Yoga is the foremost of virtues. Yoga is the very embodiment of perfection (siddhi). (37)

Thus, it is declared to be [like] the fire [that consumes the karmic] seed of incarnation, like extreme old age in regard to aging, or fatal consumption in regard to suffering, or death in regard to death itself. (38)

The great souls (maha-atman) accomplished in Yoga declare that even a mere hearing of the two syllables [of the word *yoga*], according to the rules, is sufficient for the removal of sins. (40)

Just as impure gold is inevitably purified by fire, so also the mind afflicted with the taint of [spiritual] ignorance is [purified] by the fire of Yoga. (41)

Thus, verily, Yoga is the foundation for realizing Reality (tattva), for this is ascertained through nothing else. There is nothing comparable [to Yoga]. (64)

Hence in order to realize that very Reality, the thoughtful person should always make a mighty effort. Argumentative books are of no avail. (65)

Haribhadra distinguishes between Yoga proper and what he calls preparatory service (purva-seva). The latter consists in the following practices:

1. Veneration (pujana) of the teacher, the deities, and other beings of authority, such as one's parents and elders. In the case of the deities, this involves ritual worship with flowers and other offerings. In the case of one's elders, veneration is shown by respectful bowing and general obedience to them.
2. Proper conduct (sad-acara) involves charity (dana), conformity to social mores, abstention from blaming others, the practice of praise and cheerfulness in adversity, humility, considered speech, integrity, observance of one's vows, the abandonment of lethargy, and refraining from reprehensible behavior even in the face of death.
3. Asceticism (tapas) is thought to remove one's sins and should be practiced to the utmost of one's abilities. It involves different forms of fasting, including prolonged, monthlong fasts, combined with the chanting of mantras.
4. Nonaversion toward liberation (mukty-advesha), or what in the Hindu school of Vedanta is known as the desire for liberation. This disposition is essential to success in spiritual life. The desire to transcend the ego-limitation must overwhelm all other desires and impulses. Haribhadra makes the point that ordinary people, under the spell of hedonism, find the ideal of liberation unattractive because it does not promise the usual enjoyment. In fact, they feel threatened by the prospect of a bliss that eclipses the ego. Hence it is important to cultivate right understanding.

This preparatory practice may be taken up by what the Jaina tradition calls the apunar-bandhaka, the person who has grown weary of the worldly game after numerous lifetimes and is embarking on his or her final embodiment. For Haribhadra, however, genuine Yoga practice is possible only for a spiritually more mature individual. He speaks of the samyag-drishti, the person who has correct vision or understanding, and the caritrin, who is firmly on the spiritual path.

The apunar-bandhaka is on the first of the fourteen levels of virtues, where the ego-illusion predominates. The samyag-drishti, whom Haribhadra compares to the Buddhist bodhisattva, has attained the fourth level, where fundamental spiritual insight exists but discipline is still a problem. The caritrin occupies the fifth level, which is marked by the desire to renounce the world and adopt the ascetic lifestyle.

Haribhadra speaks of five degrees of genuine Yoga, for which the caritrin alone is equipped:

1. Adhyatman, or adhyatma-yoga, is the constant remembering or pondering upon one's essential nature.
2. Bhavana, or contemplation, is the daily concentrated observance of the essential nature (adhyatman) itself, which increases the quality and time of one's dwelling in spiritually positive mental states.
3. Dhyana, or meditation, is the mind's fixation upon auspicious objects, which is accompanied by subtle enjoyment. Such meditation leads to great mental stability and the ability to control others.
4. Samata, or "sameness," is the mood of indifference toward things that one tends to feel attracted to or repelled by. Cultivation of this attitude also includes abstention from the use of psychic powers (riddhi or siddhi) and attenuates the subtle karmic forces that bind a person to worldly existence.
5. Vritti-samkshaya, or the full removal of the movements of consciousness, means the complete transcendence of karma-produced psychomental states. This leads to emancipation (moksha), which "is unobstructed and the seat of eternal bliss" (Yoga-Bindu 367).

At the core of the advanced Yoga practice is meditative absorption, which every follower of Jainism is asked to practice at least once a day for one muhurta (forty-eight minutes) in the morning. The ascetic is naturally required to dedicate most of his time to this exercise. But lay folk can take additional vows, obliging them to, say, meditate three times a day for longer periods.

There are no strict regulations about how this meditation ought to be performed; there is a choice between a variety of techniques, some of which are strongly reminiscent of Tantric exercises. In Umasvati's Tattva-Artha-Adhigama-Sutra (IX.27ff.), meditation is explained as follows:

Meditation (dhyana) is the restraint (nirodha) of the single-pointed mind (cinta) in [the case of one who possesses] the highest steadfastness . . . (27)

. . . up to one muhurta [forty-eight minutes]. (28)

[Meditation can be of four types:] disagreeable (arta), savage (raudra), virtuous (dharma), or pure (shukla). (29)

[Only] the last two [types] are the cause of liberation. (30)

The disagreeable [meditation] is when upon contacting an unpleasant experience (amano-jnana), [the practitioner] dwells on the memory [of that experience] in order to dissociate from it (31)

and [unpleasant] sensations, (32)

the reverse of pleasant experience, (33)

and the "link" (nidana) [which is the desire to fulfill a certain intention in a future life]. (34)

This [disagreeable meditation occurs] in the case of the undisciplined, partly disciplined, and the lax in restraint. (35)

The savage [meditation], [which occurs] in the case of the undisciplined or partly disciplined, is for harming, lying, theft, or the preservation of possessions. (36)

The virtuous [meditation], [which occurs] in the case of the [ascetic who is] disciplined in attentiveness, is for ascertaining the revealed order (ajna) [i.e., the sacred tradition], the diminution (apaya) [of the Self through karma], the fruition (vipaka) [of karmas], and the construction (samsthana) [of the universe]. (37)

[This meditation occurs] also in the case of those whose passions have either been pacified or vanished. (38)

[In the case of those whose passions (kashaya) have altogether vanished, there occur] also the [first] two pure [meditations]. (39)

The latter [two pure meditations occur] in the case of the transcender (kevalin). (40)

[The four forms or stages of the pure meditation are:] the consideration (vitarka) of separateness and of singleness; absorption (pratipati) in subtle activity; and the cessation of quiesced activity. (41)

This [fourfold pure meditation occurs in the case of those who respectively experience] the triple, the single, or the [purely] bodily action (yoga) [as well as those who are completely] inactive.[2] (42)

In regard to the former [two forms, which are accompanied by] consideration, [there is] a single prop [or object of meditation]. (43)

The second [of these forms accompanied by consideration, or vitarka] is beyond reflection (avicara). (44)

Consideration is [knowledge of what has been] revealed (shruta). (45)

Reflection (vicara) is the [mind's] revolving around meaning (artha), symbol (vyanjana), and activity (yoga). (46)

Meditative absorption can be practiced either sitting or standing. The Jaina scriptures mention such postures as the "bedstead" (paryanka), "half-bedstead" (ardha-paryanka), "thunderbolt posture" (vajra-asana), "lotus posture" (kamala-asana), and the tailor seat or "easy posture" (sukha-asana), which should be practiced at a suitable location. It is occasionally recommended that the place should be more disagreeable than comfortable, which reminds one of the Tantric custom of meditating on the cremation ground amidst decaying corpses—a vivid reminder of the impermanence of everything.

Some texts, like the eleventh-century Yoga-Shastra of Hemacandra, mention other postures identical to those known in Hindu Yoga, such as the "hero posture" (vira-asana), the "auspicious posture" (bhadra-asana), and the "staff posture" (danda-asana). The generic technical term for these meditative postures is *kaya-utsarga*, "casting off of the body." This is meant to suggest that the purpose of such yogic postures is not so much to cultivate the body as to transcend it.

Hemacandra recommends breath control (pranayama) as an aid to meditation, following largely the lines of Patanjali's Yoga-Sutra. However, at least one Jaina authority on Yoga, Shubhacandra, takes a different point of view. In his Jnana-Arnava he states that breath control is helpful in checking physical activity but interferes with concentration and is likely to produce disagreeable (arta) meditation experiences. Rather, the practitioner is advised to aspire to "superlative concentration" (parama-samadhi). As Kunda-Kunda puts it in his Niyama-Sara:

> What is the point of dwelling in the forest, chastising the body, observing various fasts, studying, and maintaining silence (mauna) for the renunciate (shramana) who lacks collectedness (samata)? (124)

In the same work, we find this stanza:

> If you desire independence (avashyaka), fix your steady thoughts upon the true nature of the Self. In this way, the quality of equanimity (samayika) is fully cultivated in the individual. (147)

There is a certain extremism in some of the ascetic practices recommended in Jainism, like self-starvation, which do not seem to be in keeping with the ethical code of nonharming and which have therefore invited criticism from many quarters. These excesses derive from the Jainas' attitude toward physical existence, which is experienced as a source of suffering and painful limitation. Therefore the human body-mind is constantly to be chastised through fasting and other forms of penance until the human spirit is freed from all physical bonds. Jainism, more than any other tradition, exemplifies the spirit of tapas, spoken of in Chapter 3.

Notwithstanding this justifiable criticism, Jainism can look back on a long line of noble teachers and valiant aspirants who have demonstrated the supreme value of the yogic art of taking and keeping sacred vows. Both their spiritual resoluteness and their gentleness are an inspiration particularly to modern seekers, who do not always appreciate that spiritual life is an all-demanding transformative ordeal.

योग आनन्दकल्पनः

chapter 7

Yoga in Buddhism

FROM ASCETICISM TO SPONTANEOUS
ENLIGHTENMENT: THE BUDDHA
AND HIS TEACHING

His compassion was absolute. . . . His dignity was unshakeable, his humour invariable. He was infinitely patient as one who knows the illusion of time.[1]

This is how Christmas Humphreys, the English Buddhist and popularizer of Buddhism, characterized Gautama the Buddha ("Awakened One"). The Buddha, a younger contemporary of Mahavira, was one of the great spiritual luminaries of the sixth century B.C., whose charismatic and benevolent personality speaks to us across the millennia. Like Mahavira, the founder of Jainism, Gautama rejected the Vedic revelation with its many deities and sacrificial rites. Like the Upanishadic sages, he thirsted for knowledge that would forever satisfy his heart. His teaching can be described as a pragmatic form of Yoga. The contemporary German scholar Hermann Beckh observed:

It has been pointed out that the Buddha was far removed from the behavior of the ordinary Indian yogins who only aspired after their own spiritual development and with a certain egotism shut themselves off from the world. By contrast, his concern was animated by a genuine love. . . . However, insofar as we understand Yoga to be a practical method, as opposed to mere speculative philosophy, of concentration and meditation directed toward suprasensuous goals, we can rightly regard the spiritual orientation to which the Buddha adhered as being a part of Yoga.[2]

Beckh further noted that especially in the later Sanskrit works of the Buddhist tradition, the Buddha is frequently styled a "yogin." Moreover, the sacred literature often refers to the Buddha's penchant for meditation (dhyana), which is at the heart of most schools of Yoga.

139

Buddhism is the name given to the complex religious and philosophical movement that grew around the original teaching of Gautama the Buddha, who was probably born in 563 B.C. and died at the age of eighty. Siddhartha Gautama's life is only a little better known than that of Vardhamana Mahavira, the founder of Jainism. He was of aristocratic birth, born into the Shakya clan of Koshala, a country situated at the southern border of Nepal. He grew up in the comparative luxury and security of the ruling class. Weary of his comfortable existence, he renounced the world at the age of twenty-nine and went in search of wisdom.

His quest brought him to two noted teachers who are known to us by name—Arada (or Alara) Kalama and Udraka Ramaputra. The former appears to have taught a type of early Upanishadic Yoga, culminating in the experience of the "sphere of no-thing-ness" (akimcanya-ayatana). This experience probably corresponds to the formless ecstasy (nirvikalpa-samadhi) spoken of in the Upanishads. Apparently, Gautama had no difficulty entering that state, and Arada Kalama generously offered to share with Gautama the leadership of his order of ascetics.

Feeling that he had not yet attained the highest possible realization, Gautama declined. Instead he became a disciple of Udraka Ramaputra. This sage declared the ultimate realization to be the experience of the "sphere of neither consciousness nor unconsciousness" (naiva-samjnana-asamjna-ayatana). Again, it did not take Gautama long to enter this exalted state, but once more the experience left him unsatisfied, and he intuited that it fell short of true enlightenment.

For six years he practiced the fiercest kind of self-mortification, which made his limbs look like the "joints of withered creepers." The traditional legends recount that he even rebuffed the gods when they sought to feed his emaciated body. In the end Gautama had to admit to himself that this was not the way to emancipation. He felt there must exist a middle way between ascetic self-torture and the self-indulgent life of a worldling. He resumed begging for food, as was the custom, and soon his body filled out and regained its healthy glow.

Gautama remembered a spontaneous ecstatic experience that had suddenly overwhelmed him in his youth: As he sat under a rose apple tree, his awareness had been drawn inward effortlessly, until all egoic consciousness was transcended. Inspired by the ease of that experience, Gautama now began simply to sit in meditation, resolved not to stir until he had broken through to the Unconditional beyond the ego-personality, beyond all experience. Finally his resolution bore fruit: He became an "awakened one" (buddha). He had reached "extinction" (nirvana), the cessation of all desire, signaling the transcendence of the illusion of individuation.

For seven days Gautama the Buddha sat beneath the fig tree under whose shady canopy he had won nirvana. He applied his superb intelligence, now freed from egoic desires and misconceptions, to understanding the mechanism of spiritual ignorance and bondage and the path to liberation. These deliberations were the foundation of his later teaching (dharma). After another seven days of silent contemplation and a short inner struggle, the Buddha decided to impart the newly acquired wisdom to others, to "beat the drum of the Immortal in the darkness of the world" and communicate the spiritual way.

His two teachers had recently died, and so he could not share with them his discovery. He sought out the five ascetics who had long been his traveling companions but who had left him when he abandoned his severe asceticism in favor of a meditation practice of his own design. He addressed his first sermon to them. He spoke of the "four noble truths": the prevalence of suffering; desire as the cause of that suffering; the removal of that cause through the cultivation of nonattachment; and the "noble eightfold path" as the means to enlightenment.

The Buddha's missionary activity met with such rapid success that some people thought he was using magic. For forty-five years he wandered throughout northern India, teaching to anyone who came to listen. After his death, both the monastic order and the Buddhist lay community continued to prosper. In the third century B.C. during the reign of the famous emperor Ashoka, who had converted to the Buddha's teaching, Buddhism was transformed from a local movement into a state religion.

THE PRECIOUS TEACHING OF THE MIDDLE WAY

The earliest record of the Buddha's teaching is the Pali canon, consisting mostly of his sermons and monastic rules, as compiled and edited by three successive councils of the Buddhist order.[3] The first council was convened immediately after the Buddha's death, the second about 100 years later, and the third (and most important) during Ashoka's reign. Soon afterward, Buddhism split into the two well-known traditions of Hinayana ("Small Vehicle") and Mahayana ("Large Vehicle"), both claiming to possess the true original meaning of the Buddha's gospel. The differences between them increased as both schools evolved.

The Hinayana tradition was oriented toward the individual monk or nun. It placed the personal achievement of the cessation of desire above everything else. The Mahayana adherents regarded this approach as selfish and barren. They emphasized the positive value of the emotional and social aspects of human life. In this spirit, the Mahayana teachers promoted the new ideal of the bodhisattva, the being dedicated to the enlightenment of all, who deferred his or her own ultimate liberation until all other beings had become free. Most significantly, they re-visioned the nature of the Buddhist goal itself. They no longer conceived of nirvana as an attainable goal "out there," but saw it as the ever-present substratum underlying phenomenal existence. This is epitomized in the famous Mahayana formula "nirvana equals samsara," meaning that the immutable transcendental dimension is coessential with the world of impermanence.

The nondualist teachings of the Mahayana schools offered a strong point of contact with the predominant culture of Hinduism. In fact, this growing similarity between Mahayana Buddhism and the idealistic schools of Hinduism was partly responsible for the fact that Buddhism eventually lost most of its force in India. However, the Buddha's teaching fared better abroad—in Ceylon, Indonesia, China, Japan, and Tibet—though not without being further modified.

The original teaching of the Buddha can no longer be identified with any certainty. However, considering the strong mnemonic tradition of India, there is good reason to believe that much of what has been handed down—first orally and then in written form—as the Buddha's sermons are in fact the words of that remarkable teacher.

The Four Noble Truths

The Buddha's teaching (dharma) proceeds from the statement that life is sorrowful or painful (duhkha). This is the first of his "four noble truths." The idea behind this insight, which the Buddhists share with the Hindus and Jainas, is this: Because everything is impermanent and does not afford us lasting happiness, our life is in the last analysis shot through with sorrow and pain. We compete with others and even with ourselves, always in search of greater happiness, comfort, fulfillment, or security. We feel dissatisfied even in our attainments, since there is always more to which we can aspire in the hope of being fulfilled by it. In the final analysis, suffering is the tension that is intrinsic to our effort to survive as separate, egoic personalities. But that individuality is merely a carefully maintained illusion, a convenient psychosocial convention.

In truth, declares the Buddha, there is no inner self. There are only so many factors that together constitute the human personality, giving rise to the illusion of there being a stable identity.

The doctrine of no-self (anatman) is fundamental to his teaching. No doubt the Buddha emphasized the inessential nature of the human personality and of existence in general in order to counter the idealism to which the Upanishadic teachings had given rise. By insisting that the ultimate Reality was identical with the innermost core of the human being—the Self, or atman—the Upanishadic sages indirectly encouraged the delusion of unenlightened beings that there is, after all, an immortal ego within the human personality.

The Buddha rejected all conjectures about an immutable self-essence and metaphysical speculations in general, although it is evident from his recorded sayings that he occasionally availed himself of a language reminiscent of his early Vedic background. The Buddha insisted that the truth about suffering must be deeply felt, not merely thought about abstractly. His pragmatic approach exemplifies what is best in the tradition of yogic experimentalism.

The second noble truth is that desire, or the thirst (trishna) for life, is the cause of this suffering experienced universally by human beings. To paraphrase the Buddha: Our very cells are genetically programmed to perpetuate the biological conglomerate that we call "our" body-mind. We desire to survive as individuals, and yet our very sense of individuality is the factor that complicates our existence, because we separate ourselves from everything else and then look for ways to reduce or overcome the resulting sense of isolation and fear. But we approach the matter from the wrong end. We tinker with our experiences rather than allow our understanding to penetrate to the root of our separative disposition and its accompanying survival motive.

The third noble truth affirms that it is through the elimination of that innate craving, or thirst, that we can remove all experience of suffering and penetrate to what is real and true, namely the state in which there is no ego-identity.

The fourth noble truth states that the means of eradicating our craving is the eightfold path first announced by the Buddha. That path, which will be introduced in the next section, consists in the gradual "dis-illusionment" of our egoic personality, or the step-by-step undermining of what we presume ourselves and the world to be, until the truth shines forth. Upon attaining the supreme condition of nirvana, all suffering is transcended because the illusory entity that is the source of suffering is fully abrogated. The enlightened being is no longer an individuated person, even though the personality continues to manifest its typical character.

Closely connected with the doctrine of the universality of suffering is the doctrine of moral causation (karman) and the correlated teaching of rebirth. Both hold a central position in Buddhist thought and ethics. As in Jainism, there is no God who could interfere in the nexus of birth and death or to whom beings are ultimately responsible. Instead, it is the mental activity of each individual, whether expressed in action or not, that alone determines his or her future through the moral law of causation inherent in the universe.[4]

The Buddha's denial of a transmigrating soul, or essential self, has led many students of Buddhism to the assumption that he rejected all transcendentalism outright. This is not the case. Many passages in the Pali canon describe the ultimate condition of nirvana in positive metaphysical terms. It is equated with permanence, stability, unconditionality, and immortality. It is also called "shelter," "refuge," and "security." But, more typically, the ultimate Reality, and thus also the enlightened being, is described negatively. In the words of the Buddha, recorded in the Sutta-Nipata:

> As a flame blown out by the wind goes to rest, and is lost to cognition, just so the sage (muni) who is released from "name" (nama) [or mind] and body (kaya), goes to rest and is lost to cognition. (1074)

And:

> There is no measure for him who has gone to rest, and he has nothing that could be named. When all things are abandoned, all paths of language are likewise abandoned. (1076)

Thus, the rational teaching of the Buddha terminates in the ineffable condition of nirvana. Concepts and words can be helpful to spiritual seekers until they have discovered what is Real for themselves. But language can also be a hindrance, because it entices us to "thingify" concepts, to treat words as if they were objective things. After enlightenment, however, language loses its fascination and is never again confused with reality.

THE YOGIC PATH OF THE BUDDHA

The preceding description of the theoretical foundations of Buddhism may have given the impression that the teaching of the Buddha is schematic and philosophical rather than practical; nothing could be further from the truth. The Buddha was a dedicated yogin with a passion for meditative absorption, and his doctrine was primarily designed to show a concrete way out of the maze of spiritually ignorant, and hence sorrowful, existence.

Like Patanjali's Yoga, the Yoga of the Buddha comprises eight distinct members. Hence it is known as the noble eightfold path. The Buddha referred to it as the "supramundane path" (loka-uttara-magga), because it is meant for those who are seriously committed to self-transcending practice—that is, for monks and nuns. The Buddha was convinced that a person could attain enlightenment within seven days of "setting forth"—that is, of taking up the life of a mendicant monk or nun. The eight members of the path should be cultivated simultaneously, and therefore they should not be viewed as stages or rungs of a ladder, as is often proposed. These eight constituent practices are:

1. Right vision (samyag-drishti), the realization of the transiency of conditioned existence and the understanding that there is indeed no continuous ego or self.
2. Right resolve (samyak-samkalpa), the threefold resolution to renounce what is ephemeral, to practice benevolence, and to not hurt any being.
3. Right speech (samyag-vaca), the abstention from idle and false talk.
4. Right conduct (samyak-karmanta), consisting mainly in abstention from killing, stealing, and illicit sexual intercourse.
5. Right livelihood (samyag-ajiva), the abstention from deceit, usury, treachery, and soothsaying in procuring one's sustenance.
6. Right exertion (samyag-vyayama), the prevention of future negative mental activity, the overcoming of present unwholesome feelings or thoughts, the cultivation of future wholesome states of mind, and the maintenance of present positive psychomental activity.
7. Right mindfulness (samyak-smriti), the cultivation of awareness of psychosomatic processes by means of such practices as the favorite

Theravada (Hinayana) technique of sati-patthana, consisting in the mindful observation of otherwise unconscious activities like breathing or body movement.

8. Right concentration (samyak-samadhi), the practice of certain techniques for the internalization and transcendence of the individuated consciousness.

The first two members of the noble eightfold path are said to deal with understanding (prajna); the next three with behavior (shila); and the last three with concentration (samadhi). The first five can also be grouped under the heading of socioethical regulations, while the remaining three members are specifically yogic. Exertion and mindfulness can and should be practiced throughout the entire day, but concentration (samadhi) represents a special discipline for which undisturbed quiet is essential.

Samadhi, in the Buddhist sense of intense mental collectedness, comprises the meditative phases from sense-withdrawal up to ecstatic transcendence. There are eight such stages, which are known as *jhana* in the Pali language, corresponding to the Sanskrit word *dhyana*.

1. Jhana accompanied by thoughts and the feeling of rapturous joy (priti-sukha).
2. Jhana unaccompanied by thoughts but still suffused with the feeling of joy.
3. Jhana in which the experience of joy has yielded to the subtle joy of tranquil mindfulness.
4. Jhana in which any kind of emotion is stopped and all that remains is utter mindfulness.
5. The realization of the "sphere of space-infinity," the ecstatic experience of infinitely expanded space.
6. The realization of the "sphere of consciousness-infinity," consisting in the ecstatic experience of infinitely expanded consciousness.
7. The realization of the "sphere of no-thing-ness," an elusive ecstatic experience of the absence of all forms.
8. The realization of the "sphere of neither cognition nor noncognition," a transcendental experience marked by the absence of all consciousness, yet still not identical with the ultimate condition of nirvana.

These higher yogic states are difficult to imagine, and the only key to them is direct experience. Beyond these eight levels of accomplishment lies enlightenment, or nirvana. As the Buddha has delineated it in the Udana:

[The nirvana is] a realm where there is neither the earth nor water, neither fire nor air, neither ether nor consciousness . . . neither this world nor any other world, neither sun nor moon. (80)

Nirvana is other than whatever we can affirm or deny about it. It is precisely extinction—the transcendence of thought and language, of feeling and imagination, and of the ego-personality as a whole. Because the Buddha denied the notion of a continuous entity abiding within the flux of phenomenal existence, he has been accused of nihilism, a charge against which he defended himself on several occasions.

The yogic nature of the Buddha's path is further demonstrated by the use of such techniques as posture (asana) and control of the life-force (pranayama). As opposed to some Hindu schools of Hatha-Yoga, Buddhism does not advocate the stoppage of the vital-force. The Buddhist authorities argue that forced retention of the breath does violence to the natural body. Instead they advise the practitioner to simply follow the movement of the breath with the mind. This is a particular application of the technique of mindfulness (smriti). It is known in Pali as *sati-patthana* and in Sanskrit as *smriti-pashyana*. This method is widely employed in modern Theravada Buddhism, the oldest surviving school of the Hinayana tradition.

The most commonly adopted meditative posture is the pallanka-seat (Sanskrit: paryanka), as captured in innumerable seated Buddha statues. The texts emphasize erect bodily posture (uju-kaya), undoubtedly because experience shows that in this way both breathing and mental concentration can be considerably improved.

The yogin who has penetrated all delusive phenomena by virtue of his single-mindedness in the highest stage of jhana enters nirvana. When emancipation is attained, it is no longer possible to say anything meaningful about the nature of the liberated or enlightened being—whether he exists or does not exist. Freedom is a paradox or mystery. It is to be discovered rather than talked about.

This fact did not scare the Buddha's followers into silence. Over the centuries Buddhist monks and nuns, as well as educated lay followers, have interpreted and reinterpreted the Buddha's legacy, trying to make it accessible for their own era. This effort has led to a vast literature in Pali, Sanskrit, and other languages. Not only did the Buddhist community spawn hosts of scholars, it birthed many great yogins and enlightened adepts, who periodically regenerated the spiritual basis of Buddhism. Their revitalization of the Buddha's dharma has often had effects far beyond the sphere of Buddhism. Thus, the Buddhist teachings have exerted a significant influence on many schools of Hinduism, including the tradition of Yoga.

If the Buddha was indebted to adepts who taught an early form of Yoga, Patanjali (who gave Yoga its classical philosophical shape) in turn owed an intellectual debt to Mahayana Buddhism. The long historical interplay between Buddhism and Hinduism reached its peak in the sweeping cultural movement of Tantrism, starting in the middle of the first post-Christian millennium. It gave rise to schools that are not easily identified as either Buddhist or Hindu. What they all have in common, however, is a passion for personal realization, for yogic experimentation with the hidden potential of the human body-mind.

योग आनन्दकल्पनः

chapter 8

The Flowering of Yoga

OUTLINE

The two preceding chapters have covered some of the outstanding yogic features of Jainism and Buddhism. Now we return to the rich tapestry of Hinduism. The period between the ritualistic mysticism of the earliest Upanishads, dating from the eighth century B.C., and the systematized Yoga of Patanjali of the second century A.D. was one of abundant teaching activity.

A fair number of scriptures relevant to the evolution of Yoga have survived from that early period. First is the Ramayana of Valmiki, one of India's two national epics. In its earliest form it likely antedates the Buddha. Next are such Upanishads (c. 500–300 B.C.) as the Katha, the Shvetashvatara, the Isha, and the Mundaka. At about the same time, the oldest portions of the Mahabharata epic and in particular the Bhagavad-Gita were composed. Then, in the period between 200 and 100 B.C., follow Upanishads such as the Maitrayaniya, the Prashna, and the Mandukya. Their esoteric teachings go beyond the ideology of the orthodox ritualism of the brahmins. The Upanishadic sages rejected the idea that the brahmanical rituals had the potency to save souls, though they generally conceded that external rituals had their proper function in the social order. Their main interest was in communicating the transformative vision of the transcendental Self, and to this end they put forward more or less elaborate liberation teachings.

The most important document of Yoga for that interval is undoubtedly the Bhagavad-Gita, the Song of the Lord, which, according to its colophon, is claimed to be an Upanishad. But before we examine the remarkably integral teaching of this Hindu classic, we must turn our attention to the Ramayana and the Mahabharata, India's two great national epics.

HEROISM, PURITY, AND TAPAS: THE RAMAYANA OF VALMIKI

No single literary creation has been more influential in the lives of millions of people in India and Southeast Asia than the ancient poem Ramayana ("Life of Rama"). For countless generations, this tragic love story has served as a repository of folk wisdom. Many popular sayings derive from it, and to this day it is recited and retold.

In its present form the Ramayana epic consists of around 24,000 verses distributed over seven chapters, of which the seventh is a later addition. As a whole, the Ramayana antedates the Mahabharata epic. Although the Ramayana is unquestionably the work of many authors, tradition acknowledges Valmiki as its sole composer. His name means "ant" and is connected with a colorful story. According to legend, Valmiki was born a brahmin but lived as a robber for many years. Through the intervention of some well-meaning sages, he came to recognize the wrongness of his lifestyle. He repented for his transgressions by meditating, transfixed to a single spot for thousands of years, during which time ants built a hill over his body.

The drama recorded in the Ramayana unfolds in the country of Koshala. The story begins with the aged king Dasharatha stating his intention to make his son Rama successor to the throne. One of Dasharatha's three wives, whom he owed two boons, asked for her own son, Bharata, to be appointed and for Rama to be banished for fourteen years. The king had no choice; much against his will, he exiled his son. Rama received the news with stoic equanimity and promptly repaired to the forest with his wife Sita. Upon the death of his father, Bharata refused the throne and went in search of his exiled brother. Rama, however, was intent on honoring his banishment. Instead of returning to the kingdom, he went into battle against the demons that disturbed and terrified the renouncers and sages of the forest.

Rama killed thousands of demons. The chief demon, Ravana, revenged their death by abducting beautiful Sita. With the help of the monkey king Hanumat, and after many adventures, Rama managed to slay Ravana and to free his wife, who was held captive on the island of Lanka (modern Ceylon). However, thinking that Sita had been defiled by Ravana, Rama refused to take her back. Sita swore to her innocence, and in the end insisted that Rama let the Divine decide her fate. She entered the blazing fire of a pyre that had been lit to test her. To everyone's amazement, the flames did not singe a single hair on Sita's body. Rama repented and was glad to be reunited with his brave and faithful wife. By then his exile had come to an end, and they all returned to the capital, where Rama was jubilantly welcomed. Together with his brother Bharata, he ushered in a golden age for his subjects. Rama is the ideal of the righteous hero, and Sita of the faithful and chaste wife.

But Rama is more than a hero. He is also a symbol of renunciation, equanimity, and self-discipline. The archaic spirituality of the Ramayana reflects the orientation of ancient asceticism (tapas) more than that of Yoga. The distinction between these two approaches has been made clear in Chapter 3 ("Yoga and Other Hindu Traditions"). Rama is portrayed as wandering through enchanted forests that are inhabited by sages in possession of magical powers and weapons, which they put at his disposal. With these unexpected aids, Rama fights a host of demons and monsters.

The Ramayana introduces Rama as an incarnation of God Vishnu. At the time of the composition of the Rig-Veda, Vishnu was still a minor deity, but he later served as the focal point for the religious imagination and spiritual needs of a rapidly growing community of worshippers. He became the great rival of Shiva, another minor Vedic deity who won immense popularity in later centuries. Together with God Brahma of mainline Brahmanism, Vishnu and Shiva came to form the well-known trinity (trimurti) of popular Hinduism. Here Brahma functions as the creator, Vishnu as the preserver, and Shiva as the destroyer of the universe.

Because of his benign qualities, lovingly characterized in countless popular works, Vishnu is easily the most accessible of the three aspects of the Hindu trinity. His most striking features are his incarnations (avatara), which took place in different world ages. Of his ten principal incarnations, only four were human; the others were magical animals. Vishnu's two most important human incarnations were those of Rama and Krishna.

Hindu tradition regards Rama, or Ramacandra, as having lived prior to Krishna, who served as Prince Arjuna's teacher. Over time, a religious community sprang up that made Rama its object of worship. Rama's devotees have created several Upanishads, including the Rama-Purva-Tapaniya and the Rama-Uttara-Tapaniya. Their central theological tenet is "Rama alone is the supreme Absolute, Rama alone is the supreme Reality, Shri Rama is the saving Absolute." According to the Rama-Purva-Tapaniya (I.6), Rama's name is derived, among other things, from the fact that yogins delight (ramante) in him. Another great creation by a member of the Rama community is the Yoga-Vasishtha-Ramayana, also attributed to Valmiki, which is discussed in Chapter 10. This mammoth work supplies what is missing in the original Ramayana epic, namely the yogic dimension. It portrays Rama as a renouncer who is discovering the truth behind the nondualist teachings of Vedanta.

The significance of the Ramayana for the student of Yoga lies in the moral values it promulgates so vividly. We can regard it as a consummate treatise, in narrative form, on what are known in Yoga as the moral observances (yama) and restraints (niyama). It extols virtues like righteousness (dharma), nonharming, truthfulness, and austerity. As such the Ramayana can serve as a textbook for Karma-Yoga, the Yoga of self-transcending action.

CHEATING DEATH: THE YOGA OF THE KATHA-UPANISHAD

The Katha- or Kathaka-Upanishad, which is named after an ancient Vedic school, counts as the oldest Upanishad that deals explicitly with Yoga. It was probably composed in the fifth century B.C.

This Upanishad develops its novel yogic doctrines around an old legend: A poor brahmin once offered a few old and feeble cows as a sacrificial fee to the priests. His son Naciketas, concerned about his father's afterlife, offered himself as a fit reward in place of the decrepit animals. This roused the anger of his father, who sent him to the god of death. But Yama, the ruler of the after-death world, was temporarily absent, and Naciketas had to wait for three full days without food before the god returned to his abode. Pleased with the boy's patience, Yama granted him three boons.

As his first gift the young boy asked to be returned to his father alive. For his second boon he desired to know the secret of the sacrificial fire that leads to heaven. For his third boon he insisted on knowing the mystery of life after death. Yama tried to talk the boy out of the third boon, offering all kinds of enticing substitutes—sons and grandsons, long life, large herds of cattle. When he failed to deter Naciketas, he proceeded to instruct him in the path to emancipation. On one level, the story is meant to portray the death-defying determination that the yogin must bring to his discipline.

The doctrine propounded in this scripture is called adhyatma-yoga, the "Yoga of the inmost self." Its target is the Supreme Being, which lies hidden in the "cave" of the heart.

> The sage (dhira) relinquishes exhiliration and grief, realizing, by means of the Yoga of the inmost self (adhyatman), that ancient subtle God (deva) who is difficult to behold, immanent, seated in the cave [of the heart] residing in the body. (II.12)
>
> This Self (atman) cannot be attained through study, nor by thought, nor by much learning. It is attained by the one whom it chooses. This Self reveals its own form. (II.23)

Here it is stated that the Self is not an object like other objects we can experience or analyze. It is in fact the transcendental Subject of everything. Thus, there is really nothing anyone can do to "acquire" the Self. On the contrary, Self-realization must be a matter of the Self disclosing itself of its own accord. This means Self-realization is dependent on grace. As the Katha-Upanishad has it, the Self is "attained by whom it chooses." It is clear from the context, however, that there is something the spiritual aspirant can do: He or she can undergo the necessary preparation for the event of grace.

In the third chapter of the Katha-Upanishad, the anonymous composer explains that the Self is at the top of a hierarchy of levels of existence. He employs the following metaphor:

Know that the Self is the charioteer, and the body is the chariot. Know further that the wisdom-faculty (buddhi) is the driver, whereas the mind (manas) is the rein. (III.3)

The senses, they say, are the horses, and the sense-objects are their arena. The sages call that [Self] the enjoyer (bhoktri) when united with the body (atman), the senses, and the mind. (III.4)

He whose mind is constantly unyoked, lacking in understanding—his senses are uncontrollable like the unruly horses of a driver. (III.5)

But he whose mind is always yoked, his senses are controllable like the obedient horses of a driver. (III.6)

And he who is devoid of understanding, mindless (amanaska), and always impure—he never attains that [lofty] goal, but moves around in the cycle [of repeated births and deaths]. (III.7)

But he who understands, always with a pure mind, verily reaches that goal, whence one is not born again. (III.8)

The man who has understanding for his driver, with the mind as his [well-controlled] rein—he reaches the end of the journey, [which is] Vishnu's supreme Abode. (III.9)

The Katha-Upanishad understands spiritual practice as a progressive involution or retracing in consciousness, in reverse order, the stages of the evolutionary unfolding of the world. The text distinguishes seven stages or levels that make up the Chain of Being:

1. The senses (indriya)
2. The sense-objects (vishaya)
3. The mind (manas)
4. The wisdom-faculty (buddhi)
5. The "great self" (maha-atman), or "great one" (mahat), a kind of collective entitity composed of the individuated selves
6. The unmanifest (avyakta), the transcendental ground of Nature (prakriti)
7. The Self (purusha), the true Identity of the human being

Only the Self is eternally beyond the dynamics of Nature (prakriti) in its manifest and unmanifest dimensions. Such ontological schemes, or models of the different modes of existence, are characteristic of the Samkhya tradition and of the earlier Samkhya-Yoga schools. They were never intended as mere philosophical speculations, but they served as maps for the yogic process of involution, the climbing of consciousness to ever higher levels of being, terminating with the omnipresent Being, the purusha, itself.

It is the purusha, the transcendental Self, that is the goal of the yogin's psychospiritual work. But that sacred work, or transformative alchemy, begins very humbly. This is clear from the definition of Yoga furnished in the second chapter of the Katha-Upanishad:

> This they consider to be Yoga: the steady holding (dharana) of the senses. Then [the yogin] becomes attentive (apramatta); for, Yoga can be acquired and lost. (VI.11)

In other words, Yoga means the condition of inner stability or equilibrium that depends on one's fixity of attention. When the mind is stabilized, then one can begin to discover the wonders of the inner world, the vast horizons of consciousness. But, ultimately, as we have seen, even this exploration of inner space does not lead to liberation. It is merely a precondition for the event of grace—when the light of the transcendental Self shines through into the finite body-mind.

The teachings of the Katha-Upanishad represent an important break-through in the tradition of Yoga. In beautiful poetic form, we find expressed some of the fundamental ideas underlying all yogic practice. Better than any other scripture, this Upanishad marks the transition between the proto-yogic esotericism of the early Upanishads and Pre-Classical Yoga proper. With this work, Yoga became a recognizable tradition in its own right.

THE SECRET DOCTRINE OF THE WHITE-HORSED SAGE: THE SHVETASHVATARA-UPANISHAD

The Shvetashvatara-Upanishad, which is appraised to be one of the more beautiful creations of this genre, gets its mysterious name from the sage who composed it. *Shvetashvatara* means literally "the whitest horse." According to Shankara, who wrote a learned commentary on this scripture in the early ninth century A.D., this is not the name but the title of a sage. He explains that *ashva,* which ordinarily means "horse," has also an esoteric significance, and that in initiate circles the term refers to the senses. Thus, the title *shveta-ashva-tara* is given to someone whose senses are purified and under control.

Ordinarily we are at the mercy of our senses. We make this discovery quickly when we learn to meditate. At first, every sound or movement interferes with our concentration, and almost against our will we follow after every sensation that enters into our consciousness. Only very gradually do we learn to disregard the input from our senses. Then we still have the overactive mind to deal with. The Pre-Classical Yoga and Samkhya schools regard the mind (manas) as a sixth sensory instrument (indriya). In effect, it is the relay station of the senses, where the input from the five sense organs is gathered and then forwarded to the higher mind, called buddhi, for further processing.

The author of the Shvetashvatara-Upanishad was manifestly an adept of sense-withdrawal and meditation. In his work, which is clearly informed by rich yogic experience, he expounds a Yoga that is characteristic of the panentheistic teachings of the epic age. The Greek-derived term "panentheism" refers to the religious philosophy that sees all of Nature as arising in the Divine. In distinction to this, the better-known term "pantheism" denotes the philosophical position that simply equates Nature with God.

That metaphysical equation is implicitly rejected by the sage composer of the Shvetashvatara-Upanishad, who hails the Lord (isha, ishvara) as dwelling eternally above his own creation.

> Following the Yoga of meditation (dhyana), they perceived the self-power (atma-shakti) of God (deva) hidden by His own qualities. He is the One who presides over all the causes connected with time and the self (atman). (I.3)

> The Lord (isha) supports this universe, composed of the perishable and the imperishable, the manifest and the unmanifest. The [individuated] self (atman), [which is] not the Lord, is bound by [its wrong notion of] being the enjoyer. But on knowing God, it is released from all fetters. (I.8)

> The foundation (pradhana) [i.e., Nature] is perishable. Hara [i.e., God Shiva] is immortal and imperishable. The one God rules over the perishable [Nature] and the [individuated] selves. By meditating on Him, by uniting with, and becoming the Real (tattva), there is finally the cessation of all illusion (maya). (I.10)

> By knowing God, the falling away of all fetters [is accomplished]. Upon the waning of the afflictions (klesha) [i.e., spiritual ignorance and its results], the falling away of birth and death [is accomplished]. By meditating on Him, there is a third [state], universal lordship, upon separating from the body. [Thus, the yogin becomes] the solitary (kevala) [Self], whose desires are satisfied. (I.11)

The Shvetashvatara recommends meditation by means of the recitation of the sacred syllable *om,* called the pranava. The meditative process is described as a kind of churning by which the inner fire is kindled, leading to the revelation of the Self's splendor. The instructions imply knowledge of breath control (pranayama). On a more elementary level, advice is given about correct meditation posture, which should be straight, undoubtedly in order to allow the free circulation of the bodily energies. When the vital-forces (prana) in the body have quietened down, conscious breathing should begin as a prelude to mental concentration. The Upanishad even pays attention to the right environmental conditions, recommending that one should engage in this Yoga practice in quiet caves and other pure places.

When the mind is stilled, all kinds of internal visions can appear, which must not be confused with God-realization. Among the first signs of successful Yoga practice are lightness, health, steadiness, clearness of complexion, pleasantness of voice, agreeable odor, and scanty excretions. This suggests, as the text claims, the transmutation of the body into a body "fashioned out of the fire of Yoga." But the supreme goal of this Yoga is the realization of the transcendental Self. That realization is not a mere visionary state. Enlightenment, as has been noted before, is not an experience, for experience presupposes an experiencing subject and and experienced object. Enlightenment, or liberation, is that condition of being in which the gulf between subject (mind) and object (matter) does not exist. It is the immortal state. The Upanishad records the following confession of its author:

> I know that great Self (purusha) who is effulgent like the sun beyond darkness. Realizing Him alone, one passes beyond death. There is no other way for passing [beyond the cycle of repeated births and deaths]. (III.8)

The great Being whom Sage Shvetashvatara honors is Shiva. As in the Bhagavad-Gita, where Vishnu is celebrated as the Lord of all, the yogin is not merely a dry ascetic but a devotee (bhakta), and the process of spiritual maturation and ultimate liberation is not a mechanical event but a mystery dependent on divine grace (prasada). Perhaps the Shvetashvatara-Upanishad was for the early Shiva worshippers what the Gita was and still is for the Vaishnava community—a sacred work of adoration of the Divine, edification of the heart, and instruction in the art of spiritual practice.

THE SIXFOLD YOGA:
THE MAITRAYANIYA-UPANISHAD

The central Indian tribe of the Maitrayanas converted to Brahmanism at an early period, though they never abandoned their faith in God Rudra, who was subsequently assimilated into Shiva. They were instrumental in the development of Yoga, especially meditative recitation (japa). Among other works, the Maitrayana priests created the Shata-Rudriya ("Hundred to Rudra"), a litany that was recited for protection against evil but came to be used for meditative purposes. As its title indicates, the Maitrayaniya-Upanishad was also authored in those circles. It clearly connects with archaic yogic lore. If the Shvetashvatara-Upanishad can be placed in the third century B.C., the Maitrayaniya belongs probably to the second century B.C., though it contains passages that are considerably older.

The Maitrayaniya-Upanishad begins by introducing the story of King Brihadratha, who is elsewhere known as an early ruler of Magadha and worshipper of Shiva. After installing his son as ruler, so the story goes, Brihadratha abandoned his kingdom to pursue austerities in the forest. After a thousand days (or years) of standing stock-still, with his arms raised high and staring at the sun, he was visited by the Self-realized adept Shakayanya. Finding Brihadratha worthy of instruction, Shakayanya disclosed to him the mystery of the two kinds of self—the "elemental self" (bhuta-atman), or ego-personality, and the transcendental Self.

The elemental self is constantly suffering change until it disintegrates at death. But the transcendental Self is eternally unaffected by these changes. It can be realized through study and the pursuit of one's allotted duties, including austerities, recitation, and profound contemplation. Shakayanya speaks of this realization in terms of a union (sayujya) with the Self, the Ruler (ishana). Then the sage expounds the sixfold Yoga:

The rule for effecting this [union with the Self] is this: breath control (pranayama), sense-withdrawal (pratyahara), meditation (dhyana), concentration (dharana), reflection (tarka), and ecstasy (samadhi). Such is said to be the sixfold Yoga. (VI.18)

When a seer sees the brilliant Maker, Lord, Person, the Source of [the Creator-God] Brahma, then, being a knower, shaking off good and evil, he reduces everything to unity in the supreme Imperishable. (VI.19)

The Upanishad is still more specific. It mentions the central channel, sushumna-nadi, that forms the axis of the body, along which the life-force (prana) must be forced from the base of the spine to the crown of the head and beyond. This process is accomplished by joining the breath, the mind, and the sacred syllable *om*.[1] Next Shakayanya quotes two stanzas from an unidentified authority, according to which Yoga is the joining of breath and the syllable *om*, or of breath, the mind, and the senses.

The Maitrayaniya contains many fascinating ideas, hinting at practices that suggest a further advance in the development of Yoga and that prepared the ground for Patanjali's classical formulations.

THE INTANGIBLE YOGA: THE MANDUKYA-UPANISHAD

There are a number of other Upanishads from the epic period, notably the Isha, the Mundaka, the Prashna, and the Mandukya. These scriptures are not directly connected with the Yoga tradition but belong to mainstream Vedantic nondualism, and I will therefore not discuss them here. Only the Mandukya-Upanishad deserves to be singled out, because it inspired, in the seventh century A.D., the adept Gaudapada to compose his Mandukya-Karika. Gaudapada was the teacher of the adept Govinda, who was the guru of Shankara, the most renowned philosopher of Advaita Vedanta, India's tradition of radical nondualism.

The Mandukya-Karika is a brilliant philosophical exposition of the ideas found in the Mandukya-Upanishad. In the Muktika-Upanishad it is stated that if a man cannot study all the 108 Upanishads, he can still attain liberation if he delves into the Mandukya, because it contains the quintessence of Upanishadic wisdom.

The entire Mandukya-Upanishad, which consists of only twelve stanzas, is a treatment of the esoteric symbolism of the sacred syllable *om*. As we have seen in an earlier chapter, this ancient mantra is generally thought to be composed of four units, *a, u, m,* and the nasalized echo of the *m* sound. These are symbolically related to the four basic states of consciousness, which are waking, dreaming, sleeping, and the transcendental state, which is called the "Fourth."

Gaudapada's work expounds this idea further. He introduces the concept of asparsha-yoga. The Sanskrit compound means literally the "intangible Yoga." What it stands for is the radically nondualist practice of abiding in or as the Self.

From the perspective of the Self, which is one without a second, there can be no question of contact with anything. Only the unenlightened mind, which distinguishes between subject and object, thinks in terms of contact or touch. Where there is no duality, there is also no fear. Gaudapada's Asparsha-Yoga is the realization of that fearless Condition, the "Fourth." It can be attained in every moment that the mind is obliged to relinquish the illusion that there is a world of multiplicity outside itself and, instead, is brought to rest in the native state of pure existence.

This Yoga is synonymous with Jnana-Yoga in its highest form. As such it represents the crowning achievement of the entire nondualist tradition of the Upanishads. Under Shankara's skillful hands, it became the greatest rival of Patanjali's school of Classical Yoga.

IMMORTALITY ON THE BATTLEFIELD: YOGIC TEACHINGS IN THE MAHABHARATA

The Mahabharata is a magnificent and invaluable treasure-house of mythology, religion, philosophy, ethics, customs, and information about clans, kings, and sages. It is the grand epic of India, comprising about 100,000 stanzas, which makes the Mahabharata eight times the volume of the *Iliad* and the *Odyssey* combined.

The Mahabharata was composed over many generations, and the final redaction of this work appears to have been made sometime in the second or third century A.D. But the kernel of this epic creation easily goes back to the fifth century B.C. and was kept alive by oral transmission for many centuries. Yoga and its cousin Samkhya loom large in the philosophy of the epic. Both traditions have their taproots in the time before the Buddha, but the Yoga and Samkhya schools mentioned in the epic are post-Buddhist and, with the exception of the teachings of the Bhagavad-Gita, can be placed in the centuries from 300 B.C. to A.D. 100. Some are still more recent. The earliest portions of the epic make no reference to Yoga at all but speak of asceticism (tapas) instead.

The narrative nucleus of the epic is the war between two old nations—the Pandavas (Pandu's lineage) and the Kauravas (Kuru's lineage)—which is estimated to have actually taken place at about 1000 B.C. According to this saga, Prince Yudhishthira, one of the five sons of King Pandu, lost his kingdom and his wife by a foul trick in a fateful game of dice, a favorite pastime since the ancient Vedic days. He and his four brothers, including Prince Arjuna (the hero of the Bhagavad-Gita), were banished as a result. At the end of their thirteen-year exile, the five virtuous sons of Pandu demanded the restoration of their paternal kingdom, which was now ruled by the blind

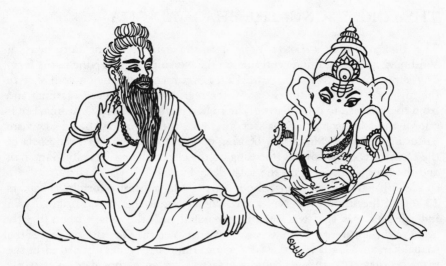

Sage Vyasa dictating the extensive text of the Mahabharata epic to the elephantine God Ganesha. According to legend, Ganesha alone was fast enough to follow Vyasa's rapid dictation.

King Dhrishtarashtra and his hundred sons, notably the power-hungry Duryodhana. When their lawful claim was dismissed, they went to war against the Kauravas, who were defeated after eighteen days of the fiercest battles.

Whatever the historical realities may have been, the Mahabharata also lends itself to symbolic and allegorical interpretations. Thus, the strife between the Pandava and Kaurava cousins has often been read in terms of the fight between good and evil in the world and in the human heart. Beyond this, the Mahabharata puts forward a mystical point of view according to which there is an unsurpassable Condition that transcends both good and evil, right and wrong. That Condition is celebrated as the highest value to which human beings can aspire. It is synonymous with freedom and immortality.

Around the epic war story, layers upon layers of instructional and legendary materials—making up no less than four-fifths of the entire epic—have been woven over the centuries. One of these additions is the famous Bhagavad-Gita, found in the sixth book of the epic. Another interpolation that is very important for our understanding of that phase in the evolution of Yoga is the Moksha-Dharma, which has been inserted into the twelfth book of the Mahabharata. I will discuss these in the next two sections.

For the Hindu, the Mahabharata epic is a treasure-house of instructive and delightful tales about heroes, rogues, and yogins; for the historian of religion, it is a mosaic of ideas, beliefs, and customs of one of the most fertile eras in the intellectual history of Hinduism. The contemporary student of Yoga can fruitfully approach the epic from both these perspectives.

THE LORD'S SONG: THE BHAGAVAD-GITA

The Bhagavad-Gita ("Lord's Song") is the earliest extant document of Vaishnavism, the tradition centering on the worship of the Divine in the form of Vishnu, specifically in his incarnation as Krishna. This religion flourished in the fifth and fourth centuries B.C. in the region of the modern Mathura and from there spread to other parts of the Indian peninsula. Today Vaishnavism is one of the five great religious sects of India, the other four being Shaivism (focusing on Shiva), Shaktism (focusing on Shakti, the female Power aspect of the Divine), the Ganapatyas (focusing on the elephant-headed deity Ganesha), and the Sauras (focusing on the solar deity Surya).

The Bhagavad-Gita is an episode of the Mahabharata, forming chapters 13–40 of the sixth book. Not a few scholars argue that it was originally an independent text that was later incorporated into the epic. Others rightly point to the apparently flawless continuity between the Gita and the rest of the Mahabharata. The date of the Gita is uncertain. It is generally placed in the third century B.C., though some scholars assign an earlier date to it while others regard it as a post-Christian work.

The Gita has enjoyed enormous popularity among Hindus for countless generations—a popularity that is epitomized in the words of Mahatma Gandhi, who said: "I find a solace in the Bhagavadgita that I miss even in the

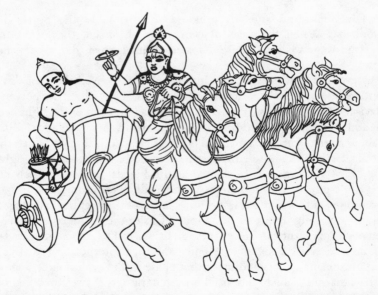

Prince Arjuna, who feels dejected about the imminent war against his kinsfolk and teachers, is instructed by the God-man Krishna. This image is charged with symbolism. The chariot represents the body, the horses stand for the unruly senses, which are controlled by Krishna, symbolizing the higher mind (buddhi), whereas Arjuna is the lower mind (manas) or ego-personality.

Sermon on the Mount. . . . I owe it all to the teachings of the Bhagavadgita."[2]

The Bhagavad-Gita is a dialogue between the incarnate god Krishna and his pupil Prince Arjuna, which took place on the battlefield of Kuru-Kshetra, located in the Gangetic plain around modern Delhi. This immortal conversation is the climax of the epic story. Its importance for the student of Yoga is obvious, since it must be regarded as the first proper Yoga scripture. Indeed, the Gita speaks of itself as a yoga-shastra, or yogic teaching, restating ancient truths.

Historically, the Bhagavad-Gita can be understood as a massive effort to integrate the diverse strands of spiritual thought prevalent within Hinduism in that period. It mediates between the sacrificial ritualism of the orthodox priesthood and such heterodox teachings as we have encountered in the esoteric doctrines of the early Upanishads as well as in the traditions of Buddhism and Jainism. Aldous Huxley, in his introduction to the Gita rendering by Swami Prabhavananda and Christopher Isherwood, called this ancient work "perhaps the most systematic statement of the Perennial Philosophy."[3]

The central message of Krishna's Song is the balancing out of conventional religious and ethical activity and other worldly ascetic goals. The gist of Krishna's teaching is given in the following stanza: "Steadfast in Yoga perform actions, abandoning attachment and remaining the same in success and failure, O Dhanamjaya. Yoga is called 'evenness' (samatva)" (II.48).

In order to win peace and enlightenment—so Krishna declares—one need not forsake the world or one's responsibilities, even when they oblige one to go into battle. Renunciation (samnyasa) *of* action is good in itself, but better still is renunciation *in* action. This is the celebrated Hindu ideal of inaction-in-action (naishkarmya-karman), which is the basis of Karma-Yoga. Life in the world and spiritual life are not in principle inimical to each other; they can and should be cultivated simultaneously. Such is the essence of a whole or integrated life.

Not by abstention from actions does a man enjoy action-transcendence (naishkarmya), nor by renunciation alone does he approach perfection. (III.4)

For, not even for a moment can anyone ever remain without performing action. Everyone is unwittingly made to act by the constituents (guna) belonging to Nature (prakriti). (III.5)

He who restrains his organs of action but sits remembering in his mind the objects of the senses, is called a hypocrite, a bewildered person (atman). (III.6)

But more excellent is he, O Arjuna, who, controlling with his mind the senses, embarks unattached on Karma-Yoga with the organs of action. (III.7)

You must [always] do the alloted action, for action is superior to inaction; not even your body's processes can be accomplished by inaction. (III.8)

This world is bound by action, save when this action is [performed as] sacrifice (yajna). With that purpose [in mind], O Kaunteya [i.e., Arjuna], engage in action devoid of attachment. (III.9)

Krishna points to himself as an example of enlightened activity:

For Me, O Partha [i.e., Arjuna], there is nothing to be done in the three worlds, nothing ungained to be gained—and yet I engage in action. (III.22)

For, if I were not untiringly ever to abide in action, people would, O Partha, follow everywhere My "track" [or example]. (III.23)

If I were not to perform action, these worlds would perish, and I would be the author of chaos destroying [all] these creatures. (III.24)

Just as the unwise perform [their deeds] attached to action, O Bharata [i.e., Arjuna], the wise should act unattached, desiring the world's welfare (loka-samgraha). (III.25)

The secret lies in the human mind as the primary source of all action. If the mind is pure, without attachment to deeds, it cannot be defiled by them even as they are performed. Only attachment, not action itself, sets in motion the law of moral causation (karma) by which a person is bound to the wheel of existence in ever new reembodiments. The mind that is polished like a mirror, freed entirely of the stain of attachment, spotlessly reveals things as they truly are. And what they truly are is the Divine, the Self. The perfected yogin always enjoys that divine vision: "Whose self is yoked in Yoga and who beholds everywhere the same, he sees the Self abiding in all beings and all beings in the Self" (VI.29).

This vision of the sameness of all things and beings is the fruit of consummate nonattachment. Nonattachment is a matter of assuming the position of the transcendental Self, the eternal witness of all processes, and of penetrating the illusion of being an acting subject, or ego. Nonetheless, actions must continue to be performed.

Acts must not only be performed in the spirit of unselfishness, or nonattachment, they must also be morally sound and justifiable. This view has not always been emphasized sufficiently in Western interpretations of the Gita. If action depended solely on one's frame of mind, it would be the best excuse for immoral behavior. The Bhagavad-Gita does not propound such a crude subjectivism. For action to be wholesome (kritsna) it must have two essential ingredients: subjective purity (i.e., nonattachment) and objective morality (i.e., moral rightness). The external factor of moral right or wrong is determined by the traditional values and the prevalent code of behavior, as well as by the growing insight into right and wrong through the practice of Yoga. The Gita builds on the foundations of the ethics of the Mahabharata. The epic is, on one level, a gigantic attempt to come to grips with the nature of what is lawful (dharma) and what is unlawful (adharma). This is echoed in the following stanzas of the Gita:

What is action? What is inaction? On this even the sages (kavi) are bewildered. I shall declare to you that action which, when understood, will set you free from ill. (IV.16)

Indeed, [a yogin] ought to understand [the nature of] action (karman), he ought to understand wrong action (vikarman), and he ought to understand inaction (akarman). Impenetrable is the way of action. (IV.17)

He who sees inaction in action and action in inaction is wise among men; he is yoked, performing whole (kritsna) actions. (IV.18)

The war into which Arjuna was drawn, on the sagacious advice of the incarnate God Krishna, was in the interest of the maintenance of a higher moral order. The Kauravas were power-hungry and corrupt rulers who had usurped the throne; the peace-loving Pandavas had the welfare of the people at heart. The Gita portrays Arjuna's qualms about going into battle even over what is obviously right and lawful. Seeing his cousins and former teachers arrayed on the opposite side of the battlefield, he was ready to cast down his bow and surrender his claims to the throne. But Krishna instructed him otherwise. His yogic teaching goes beyond both pacificism and warmongering, just as it goes beyond the mere doing of one's duty on the one hand and the neglect of one's obligations on the other. For, in the last analysis, Krishna expects his devotee to step beyond the moral realm. He makes this exhortation and solemn promise:

Relinquishing all norms (dharma), go to Me alone for shelter. I will deliver you from all sin. Do not grieve! (XVIII.66)

The Lord abides in the heart region of all beings, O Arjuna, whirling all beings [in the cycle of conditioned existence] through His power (maya), [as if they were] mounted on a machine. (XVIII.61)

To Him alone go for shelter with your whole being, O Bharata [i.e., Arjuna]! By His grace you will obtain supreme peace, the eternal Abode. (XVIII.62)

In the Bhagavad-Gita, Yoga is not yet systematically outlined. For Krishna, Yoga consists essentially in the total realignment of one's daily life to the Supreme Being. Everything that is done should be done in the light of the Divine. One's whole life must become a continual Yoga. By seeing in everything the presence of the Divine and by casting off all mundane attachments, the yogin purifies his life and no longer takes flight from it. With his mind immersed in the Supreme Being, he is active in the world, guided by the desire to promote the welfare of all beings. This is the well-known Hindu ideal of loka-samgraha, which literally means "drawing together of the world."

It is difficult to give this Yoga an appropriate label. It is not only Jnana-Yoga and Karma-Yoga but also Bhakti-Yoga. It seeks to integrate all aspects of the human being and then to employ them in the great enterprise to reach enlightenment in this very life. For this reason, Krishna's path might best be described as an early form of "integral Yoga" (purna-yoga).

The ethical activism of the Bhagavad-Gita is founded on a panentheistic metaphysics: Everything is in God, while God nevertheless transcends everything. The Supreme Being, Vishnu (as Krishna), is both the ultimate source of all existence and the manifest universe in its entire multiplicity. Vishnu encompasses Being as well as Becoming. Krishna, the incarnate God, declares:

> By Me, unmanifest in form, this entire [universe] is spread out. All beings abide in Me, but I do not subsist in them. (IX.4)

> And [yet] beings do not abide in Me. Behold My lordly Yoga: My Self sustains [all] beings, yet not abiding in beings, causes beings to be. (IX.5)

Vishnu is the all-embracing Whole (purna), the One and the Many. Since He is everywhere and in everything, we do not have to shun the world in order to find Him, but merely need to cultivate our higher wisdom (buddhi), the "eye of gnosis" (jnana-cakshus), to be able to apprehend the omnipresent Being-in-Becoming.

The Bhagavad-Gita knows of two types of emancipation, which are more accurately two successive stages of completeness. The first kind, called brahma-nirvana, is the "extinction in the world-ground." Here the yogin transcends the space-time continuum and abides in his essential nature. But this state is without outflowing love, and the divine personality of Krishna remains concealed from him. The Supreme Person (purusha-uttama) is realized only in the higher form of emancipation when the yogin awakens in God.

> That man who, having forsaken all desires, moves about devoid of longing, devoid of [the thought of] "mine," without ego-sense—he approaches peace (shanti). (II.71)

> This is the state of the Absolute (brahman), O Partha [i.e., Arjuna]. Attaining this, one is no [longer] deluded. Abiding therein also at the end-time [i.e., at death], one attains extinction (nirvana) in the Absolute (II.72)

> He who has inner joy, inner rejoicing, and inner light is a yogin. Having become the Absolute, he approaches extinction in the Absolute. (V.24)

> Thus ever yoking the self, the yogin of restrained mind approaches peace, the supreme extinction that subsists in Me. (VI.15)

> He who is intent on oneness (ekatva) and loves Me, abiding in all beings, in whatever [state] he exists—that yogin dwells in Me. (VI.31)

Love (bhakti) is a key element in Krishna's teaching. On the finite plane, it is the surest mechanism by which the yogin-devotee bonds himself to the Divine Person and thereby wins grace. On the ultimate level, love is the very nature of the liberated Condition. Thus Krishna declares: "Of all yogins, he who loves Me with faith and whose inner self is absorbed in Me—him I deem to be most yoked" (VI.47).

How may we understand the transcendental love in which the liberated yogin participates? Elsewhere I proposed this answer:

The love that flourishes eternally between God and the Self-particles who have awakened to His presence is one of ineffable divine creativity: The Whole communing with Itself. The logical mind shrinks back from this paradox. It fails to gain a foothold in that realm in which all opposites coincide. The ultimate test must be unmediated experience. This transcendental love (para-bhakti) is an essential part of God and can be fully realized only in and through God. This love is . . . unconditional and without object.[4]

The Gita's teaching of the eternal love that flows from the Divine Person to the devotee and to all creation is one of the most momentous innovations in the history of Indian religiosity. The Yoga taught by Krishna, the avatara (divine descent), infused Hinduism with a rare emotionality that had until then been absent from the largely ascetic efforts of the Hindu seers and sages. Suddenly the spiritual seeker was empowered to relate to the Divine in personal terms, from the heart and not merely through the exercise of the will. The tentative beginnings of this teaching can be seen in the early Upanishads, but with the Gita it entered the popular consciousness and became a vehicle for the simple spiritual aspirations of countless millions.

THE LIBERATING GOSPELS OF THE EPIC: THE MOKSHA-DHARMA

Next to the Bhagavad-Gita, the most significant materials on Yoga in the Mahabharata are found in the Moksha-Dharma section, which comprises chapters 168–353 of the twelfth book. Here a host of traditions are given voice. Besides the orthodox brahmanical schools represented by Vedanta, we encounter several other traditions, notably the Pancaratra religion (an early form of Vaishnavism), the Pashupata religion (a form of Shaivism), Pre-Classical Samkhya, and pre-Patanjali Yoga. These diverse teachings have sometimes been looked upon as being merely a corrupt jumble crafted onto the nondualistic metaphysics of Vedanta. Nothing could be further from the truth.

The liberation gospels represented in the Moksha-Dharma give us important clues especially about Samkhya and Yoga in their "epic" forms prior to their systematizations at the hands of Ishvara Krishna (c. A.D. 350) and Patanjali (c. A.D. 200) respectively. What emerges from a careful study of the Moksha-Dharma is that, notwithstanding the great similarities between Samkhya and Yoga, these two traditions were already distinct and independent developments at the time of the final composition of the Mahabharata. This is epitomized in the following statement: "The method of the Yogas is perception, [whereas] of the Samkhyas it is scriptural tradition" (XII.289.7). "These are not the same," as the epic affirms two stanzas later. The distinction made here is between the pragmatic-experimental approach of the yogins (called yogas), and the reliance on the traditional revelation (accompanied by rational inquiry into the nature of human existence) that typifies the followers of Samkhya. But epic or Pre-Classical Yoga is not simply practice, as opposed to Samkhya theory. Both traditions have their specific theoretical frameworks and psychotechnology.

Epic Samkhya arose out of the Upanishadic speculations about the levels of existence and consciousness as they disclosed themselves to the penetrating meditations of the sages. But by the time of the Moksha-Dharma, Samkhya and Vedanta had become distinct traditions. Yet, like some schools of Vedanta, epic Samkhya espoused a form of nondualism. This is also true of the epic schools of Yoga. What distinguishes epic Samkhya and Yoga from their classical formulations is, above all, their theistic orientation. The atheism of Classical Samkhya and the quasi theism of Classical Yoga must be understood as deviations from a strongly theistic base, reflected in the Upanishads.

The reason for this shift away from the original panentheism of Samkhya and Yoga was a felt need to respond to the challenge of such vigorously analytical traditions as Buddhism by systematizing both Samkhya and Yoga along rationalistic philosophical lines. In both cases, this effort led to a metaphysical dualism that is barely convincing and that limps behind the nondualistic interpretations of Vedanta in philosophical sophistication.

There were important differences between the epic or preclassical schools of Samkhya and Yoga on metaphysical-theological matters. The epic Samkhya teachers maintained that there is an essential identity between the individuated or empirical self, called budhyamana or jiva, and the universal Self, called buddha or atman. By contrast, the Yoga tradition asserted that there is more of a rift between the transcendental Self and the many empirical selves or ego-personalities. Also, according to the adepts of Yoga there is a supreme Being, or Divinity, above the collective of transcendental Selves. In comparison with that Absolute, which is known as the buddha, or "awakened" principle, or as "Lord" (ishvara), even the liberated beings are still unenlightened (abuddhiman). Thus, the epic yogins allowed twenty-six fundamental categories of existence, called principles (tattva), whereas the Samkhya followers allowed only twenty-five. These principles will be discussed in Chapter 9 ("Yoga as Philosophy and Religion").

The epic schools of Samkhya and Yoga gave rise to the Samkhya-Yoga syncretism. For the historian of Indian philosophy and spirituality, these developments, which have for so long been misunderstood, form one of the most exciting areas of inquiry. For the student of Yoga, it is important to know that Patanjali's Yoga-Sutra was preceded by centuries of lively experimentation and thought about the great matter of self-transcendence. Patanjali's work, impressive as it is as a concise statement of Yoga philosophy and practice, scarcely betokens the immense ingenuity and spiritual creativity on which it was built.

When we read the Moksha-Dharma, we encounter all kinds of more or less elaborate and more or less abstruse teachings. In terms of actual practice, the Yoga authorities who make their appearance in the epic insist on solid moral foundations. They demand such virtues as truthfulness, humility, nonpossessiveness, nonviolence, forgiveness, and compassion, which also form the bedrock of later Yoga.

Lust, anger, greed, and fear are frequently listed as the yogin's greatest enemies. There are also references to dreaming and sleep, infatuation and "mental diarrhea" (bhrama), as well as doubt and discontent, which are all deemed to be severe obstacles on the spiritual road. Another considerable obstruction is said to be the psychic powers (siddhi or vibhuti). They can distract the yogin from his real concern, which is to transcend the self, or ego-personality. These powers are a natural by-product of the yogin's meditation practice. Yet, as Patanjali observes in his Yoga-Sutra (III.37), they are accomplishments only from the point of view of the egoic consciousness. Their exercise prevents the ecstatic state (samadhi), precisely because the deployment of these powers presupposes that we pay attention to the external world and its concerns. This, in turn, means that we reinforce the habit of assuming that we are ego-personalities rather than the transcendental Self.

The Moksha-Dharma teachers also provide useful instructions about right diet and fasting, as well as suitable environments for yogic practice. They also knew of the value of breath control (pranayama) and distinguished between the five types of life-force (prana) circulating in the body. Breath control prepares the mind for the next stage of the process of gradual introversion, which is the withdrawal (pratyahara) of the senses from the external world.

Most of the Pre-Classical or epic schools of Yoga subscribe to the model of what the Moksha-Dharma calls nirodha-yoga, the "Yoga of cessation." This approach consists in the progressive disowning of the contents of consciousness—from sensations, to thoughts, to higher experiences—until the transcendental Self shines forth in its full glory. Thus, sense-withdrawal, concentration, and meditation are considered the primary means of Yoga. In one section (XII.188.15ff.) several degrees of meditation are distinguished that remind one of Patanjali's terminology.[5] The yogin who is successful at nirodha-yoga enters the state of complete inner stillness, "windlessness" (nirvana), which is accompanied by the total absence of sensory input. The body of such a yogin is said to appear to others like a stone pillar.

Another type of Yoga discussed in the Moksha-Dharma is known as jnana-dipti-yoga, the "Yoga of the effulgence of wisdom." It consists in prolonged concentration upon progressively more subtle objects. For instance, a person may first fix attention on one of the five material elements, followed by concentration on the mind (manas) or the higher mind (buddhi). Or a yogin may start out by concentrating on different points in the body, such as the heart, the navel, or the head, and subsequently concentrate on the Self itself. These concentration practices are called dharana.

In one passage, Yoga is likened to a faultless jewel that first gathers in and then emits the bright light of the sun. The sun, of course, is a universal symbol for the Self, which is experienced as a dazzling effulgence. This metaphor describes well the essential yogic process of concentration. Dharana gathers in the "rays" or whirls of the mind and focuses them on the Self within, until the radiance of the Self becomes manifest in the state of ecstasy (samadhi) and transforms the yogin's being.

The fact that such teachings came to be included in the Mahabharata demonstrates their immense popularity during the period under review. In the centuries just before and after the beginning of the Christian calendar, Yoga had manifestly become a vociferous contender in the philosophical and spiritual arena of Hinduism. It was only a matter of time before an educated adept of Yoga would create a work of lasting success, in which the philosophy and practice of Hindu Yoga was coherently formulated. That work was the Yoga-Sutra of Patanjali, to which we will turn in Chapter 9 ("Yoga as Philosophy and Religion").

MORALITY AND SPIRITUALITY: PRE-CLASSICAL YOGA IN THE ETHICAL LITERATURE

In addition to the epics and Upanishads, elements of Pre-Classical Yoga are also found in a number of other semireligious works of Hinduism, notably the ethical-juristic literature known as dharma-shastra. Why is there this connection between ethics (dharma) and spirituality (yoga)? According to an old brahmanical model of human motivation, there are four great values to which people can dedicate themselves. These are known as the human goals (purusha-artha): material welfare (artha), pleasure (kama), morality (dharma), and liberation (moksha). They form a hierarchical continuum, with liberation as the highest possible value to which we can aspire. Morality and the quest for emancipation, or spiritual freedom, stand in a special relationship to each other, for the higher spiritual life can blossom only when it is securely founded on morality.

Thus, it is not surprising that we should find many references to Yoga in the manuals on ethics and law, which regard liberation as the highest possible virtue, just as the Yoga scriptures mention all kinds of moral virtues in which the yogin must be established or which he must cultivate. For instance, in his Yoga-Sutra (II.30–31), Patanjali lists the five virtues that comprise the great vow (maha-vrata) as follows: nonharming, truthfulness, nonstealing, chastity, and greedlessness. These compose the first of the eight limbs of Classical Yoga.

In the Manu-Smriti (VI.70ff.), an important pre-Christian work on morality and law, there is a passage that speaks of the benefits of breath control (pranayama). It is meant to be performed with the appropriate Vedic mantras, especially the syllable *om*. This is considered the highest form of austerity, which "burns away" all kinds of physical and psychic blemishes. This work also recommends concentration (dharana) as a means of atoning for one's sins, and meditation (dhyana) for combating such undesirable emotions as anger, avarice, and jealousy.

Similar statements are found, for instance, in the Baudayana-Dharma-Sutra, a much-respected juridical work from the same period. The Shankhayana-Smriti (XII.18–19), another ancient scripture dealing with Hindu law and custom, makes the exaggerated claim that sixteen daily cycles of breath control absolve even the slayer of a brahmin from his heinous sin.

The author of the Apastamba-Dharma-Sutra (I.5.23.3ff.), which belongs to the fourth century B.C., quotes a verse from an unidentified work, according to which the wise person eliminates all taints (dosha) of character through the practice of Yoga. He enumerates fifteen such taints, or defects, including anger, greed, hypocrisy, and even exuberance.

The Yajnavalkya-Smriti ranks next in importance to the Manu-Smriti, though it was composed several centuries later. This scripture is attributed, probably wrongly, to the illustrious Sage Yajnavalkya, whose teachings are recorded in the Brihad-Aranyaka-Upanishad. However, it contains a passage (III.305) in which a hundred cycles of breath control are prescribed to bring about the removal of the ill effects of one's immoral deeds. Another passage (III.195ff.) describes the entire yogic process—from assuming the right posture, to withdrawing the senses from the external world, to performing breath control, to concentration and meditation. This work also lists (III.202f.) several of the yogic powers (siddhi), such as the ability to become invisible, to remember past lives, and to see the future.

The juristic or dharma-shastra literature of Hinduism is quite extensive and so far has barely been studied from the point of view of the history of Hindu spirituality. What is clear from even a cursory glance at the manuals on right behavior by such juristic and spiritual authorities as Gautama, Apastamba, Baudhana, and Yajnavalkya, is that Yoga was already an integral part of India's cultural and moral life in pre-Christian times. Even if Yoga originated largely outside orthodox brahmanical circles, by the beginning of the Christian era it had become so far-flung a tradition that even the lawgivers of the priestly orthodoxy could not ignore it.

With the acceptance of Yoga into mainstream Brahmanism, this once heretical tradition was destined to play an ever more important role in the emergence of the great religious culture of so-called Hinduism. The practical orientation of Yoga proved a constant grounding force for the metaphysical flights, as well as the continuing ritual preoccupations, of the Hindu elite. At the same time, the emphasis on personal experience in Yoga, especially such approaches as Karma-Yoga and Bhakti-Yoga, appealed to the religious-minded individual who was not born into the brahmin caste with its privileged access to the sacred scriptures. Especially with the rise of Tantrism, caste barriers began to be torn down in the field of spirituality. Everyone, regardless of social status or skin color, was, at least in principle, granted access to the highest teachings. The only qualification was that of spiritual readiness.

In the post-Christian era, the person who has done more than anyone else to make Yoga respectable in the eyes of the brahmanical orthodoxy is Patanjali. We will turn to him and his famous aphorisms next.

योग श्रानन्दकल्पनः

chapter 9
Yoga as Philosophy and Religion: Classical Dualist Yoga

PATANJALI: PHILOSOPHER AND YOGIN

Most yogins, like most people, do not have an intellectual bent of mind. But yogins, unlike ordinary people, turn this into an advantage by cultivating wisdom and the kind of psychic and spiritual experiences that the rational mind tends to deny and block out. Yet there has always been a handful of Yoga practitioners who were also brilliant intellects. Thus, Shankara of the early eighth century A.D. is not only remembered as the greatest proponent of Hindu nondualism, or Advaita Vedanta, but also as an adept of Yoga. The Buddhist teacher Nagarjuna, who lived in the second century A.D., was not only a celebrated Tantric alchemist but also a philosophical genius of the first order. In the sixteenth century A.D., Vijnana Bhiksu wrote profound commentaries on all the major schools of thought. He was a noted thinker who greatly impressed the German pioneering indologist and founder of comparative mythology Max Müller. At the same time he was a spiritual practitioner, following Vedanta.

Similarly, Patanjali, the author of the Yoga-Sutra, was obviously a Yoga adept who also had a head on his shoulders. The Yoga of Patanjali represents the climax of a long development of yogic technology. Of all the numerous schools that existed in the early Christian era, Patanjali's was the one to become acknowledged as the authoritative system (darshana) of the Yoga tradition.

Disappointingly enough, we know next to nothing about Patanjali. Hindu tradition identifies him with the famous grammarian of the same name who lived in the second century B.C. The consensus of scholarly opinion, however, considers this unlikely. Both the contents and the terminology of the

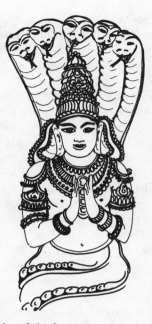

Patanjali, compiler of the famous Yoga-Sutra (after a statue).

Yoga-Sutra suggest the second century A.D. as a probable date for Patanjali, whoever he may have been.

Hindu tradition has it that Patanjali was an incarnation of Ananta, or Shesha, the thousand-headed ruler of the serpent race, which is thought to guard the hidden treasures of the earth. The name Patanjali is said to have been given to Ananta because he desired to teach Yoga on earth and fell (*pat*) from heaven onto the palm (*anjali*) of a virtuous woman named Gonika. Iconography often depicts Ananta as the couch on which God Vishnu reclines. The Lord of Serpents' many heads symbolize infinity or omnipresence. Ananta's connection to Yoga is not difficult to uncover, since Yoga is the secret treasure, or esoteric lore, par excellence. To this day, many yogins bow to Ananta before they begin their daily round of yogic exercises.

In the benedictory verse at the beginning of the Yoga-Bhashya commentary to the Yoga-Sutra, the lord of serpents, Ahisha, is saluted as follows:

> May He who, giving up His original [unmanifest] form, rule to favor the world in many ways — He who is beautifully coiled and many-mouthed, endowed with lethal poisons and yet removing the host of afflictions (klesha), who is the source of all wisdom (jnana) and whose circle of attendant serpents constantly generate pleasure, who is the divine Lord of Serpents: may He, the bestower of Yoga, yoked in Yoga, protect you with His pure white body.

Whatever we can say about Patanjali is purely speculative. It is reasonable to assume that he was a great Yoga authority, most probably the head of a school in which study (svadhyaya) was regarded as an important aspect of spiritual practice. In composing his aphorisms (sutra) he availed himself of existing works. His own philosophical contribution, as far as it can be gauged from the Yoga-Sutra itself, was modest. He appears to have been a compiler and systematizer rather than an originator. It is of course possible that he wrote other works that have not survived.

Western Yoga enthusiasts often regard Patanjali as the father of Yoga, but this is misleading. According to Post-Classical traditions, the originator of Yoga was Hiranyagarbha. Although some texts speak of Hiranyagarbha as a Self-realized adept who lived in ancient times, this tradition is doubtful. The name means "Golden Germ" and in Vedanta cosmo-mythology refers to the womb of creation, the first being to emerge from the unmanifest ground of the world and the matrix of all the myriad forms of creation. Thus, Hiranyagarbha is a primal cosmic force rather than an individual. To speak of him—or it—as the originator of Yoga makes sense when one understands that Yoga essentially consists in altered states of awareness, through which the yogin tunes into nonordinary levels of reality. In this sense, then, Yoga is always revelation. Hiranyagarbha is simply a symbol for the power, or grace, by which the spiritual process is initiated and revealed.

Later Yoga commentators believed that there was an actual person called Hiranyagarbha who had authored a treatise on Yoga. Such a work is indeed referred to by many other authorities, but this does not necessarily say anything about Hiranyagarbha. The most detailed information about that scripture is found in the twelfth chapter of the Ahirbudhnya-Samhita (Collection of the Dragon of the Deep), a medieval work of the Vaishnava tradition. According to this scripture, Hiranyagarbha composed two works on Yoga, one on nirodha-yoga ("Yoga of restriction") and one on karma-yoga ("Yoga of action"). The former apparently dealt with the higher stages of the spiritual process, notably the ecstatic states, whereas the latter is said to have been concerned with spiritual attitudes and forms of behavior.

There may well have been a work on Yoga of this nature, and it may have antedated Patanjali's compilation. The fact is, however, that Patanjali's Yoga-Sutra has eclipsed all earlier Sutra compositions within the Yoga tradition, perhaps because it was the most comprehensive or systematic.

THE CODIFICATION OF WISDOM: THE YOGA-SUTRA

Patanjali gave the Yoga tradition its classical format, and hence his school is often referred to as Classical Yoga. He composed his aphoristic work in the heyday of philosophical speculation and debate in India, and it is to his credit that he supplied the Yoga tradition with a reasonably homogeneous framework that could stand up against the many rival traditions, such as Vedanta, Nyaya, and (not least) Buddhism. His composition is in principle a systematic treatise concerned with defining the most important elements of Yoga theory and practice. At one time, Patanjali's school was enormously influential, as can be deduced from the many references to the Yoga-Sutra, as well as the criticisms of it, in the scriptures of other philosophical systems.

Each school of Hinduism has produced its own Sutra. The Sanskrit word *sutra* means literally "thread," and a Sutra composition is a work consisting of aphoristic statements that together furnish the reader with a thread stringing together all the memorable ideas characteristic of that school of thought. A sutra, then, is a mnemonic device, rather like a knot in one's handkerchief or a scribbled note in one's appointment book.

Just how concise the sutra style of writing is can be gauged from the following opening aphorisms of Patanjali's compilation:

> I.1: *Atha yoga-anushasanam.*
> "Now [commences] the exposition of Yoga."
> I.2: *Yogash citta-vritti-nirodhah.*
> "Yoga is the restriction of the whirls of consciousness."
> I.3: *Tada drashthuh svarupe'vasthanam.*
> "Then [i.e., when that restriction has been accomplished] the 'Seer' [i.e., the transcendental Self] appears."

Of course, such terms as *citta* (consciousness), *vritti* ("whirl"), and *drashtri* ("seer") are themselves highly condensed expressions for rather complex concepts. Even such a seemingly straightforward word as "now" (*atha*), which opens most traditional Sanskrit works, is packed with meanings, as is evident from the many pages of exegesis dedicated to it in some of the commentaries on the Yoga-Sutra.

In his monumental *History of Indian Philosophy,* Surendranath Dasgupta made the following observations about this style of writing:

> The systematic treatises were written in short and pregnant half-sentences (*sutras*) which did not elaborate the subject in detail, but served only to hold before the reader the lost threads of memory of elaborate disquisitions with which he was already thoroughly acquainted. It seems, therefore, that these pithy half-sentences were like lecture hints, intended for those who had had direct elaborate oral instructions on the subject. It is indeed difficult to guess from the sutras the extent of their significance, or how far the discussions which they gave rise to in later days were originally intended by them.[1]

Our knowledge of Patanjala-Yoga is primarily, though not entirely, based on the Yoga-Sutra. As we will see, the many commentaries that have been written on it aid our understanding of this system. But, as scholarship has demonstrated, these secondary works do not appear to have come out of Patanjali's school itself, and therefore their expositions need to be taken with a good measure of discrimination.

The Yoga-Sutra itself consists of 195 aphorisms distributed over four chapters:

1. Samadhi-pada, chapter on ecstasy—51 aphorisms
2. Sadhana-pada, chapter on the path—55 aphorisms
3. Vibhuti-pada, chapter on the powers—55 aphorisms
4. Kaivalya-pada, chapter on liberation—34 aphorisms

This division is somewhat arbitrary and appears to be the result of inadequate reediting of the text. A close study of the Yoga-Sutra shows that in its present form it cannot possibly be considered as a uniform creation. For this reason various scholars have attempted to reconstruct the original by dissecting the available text into subtexts of supposedly independent origins. These efforts, however, have not been very successful, because they left us with inconclusive fragments. It is, therefore, preferable to take a more generous view of Patanjali's work and grant the possibility that it is far more homogeneous than Western scholarship has tended to assume.[2]

At any rate, these scholarly quibbles do not detract from the merit of the work as it is extant today. Now as then, the Yoga practitioner can benefit greatly from the study of Patanjali's compilation.

THE ELABORATION OF WISDOM: THE COMMENTARIAL LITERATURE

Sutras were not created in the first blush of a tradition or school of thought. Rather, they were authoritative summaries that drew on many generations of thinking and debating. But their conciseness proved both a stumbling block and an advantage. On the one hand, the Sutra style gave rise to much ambiguity: As the oral transmission of the teachings became weak, the original ideas and formulations were gradually lost from sight, which encouraged the surfacing of sometimes widely divergent interpretations. For instance, the Brahma-Sutra of Badarayana, a key scripture of Vedanta composed around A.D. 200, was cited in support of nondualistic (advaita) as well as dualistic (dvaita) schools of metaphysics. On the other hand, the inbuilt ambiguity in the Sutra works allowed just such refreshing variation.

Even the most creative minds of traditional India were obliged to weave their innovative thoughts within the framework of their own tradition, whether it was Vedanta, Buddhism, Jainism, or Yoga. They had to take existing authoritative opinion into account or at least pay lip service to it. At any rate, rather than hemming creativity, the Sutras stimulated discussion and dissent. They gave rise to commentaries, which occasioned new commentaries, subcommentaries, and glosses thereon. Patanjali's Yoga-Sutra, too, inspired later generations to produce a considerable commentarial literature.

The Yoga-Bhashya of Vyasa

The oldest extant commentary on the Yoga-Sutra is the Yoga-Bhashya ("Discussion on Yoga") by Vyasa. It was probably composed in the fifth century A.D. Its author is allegedly the same person responsible for the Mahabharata epic, the numerous Puranas (popular encyclopedias), and a host of other works. This idea has no basis in reality. The name Vyasa means "Collector" and was probably more a title than a personal name. In other words, we know as little about Vyasa as we do about Patanjali.

According to legend, Vyasa was the son of the sage Parashara and the nymph Satyavati, whom Parashara had seduced. In appreciation of her beauty and love, the sage not only restored her virginity by magical means but also relieved her of the fishy smell she had inherited from her mother. Vyasa was brought up in secret. Later Satyavati's beauty caught the eye of the aged king Santanu, who promptly fell in love with her. He asked for Satyavati's hand, which her father granted on the condition that it must be her children who would succeed to the throne, not the remaining child from the king's first marriage. Santanu agreed after his grown son Bhishma, whose heroic exploits are told in the Mahabharata, renounced his hereditary rights. The couple lived happily for almost twenty years and had two sons. After Santanu's death the first-born duly ascended the throne, but died during a military adventure. Then his brother, who was married to two women, was crowned. Alas, his rule was also short-lived, for he soon died of consumption. Custom demanded that since he had left no offspring, the nearest male relative should sire a child with either of the two widows. Bhishma disqualified because he had sworn never to have children.

Satyavati called Vyasa to the court to perform this noble duty. The two ladies had expected the stately Bhishma to do the honors. They were shocked when Vyasa, in the scant attire of a hermit, visited their chambers. Vyasa made love first to one widow, then the other. In this way he fathered the blind Dhrishtarashtra and the pale Pandu. On that evening Vyasa also sired a third child—by a maid who acted as a substitute when he wanted to repeat his duty with one of the widows. Dhrishtarashtra was born blind because his mother closed her eyes in shock upon sight of Vyasa, whereas Pandu was born pale because all blood drained from his mother's face when Vyasa approached her. The sage Vyasa, then, is the reason for the great war reported in the Mahabharata between the sons of Dhrishtarashtra and Pandu. We can see in this an ingenious device by which the creator of the Mahabharata epic inserted himself into the story.

Whoever the author of the Yoga-Bhashya may have been, this work contains the key to many of the more enigmatic aphorisms of Patanjali's scripture. However, we have to use it with caution, since several centuries separate the two Yoga authorities. Even though Vyasa was in all likelihood a yogin of considerable attainment, since he writes with great authority about rather esoteric matters, he does not appear to have been in the direct lineage of Patanjali. Some of his interpretations and terminology are at variance with the Yoga-Sutra.

Other Commentaries

The next available commentary is Shankara Bhagavatpada's Vivarana ("Exposition") on the Yoga-Bhashya. Although this is a subcommentary, it is a remarkably original work showing an uncommon exegetical independence. Its author, according to tradition, is none other than the adept Shankara himself, who lived in the eighth century A.D. Western scholarship has been skeptical about this identification, but recent research tends to support this belief, and the very originality of the text speaks for itself. Shankara, who was the greatest spokesman for Advaita Vedanta, was more than a learned pundit; he was also a renowned practitioner of Yoga. It seems likely that prior to his conversion to the nondualist philosophy of Advaita Vedanta, Shankara was a Vishnu devotee and an adherent of the Yoga tradition. He must then have met his teacher Govinda, who expounded to him the "intangible Yoga" (asparsha-yoga) of nondualism taught by Gaudapada, the author of the Mandukya-Karika. It is certainly interesting that of all his writings, Shankara's commentary on the Karika contains the most references to the Yoga tradition.

In contrast to Shankara, Vacaspati Mishra, author of the subcommentary known as Tattva-Vaisharadi ("Clarity of Truth"), was a pundit through and through. Living in the ninth century A.D., he wrote outstanding commentaries on the six classical systems of Hindu philosophy—Yoga, Samkhya, Vedanta, Mimamsa, Nyaya, and Vaisheshika. But his knowledge was theoretical rather than practical. Hence in his gloss on the Yoga-Bhashya, he tends to expand on philological and epistemological matters while leaving important practical considerations unexplained. A story that is told about him suggests how much of a scholar Vacaspati Mishra was. When he had completed his major work, the Bhamati commentary on the Brahma-Sutra, he apologized to his wife for neglecting her for so many years—by dedicating the commentary to her, a truly scholarly recompense. Nonetheless, his work offers many useful clues to some of the more difficult passages of the Yoga-Bhashya.

From the eleventh century, we have two important works. The first is the Arabic translation of the Yoga-Sutra prepared by the renowned Persian scholar al-Biruni—a rendering that may well have exercised a lasting influence on the development of Persian mysticism. The other is the subcommentary known as Raja-Martanda ("Royal Sun-Bird") by King Bhoja of Dhara, an adherent of

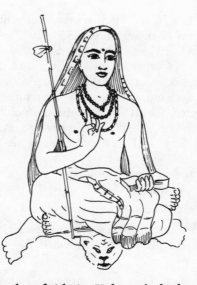

Shankara, the greatest teacher of Advaita Vedanta (radical nondualism), was also a renowned authority on Yoga.

Shaivism. The value of this work is more historical than exegetical. Although Bhoja criticized previous commentators for their arbitrary interpretations, his own efforts are often no less capricious and perhaps less original than he made them out to be. King Bhoja was a great patron of the arts and spiritual traditions, and we must assume that his interest in Yoga was not purely theoretical either.

From the fourteenth century, we have an admirable systematic account of Classical Yoga in Madhava's Sarva-Darshana-Samgraha. As the title indicates, this is a compendium of all the major philosophical systems of medieval India. In the sixteenth century, outstanding commentaries on the Yoga-Bhashya were written by Ramananda and Vijnana Bhikshu. The former's work is entitled Mani-Prabha ("Jewel Lustre"). The latter has authored an elaborate commentary called Yoga-Varttika ("Tract on Yoga") and the Yoga-Sara-Samgraha ("Compendium of the Essence of Yoga"), a digest of his voluminous treatise. Vijnana Bhikshu was a renowned scholar who interpreted Yoga from a Vedantic point of view.

Among the later commentaries on the Yoga-Sutra, we must mention Bhava Ganesha's Dipika ("Torch"), Nagesha's Chaya-Vyakhya ("Explanation of Reflection"), Baladeva Mishra's Pradipika ("Lamp"), Narayana Tirtha's Candrika ("Moonlight") and Sutra-Artha-Bodhini ("Illumination of the Meaning of the Aphorisms"), Sadashiva Indra's Sudhakara ("Mine of Ambrosia"), Nagoji Bhatta's Vritti ("Commentary"), Raghavananda's Patanjala-Rahasya ("Secret of the Patanjala"), Ramabhadra Dikshita's Patanjali-Carita

("Patanjali's Way of Life"), and Hariharananda's twentieth-century Bhasvati ("Elucidation"). Swami Hariharananda (1869–1947) was head of the Kapila Matha in Madhupur (Bihar) and a practitioner of Samkhya-Yoga.

There are a number of other, lesser-known works, known by name only. On the whole, these secondary commentaries do not excel in originality, relying largely on Vyasa's old scholium. The literature of Classical Yoga tends to be dry and repetitive, which drives home the point that Yoga has always been an esoteric discipline, taught by word of mouth. It is definitely not a tradition of book learning. As Dattatreya states in his Yoga-Shastra:

> There will be success for the practitioner (kriya-yukta). [But] how can there be [success] for the nonpractitioner? (83)
>
> Success is never gained through mere reading of books. (84)
>
> Those who [merely] talk about Yoga and wear the apparel [of a yogin] but lack all application and live for their bellies and their dicks—they cheat people. (92–93)

If the Yoga tradition is, by comparison with Vedanta or Buddhism, weak in philosophical acuity and elaboration, it is nevertheless strong in spiritual practice.

THE CHAIN OF BEING: SELF AND WORLD FROM PATANJALI'S PERSPECTIVE

When describing the Buddhist approach to life, the late Lama Anagarika Govinda ventured the following observation:

> Psychology can be studied and dealt with in two ways: either for its own sake alone, i.e. as pure science, which leaves entirely out of account the usefulness or non-usefulness of its results—or else for the sake of some definite object, that is, with a view to practical application. . . .[3]

These remarks apply not only to Buddhism but equally to Yoga. As a form of psychotechnology, Yoga deals first and foremost with the human mind or psyche. But, according to the yogic visionaries, our inner world parallels the structure of the cosmos itself. It is made up of the same fundamental layers that compose the hierarchy of the external world. Hence the "maps" put forward by Patanjali and other spiritual authorities are psychocosmograms, or guides to both the inner and the outer universe. Their principal purpose, however, is to point beyond the levels, or layers, of psyche and cosmos. For the essential nature of the human being, the Self, is held to be an utterly transcendental reality.

The idea of a multilayered or hierarchical cosmos is alien to the reigning paradigm of scientific materialism. Yet it is a vitally important notion in ancient and modern religious and spiritual traditions.

Vast chain of being! which from God began,
Nature's aethereal, human, angel, man,
Beast, bird, fish, insect . . .
. . . from Infinite to thee,
From thee to nothing. —On superior pow'rs
Were we to press, inferior might on ours;
Or in the full creation leave a void,
Where, one step broken, the great scale's destroy'd;
From Nature's chain whatever link you strike,
Tenth, or ten thousandth, breaks the chain alike.

Thus Pope, in his *Essay on Man,* gave poetic expression to the premodern intuition of the hierarchic connectedness of things—the chain of being.

Yoga philosophy shares the same view: The cosmos is a vast structure of interlocking and nested wholes. On the one end of the scale of nature are the material forms, on the other end is the transcendental ground of Nature itself. Beyond that is the dimension of Consciousness, in the form of the formless transcendental Selves (purusha). Yoga philosophy in its function as ontology— science of being—provides the yogin with a map that allows him to traverse the different levels of existence until at the moment of liberation, he leaves the orbit of Nature altogether.

Different schools have devised different maps of the cosmic hierarchy. Patanjali's particular map has frequently been belittled as a borrowing from Classical Samkhya, as formulated about A.D. 350 by Ishvara Krishna in his Samkhya-Karika. The historically accurate view is that Classical Yoga and Classical Samkhya are extreme rationalistic expressions of divergent developments that occurred in the late pre-Christian, or epic, era. As we have seen in connection with the Mahabharata (notably the Moksha-Dharma section), it was in the period around 200 B.C. that Yoga and Samkhya assumed separate identities from their common Vedantic base. Moreover, the Yoga-Sutra is older than the Samkhya-Karika, and therefore if any borrowing has occurred it must surely be on the part of Ishvara Krishna.

There are numerous philosophical differences between Classical Yoga and Classical Samkhya. I have elsewhere proposed that these derive from the different methodologies adopted by these two schools of thought.[4] Whereas Classical Samkhya relies primarily on the exercise of discernment (viveka) and renunciation, Classical Yoga stresses the necessity for the cultivation of ecstatic states (samadhi), in which insight can penetrate the deeper levels of consciousness and the world.

The psychocosmological map put forward by Patanjali is profoundly informed by the territory he discovered in the course of his own explorations of the human psyche—the vast spaces of consciousness, which are correlated to the dimensions of Nature. On the other side, Ishvara Krishna's map gives one the impression of having been sketched on the basis of theoretical considerations and with the hindsight of many centuries of metaphysical speculations within the Samkhya tradition. Both maps, of course, were intended to guide the practitioner to Self-realization. Yet, in the case of Patanjali's map, we are dealing with a device whose ingenuity becomes obvious only when we follow the psychoexperimental path of Yoga and begin to discover the landscapes of our own consciousness through regular meditation—and, if we are so fortunate, occasional plunges into the unified condition of samadhi. Then we also develop an appreciation for the fact that the ancient notion of the chain of being is, contrary to the atomistic ideology of scientific materialism, not merely gray theory.

The Transcendental Self and the Mind

At the apex of that hierarchy of being is the transcendental Reality, the Self (purusha). For Classical Yoga, as for the other schools of Indian spirituality, the Self is the principle of pure Consciousness (cit), or sheer Awareness. It is absolutely distinct from the ordinary consciousness (citta), with its turbulence of thoughts and emotions, which Patanjali explains as the product of the interaction between the transcendental Self (purusha) and insentient Nature (prakriti): The Self's proximity to the highly evolved human organism creates the phenomenon of consciousness. But Nature itself—the human body-mind on its own—is utterly unconscious.

How this absolutely transcendental Self, or pure Awareness, should have any effect on the ongoing processes of Nature is a philosophical problem that none of the spiritual traditions of the world has solved. In particular, Patanjali's radical dualism between Self and Nature does not lend itself to such a solution. Patanjali himself tries to overcome the problem by suggesting that there is some kind of connection, which he calls correlation (samyoga), between the Self and Nature—that is, between pure Awareness and the complex of the body and personality.

That connection is made possible because at the highest level of Nature we find a predominance of the sattva component. The transparency of the sattva factor of Nature is analogous to the transparency or luminosity of the Self. Therefore, Nature (in the form of the psyche or mind) in its sattvic state acts like a mirror for the "light" of the Self.

Since both the Self (or rather the many Selves) and Nature are eternal and omnipresent, the connection between them is also without beginning. For Patanjali this correlation is the real source of all human malaise (duhkha), because it gives rise to the illusion that we are the individuated body-mind, or personality complex, rather than the transcendental Self. Thus, spiritual ignorance (avidya) is at the root of our mistaken identity as the finite egoic body-mind. It is, secondarily, also the source of our attachments and aversions as well as our general hunger for life (the survival instinct). Their attenuation and ultimate transcendence is the objective of the psychotechnology of Yoga.

The Yogic Concept of the Unconscious

The path to Self-realization has two main aspects. The first is dispassion (vairagya), which consists in our disidentification with what is not the Self—that is, with everything that belongs to the realm of Nature. The second aspect is the practice (abhyasa) of identifying with the Self through repeated meditative absorption and ecstasy (samadhi).

Every experience leaves its impression on the psyche, or mind. Ego-derived experiences reinforce the ego-illusion, whereas moments of self-transcendence, in daily life or in the ecstatic state, strengthen the spiritual impulse toward Self-realization.

The carriers of this process of either "egoification" or "spiritualization" are the traits (vasana). These make up the very depth of the human mind. If we liken the psyche to soft wax, then these vasanas are the karmic imprints left behind by our psychic activities. Every single time we sense, feel, think, will, or do anything at all, we create what the yogic authorities style a subliminal activator (samskara). We can picture this as an atom that is added to a string of atoms making up a molecule.

The vasanas, then, are whole chains of similar activators. They are responsible for renewed psychomental activity, in the form of the five types of fluctuations or "whirls" (vritti) spoken of by Patanjali.[5] The activators, combining into complex traits or habit patterns, are the hidden forces behind our conscious life and form the soil of our destiny. For this reason, Patanjali also uses the term "action deposit" (karma-ashaya), or karmic stock, for these stored impressions.

The following example will make this doctrine a little clearer: In entering this passage into my computer, I first of all perform the relatively complex movements of my fingers over the keyboard. In doing so, I exercise a skill I acquired many years ago. I am also aware that I constantly reinforce

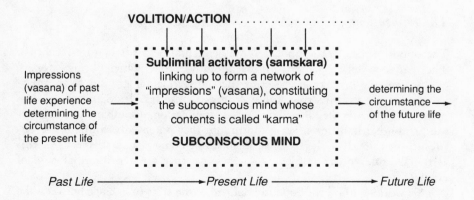

VOLITION/ACTION . . . .

Subliminal activators (samskara)
linking up to form a network of
"impressions" (vasana), constituting
the subconscious mind whose
contents is called "karma"
SUBCONSCIOUS MIND

Impressions (vasana) of past life experience determining the circumstance of the present life

determining the circumstance of the future life

Past Life —————→ *Present Life* —————→ *Future Life*

The Yoga theory of the subconscious is one of the earliest models of depth psychology.

several bad habits, such as the tendency to tighten my shoulder muscles and to squint at the screen. This is a form of karmic conditioning on the simplest level. I am likely to behave similarly the next time I sit down to write.

On a different level, I think about what I am going to write, drawing on my learning and active vocabulary. This too has its karmic aspect, for I am continually propelling my mind to think, and to think in a certain way. From a conventional point of view, this is a desirable activity, because I am said to train and refine my mind. From a spiritual point of view, however, rational thinking coincides with a particular state of being that is not authentic of "me," because "I" am the transcendental Witness-Consciousness, not the contracted ego. "To be in one's head" means not to be present as the entire body. But only when one is bodily present and open at the heart is the Self beyond the ego likely to reveal itself. Therefore, when thinking becomes chronic, because of the subliminal traits set up by the constant exercise of thought, it runs counter to Self-realization.

On a further level, my actions as a writer are imbued with all kinds of spoken and unspoken expectations and motivations, which generate their own karmic impressions. For a subliminal activator to be produced, I need not even be fully aware of my own feelings or moods. Hence even sleep is not exempt from this inexorable process of karmic self-duplication.

In this theory of subliminal activators, Yoga anticipated the modern notion of the unconscious. But it went beyond the insights and goals of psychoanalysis in developing means by which the entire unconscious content can be uprooted. As we learn from the Yoga-Sutra (I.50), unless the traits of subliminal activators are completely transcended through the repeated practice of supraconscious ecstasy (asamprajnata-samadhi), we are trapped in the circle of our own egoic experiences, forever alienated from the Self, which is our true identity.

The Dimensions of Nature

The opposite pole to the multiple transcendental Selves is Nature (prakriti). The Sanskrit term prakriti means literally "that which brings forth" or "procreatrix" and refers to both the transcendental ground of the myriad of manifest forms and those forms themselves. In Samkhya philosophy, the former is also known as foundation (pradhana), which is the primordial undifferentiated continuum that potentially contains the entire universe in all its levels and categories of being. Patanjali speaks of this as the Undifferentiate (alinga), in which we may see a primordial field of energy.

This world-ground is frequently defined as the state of balance between the three types of primary constituents (guna) of Nature, which I will explain shortly. When this primordial balance is disturbed, the process of creation occurs. Then Nature unfolds according to a definite ground plan, whereby simpler principles give birth to ever more complex configurations (called tattva). This theory of cosmic evolution bears the technical name *sat-karya-vada* and also *prakriti-parinama-vada*. The former phrase implies that the effect (karya) is preexistent (sat) in its cause, whereas the latter signifies that the effect is a real transformation (parinama) of Nature, not merely an illusory change as is thought in the idealistic schools of Vedanta and Mahayana Buddhism.

What this position implies is that whatever comes into existence is not a completely new production—out of nothing, as it were—but rather the manifestation (avirbhava) of latent possibilities. Furthermore, the disappearance of an existing object does not mean its total annihilation but merely its becoming latent again—a state that is designated tirobhava. This theory may well have been derived from the kind of metaphysical speculation that we find, for instance, in the Bhagavad-Gita, where Krishna instructs Arjuna about the deathless nature of the transcendental Self. He argues that it is deathless precisely because it is never born; that is, it cannot be destroyed, for it is immune to change.

> Of the nonexistent (asat) there is no coming-into-being (bhava). Of the existent (sat) there is no nonbecoming (abhava). Also, the boundary between these two is seen by the seers of Reality. (II.16)
>
> Yet, know as indestructible that by which this entire [universe] is spread out. No one is able to accomplish the destruction of that which is immutable. (II.17)
>
> Finite, it is said, are these bodies ["owned" by] the eternal embodier [i.e., the Self], the Indestructible, the Incommensurable. Hence fight, O Bharata! (II.18)
>
> He who thinks of It as slayer and he who thinks [that the Self can be] slain—these both do not know. It does not slay nor is It slain. (II.19)
>
> Never is It born or dies. It did not come-into-being, nor shall It ever come to be. This primeval [Self] is unborn, eternal, everlasting. It is not slain when the body is slain. (II.20)

Like the Self, the transcendental core of Nature—pradhana or alinga—is also indestructible. Yet it has the capacity to modify itself, and it does so in the process of creation, or manifestation, during which it gives birth to the multidimensional universe. But Yoga reminds the spiritual practitioner that even though his or her body-mind is a composite of the forces of Nature and is merely a temporary modification, it is also associated with an eternal transcendental aspect, the Self. Upon death, the material and psychic constituents of the body-mind are resolved into their hierarchically simpler forms, until there is only the transcendental ground of Nature. The challenge, both during life and at the moment of death, is to awaken *as* the Self beyond Nature.

Those who fail to do so continue to exist in simpler form on different levels of manifestation until "they" are reborn. At best, they merge into the transcendental ground of Nature, in which case they are known as the Nature-absorbed (prakriti-laya), which is a state of pseudoliberation. Only Self-realization is genuine enlightenment and emancipation.

Cosmic Evolution and the Theory of the Gunas

The Self transcends the primary constituents (guna) of Nature. As has been noted in the discussion of the relationship between Yoga and other Hindu schools of thought in Part One, the guna theory is one of the most original contributions of the Yoga-Samkhya tradition.

The gunas, which can be looked upon as three phases within the same homogeneous field of Nature, produce by their interplay the entire structure of the cosmos, including the psyche. Classical Yoga recognizes four hierarchic levels of existence, whose character is determined by the relative preeminence of any of the three gunas:

1. The Undifferentiate (alinga)
2. The Pure Differentiated (linga-matra)
3. The Unparticularized (avishesha)
4. The Particularized (vishesha)

The Undifferentiate is the transcendental core of Nature, which is pure potentiality. It is without any "mark" (linga), or identifiable characteristic. It simply *is*. Although Patanjali does not state so explicitly, the Undifferentiate is the perfect balance of the three gunas.

Out of the Undifferentiate emerges the Pure Differentiated, or linga-matra, as the first cosmic principle or level of existence. Viewed from a psychological point of view, this is also known as "Pure I-am-ness" (asmita-matra), the *cosmic* sense of individuation. It has its analog in the "I-maker" (ahamkara) or "I-am-ness" (asmita) on the microcosmic or individual human level. From this cosmic sense of individuation evolve the five types of fine structures (tanmatra), or potentials, of sensory experience—sound, touch, form, taste, and smell. These, in turn, give rise to eleven types of senses (indriya) on the one side and the five types of material elements (bhuta) on the other. In other words, it is the principle of Pure I-am-ness that produces both the psycho-mental and the physical realities.

Outside this evolutionary dynamics abide, in perfect autonomy, the numerous transcendental Selves, which are all omnipresent and omnitemporal. But their transcendental status is not obvious to the unenlightened or egoic personality, which confuses the body-mind (a product of unconscious Nature) with the Self. Yoga is a tour de force designed to undermine this confusion and guide us toward authentic existence.

In our journey toward the Self, we must inevitably cross the "ocean" of the conditional reality. This passage takes place not in ordinary space-time but vertically, as it were, through the depths of our multilayered universe. The ontology of Classical Yoga is a rough sketch of the psychocosmic features that the yogin can expect to encounter on his pilgrimage to the Self.

THE EIGHT LIMBS OF THE PATH OF SELF-TRANSCENDENCE

Patanjali's practical spirituality comprises eight aspects, known as the limbs (anga) of Yoga. These are:

1. Restraint (yama)
2. Discipline (niyama)
3. Posture (asana)
4. Breath control (pranayama)
5. Sense-withdrawal (pratyahara)
6. Concentration (dharana)
7. Meditation (dhyana)
8. Ecstasy (samadhi)

One limb builds upon the other, so the eightfold path has sometimes been depicted as a ladder, leading from the common life of self-involvement to the uncommon realization of the Self beyond the ego-personality. This progression can be looked at from a number of perspectives. Seen from one angle, it consists in the growing unification of consciousness; from another angle, it presents itself as a matter of progressive purification. Both viewpoints are present in the Yoga-Sutra.

Ethics

The foundation of Yoga, as of all authentic spirituality, is a universal ethics. Patanjali's first limb, therefore, is not posture or meditation but restraint (yama). This practice includes five important moral obligations, which can be considered the property of all major religions. These are:

1. Nonharming (ahimsa)
2. Truthfulness (satya)
3. Nonstealing (asteya)
4. Chastity (brahmacarya)
5. Greedlessness (aparigraha)

These constitute the great vow (maha-vrata) which, according to the Yoga-Sutra (II.31), must be practiced irrespective of place, time, circumstance, or a person's particular social status. These moral attitudes are meant to bring our instinctual life under control. Moral integrity is an indispensable prerequisite of successful yogic practice.

The most fundamental of all moral injunctions is nonharming, ahimsa. This word is frequently translated as "nonkilling," but this fails to convey its full meaning. Ahimsa is, in fact, nonviolence in thought and action. It is the root of all the other moral norms. The Mahabharata (III.312.76) employs the word *anrishamsya* ("nonmaliciousness") as a synonym of ahimsa.

The physician Caraka, one of the great lights of the naturopathic medicine native to India, observed that doing harm to others reduces one's own life-span, whereas the practice of ahimsa prolongs it because it represents a positive, life-enhancing state of mind. While this is likely to be true, the yogin's motive for cultivating this virtue is a higher one: The desire not to harm another being springs from the impulse toward unification and ultimate transcendence of the ego, which, as the contemporary Western teacher Da Free John observed, is always at war with itself. The yogin seeks to nurture those attitudes that will gradually help him realize what the Bhagavad-Gita (XIII.27) calls the vision of sameness (sama-darshana)—a vision that penetrates beyond the apparent differences between beings, to their transcendental Self-nature.

Truthfulness, satya, is often exalted in the ethical and yogic literature. For instance, in the Mahanirvana-Tantra, we are told:

No virtue is more excellent than truthfulness, no sin greater than lying. Therefore, the [virtuous] man should seek refuge in truthfulness with all his heart. (IV.75)

Without truthfulness the recitation [of sacred mantras] is useless, without truthfulness austerities are as unfruitful as seed on barren land. (IV.76)

Truthfulness is the form of the supreme Absolute (brahman). Truthfulness truly is the best asceticism. All deeds [should be] rooted in truthfulness. Nothing is more excellent than truthfulness. (IV.77)

Nonstealing, asteya, is closely related to nonharming, since the unauthorized appropriation of things of value violates the person from whom they are stolen.

Chastity, brahmacarya, is of central importance in all spiritual traditions, though it is differently interpreted. In Classical Yoga it is defined as abstention from sexual activity, whether in deed, thought, or words. Some authorities, like the Darshana-Upanishad, relax this rule for the married yogin. Moreover, in the medieval tradition of Tantrism, as we will see, a more sex-positive orientation came to the fore, which revolutionized both Hinduism and Buddhism. But even here no unbridled hedonism is embraced. Generally speaking, sexual stimulation is thought to interrupt the yogin's impulse toward enlightenment, or liberation, by feeding his hunger for sensory experience.

Greedlessness, aparigraha, is defined as the nonacceptance of gifts, because they tend to generate attachment and the fear of loss. Thus the yogin is encouraged to cultivate voluntary simplicity. Too many possessions are thought to only distract the mind. Renunciation is an integral aspect of the yogic lifestyle.

Each of these five virtues is said to procure, when fully mastered, certain extraordinary powers (siddhi). For instance, perfection in nonharming creates an aura of peace around the yogin that neutralizes all feelings of enmity in his presence, even the natural hostility between animal species like the cat and the mouse or, as the Yoga commentaries put it, the snake and the mongoose. Through perfect truthfulness the yogin acquires the power of having his words always come true. Perfection in the virtue of nonstealing brings him effortlessly treasures of all kinds, while greedlessness is the key to understanding his present and former births. The reason for this is, presumably, that attachment to the body-mind is a form of greed, whereas greedlessness implies a high degree of nonattachment to material things, including the body, and this loosens the forgotten memories about former existences.

Finally, when the yogin is established in the virtue of chastity, he gains great vigor. All Yoga scriptures agree that sexual abstinence does not turn the yogin into a weakling but, on the contrary, invigorates his body and makes him especially attractive to the opposite gender—a fact that, as some yogins have discovered, can be either a blessing or a curse.

Some later Yoga texts mention an additional five moral precepts:

1. Compassion (daya), active love
2. Uprightness (arjava), moral integrity
3. Patience (kshama), the ability to assume the witnessing consciousness and allow things to unfold as they will
4. Steadfastness (dhriti), the ability to remain true to one's principles
5. Sparing diet (mitahara), which can be considered a subcategory of nonstealing, since overeating is a form of theft from others and from Nature

In a way, all these are subsumed under the five categories of yama, restraint. This creative regulation of one's outgoing energies results in a surplus of energy, which can then be used for the spiritual transformation of the personality.

Self-Discipline

The norms of restraint (yama) are intended to check the powerful survival instinct and rechannel it to serve a higher purpose, regulating the yogin's social interactions. The second limb of Patanjali's eightfold path continues to harness the psychophysical energy freed up by the regular practice of restraint. The constituent elements of discipline (niyama) are concerned with the yogin's inner life. If the five rules of yama harmonize his relationship with other beings, the five rules of niyama harmonize his relationship to life at large and to the transcendental Reality. The five practices are:

1. Purity (shauca)
2. Contentment (samtosha)
3. Austerity (tapas)
4. Study (svadhyaya)
5. Devotion to the Lord (ishvara-pranidhana)

"Cleanliness is next to godliness," preached John Wesley, and Indian puritanism resonates with this judgment perfectly. Purification is a key metaphor of yogic spirituality, and hence it is not suprising that purity should be listed as one of the five disciplines. What is meant by purity is explained in Vyasa's Yoga-Bhashya (II.32), which distinguishes external cleanliness from inner (mental) purity. The former is achieved by such means as baths or proper diet, whereas the latter is brought about by such means as concentration and meditation. Ultimately, the personality in its highest, or sattva, aspect must be so pure that it can mirror the light of the transcendental Self without distortion. From the Maitrayaniya-Upanishad we learn about mental purity:

> The mind is said to be twofold: pure or impure. It is impure from contact with desires; pure when free from desire. When one has liberated the mind from sloth and heedlessness and made it immovable and then attains to the mindless [state], this is the supreme estate. The mind should be restrained within until such time as it becomes dissolved. This is gnosis and salvation; all else is but book knowledge. He whose mind has become pure through absorption and entered the Self, he experiences a bliss impossible to describe in words and only intelligible to the inner instrument [i.e., the psyche]. (VI.34)

Contentment (samtosha) is a virtue praised by sages around the world. In his Yoga-Bhashya (II.32), Vyasa explains it as not coveting more than what is at hand. Contentment is thus a virtue diametrically opposed to our modern consumer mentality, which is driven by the need to acquire ever more to fill the vacuum within. Contentment is an expression of renunciation, the voluntary sacrifice of what is destined to be snatched from us anyway at the moment of death. Contentment is closely allied with the attitude of indifference that has the yogin look upon a lump of earth and a piece of gold with the same coolheadedness. This allows the yogin to experience success or failure, pleasure or sorrow, with unshakable equanimity.

Austerity (tapas), the third component of niyama, comprises such practices as prolonged immobilized standing or sitting; the bearing of hunger, thirst, cold, and heat; formal silence; and fasting. As we have discussed already, the word *tapas* means "glow" or "heat" and refers to the great psychosomatic energy produced through asceticism, which is often experienced as heat. The yogin uses this energy to heat the caldron of his body-mind until it yields the elixir of higher awareness. According to the Yoga-Sutra (III.45), the fruit of such asceticism is the perfection of the body, which becomes robust like a diamond. Tapas must not be confused with harmful self-castigation and fakiristic self-torture.

In the Bhagavad-Gita, three kinds of asceticism are distinguished, depending on the predominance of one or another of the three constituents (guna) of Nature:

Worship of the gods, the twice-born ones [i.e., the members of the priestly caste, the warrior caste, and the merchant caste], the teachers, and the wise, as well as purity, uprightness, chastity, and nonharming—[these are] called asceticism of the body. (XVII.14)

Speech that causes no disquiet and is truthful, pleasant, and beneficial, as well as the practice of study (svadhyaya)—[these are] called asceticism of speech. (XVII.15)

Serenity of mind, gentleness, silence, self-restraint, and purification of the [inner] states—these are called mental asceticism. (XVII.16)

This threefold asceticism practiced with supreme faith by men [who are] yoked and not longing for the fruit [of their deeds] is designated as sattva-natured. (XVII.17)

Asceticism that is performed for the sake of [gaining] good treatment [from others], honor and reverence, or with ostentation—that is called here [in this world] rajas-natured. It is fickle and unsteady. (XVII.18)

Asceticism that is performed out of foolish conceptions [with the aim] of torturing oneself or that has the purpose of ruining another—that is called tamas-natured. (XVII.19)

Study (svadhyaya), the fourth member of niyama, is a significant aspect of yogic praxis. The word is composed of *sva* ("own") and *adhyaya* ("going into") and denotes one's own going into, or delving into, the hidden meanings of the scriptures. The Shata-Patha-Brahmana ("Brahmana of the Hundred Paths"), a pre-Buddhist work, contains the following passage, which vividly describes the extraordinary esteem in which study of the sacred lore was held:

The study and the interpretation [of the sacred scriptures] are [a source] of joy [for the serious student]. He becomes of yoked mind and independent of others, and day by day he gains [spiritual] power. He sleeps peacefully and is his own best physician. He controls the senses and delights in the One. His insight and [inner] glory (yashas) grow, [and he acquires the ability] to promote the world (loka-pakti) [lit., "world-cooking"]. (XI.5.7.1)

Svadhyaya is not intellectual learning; it is absorption into ancient wisdom, or the meditative pondering of the truths revealed by the seers and sages who have walked the spiritual path to those remote regions where the mind cannot follow but only the heart receives and is changed.[6]

The final component of niyama is devotion to the Lord (ishvara-pranidhana), which deserves our special attention. The Lord (ishvara), as has already been stated, is one of the multiple but coalescing transcendental Selves (purusha). According to Patanjali's definition, the Lord's extraordinary status among the many Selves is due to the fact that He can never be subject to the illusion that He is deprived of His omniscience and omnipresence, whereas the other free Selves have at one time experienced this loss, when they deemed themselves to be a particular egoic personality, or finite body-mind. All Selves are of course inherently free, but only the Lord is forever aware of this truth.

The Lord is not a Creator like the Judeo-Christian God, nor the kind of universal Absolute taught in the Upanishads or in the scriptures of Mahayana Buddhism. This has prompted some critics to regard the ishvara as an intruder into Classical Yoga. However, the assertion that the Lord has found His way surreptitiously into the dualistic metaphysics of Patanjali's Yoga is not warranted. It overlooks the entire history of Pre-Classical Yoga, which was clearly theistic. A more reasonable reading of the situation would be that, in his effort to furnish a rational framework for Yoga, Patanjali gave the concept of ishvara a definitional twist that allowed him to incorporate it into his dualistic system. That his solution was barely satisfactory can be gathered from the many criticisms of it in other traditions, and from the fact that Post-Classical Yoga returned to the pantheistic conceptions of the pre-Patanjali schools.

Why did Patanjali pay any attention at all to the ishvara doctrine? The reason is, very simply, that the Lord was more than a mere concept to him and the yogins of his time. It makes sense to assume that the Lord, on the contrary, corresponded to an experience they shared. The idea of grace (prasada) has been an integral element of Yoga from the earliest beginnings, but especially since the rise of such theistic traditions as the Pancaratra, epitomized in the Bhagavad-Gita.

The religious mind is naturally bent to worship the higher Reality. As Swami Ajaya (Allan Weinstock) remarked:

As long as we are engrossed in our own needs, in "I" and "mine" we will remain insecure. . . . Cultivating surrender and devotion replaces such self-preoccupation with a sense of our connection with that which sustains this entire universe. A sense of devotion and surrender opens us to experiences of being nurtured. We also learn that we have the capacity to become instruments of higher consciousness, serving and giving what we can to help others in their own awakening.[7]

Devotion to the Lord is a heart-opening to the transcendental Being who, for the unenlightened individual, is an objective reality and force but who, upon enlightenment, is found to coincide with the yogin's transcendental Self. This is not spelled out in the Yoga-Sutra, but it is implied in the doctrine that all the transcendental Selves, including the ishvara, are eternal and omnipresent; hence even though they are spoken of as many, they must coincide with each other.

In the Yoga-Bhashya (I.23), the mechanics of this process of devotion and grace is explained as follows:

> On account of devotion, [that is,] through a particular love (bhakti) [toward Him], the Lord inclines [toward the yogin] and favors him alone by reason of his disposition. By this disposition only, the yogin draws near to the attainment of ecstasy (samadhi) and the fruit of ecstasy, [which is liberation].

Self-discipline (niyama), in its five forms, is thus more than self-effort, because it entails the element of grace. The yogin does his utmost to understand and transcend the many ways in which the conventional ego-personality endeavors to perpetuate itself. But, in the last instance, the leap from individuated experience to ecstatic Self-realization is a matter of divine intervention.

Posture

The first two limbs, yama and niyama, regulate the yogin's social and personal life in an effort to reduce the production of unwholesome volition, which would only increase his karmic stock. The yogin's goal is to eliminate all karma—that is, all the subliminal activators (samskara) embedded in the depths of his psyche. For this transformation of consciousness to be successful, he has to create the right environmental conditions, within and without. Yama and niyama can be seen as the first steps in this direction. Posture, or asana (lit., "seat"), takes this effort to the next level, that of the body.

For Patanjali, posture is essentially the immobilization of the body-mind. The profusion of postures for therapeutic purposes belongs to a later phase in the history of Yoga. According to the Yoga-Sutra (II.46), one's posture should be stable and comfortable. By folding together his limbs, the yogin achieves an immediate change of mood: He becomes inwardly quiet, which greatly facilitates his endeavor to concentrate the mind. A certain group of postures, known as seals (mudra), are especially potent in altering one's mood because they have a more intense effect on the body's endocrinal system. Beginning Yoga practitioners sometimes find it difficult to detect these inner changes, perhaps because they are paying too much attention to the tensions in the musculature. But with sufficient practice, anyone can discover the mood-altering effects of the different asanas, and then the real inner work can begin. For, as Patanjali tells us, the proper execution of posture makes the yogin insensitive to the impact of the "pairs of opposites" (dvandva), such as heat and cold, light and darkness, quiet and noise.

Breath Control

The whole adventure of Yoga is but a play of the Pranic force. . . .[8]

This quote spells out the signal importance of prana, the life-force, in the adventure of Yoga. When the yogin has become sufficiently aware of his inner environment and is no longer distracted by muscular tensions and external stimuli, he begins to become more and more attuned to the life-force as it circulates in the body. The next step consists in energizing the inner continuum—the experienced body-mind—through the practice of pranayama. Prana, as has often been pointed out, is not merely the breath. The breath is only an external aspect, or a form of manifestation, of prana, which is the life-force that interpenetrates and sustains all life.

The technique of pranayama (lit., "extension of prana") is merely the most obvious way in which the yogin seeks to influence the bioenergetic field of the body. Even the practice of the moral disciplines and the techniques of sensory inhibition and mental concentration are forms of manipulating the pranic force.

Although different researchers have at different times made a case for the existence of prana, their ideas have had little impact on the medical establishment. Some, like the Austrian physician Anton Mesmer (the gray eminence of hypnotism) and the American psychiatrist Wilhelm Reich (inventor of the orgone box), were ridiculed and even persecuted for their innovative ideas. But the idea of bioenergy can be found in many cultures: the Chinese call it chi, the Polynesians mana, the Amerindians orenda. Modern researchers speak of bioplasma. Whatever prana turns out to be—and manifestly a lot more research has to be done before it will be accepted by modern science as reality—it is an experienceable fact for the practitioner of Yoga.

The yogin knows there is an intimate link between the life-force, the breath, and the mind. The Yoga-Shikha-Upanishad declares:

Consciousness (citta) is connected with the life-force indwelling in all beings. Like a bird tied to a string: so is the mind. (59)

The mind is not brought under control by many considerations. The means for its control is nothing else but the life-force. (60)

Through the regulation of the breath, combined with concentration, the life-force of the body-mind can be stimulated and directed. The usual vector is toward the head or, more precisely, the centers of the brain. This will be discussed in more detail in Chapter 13 ("Yoga as Spiritual Alchemy"). At any rate, prana is the vehicle for the ascent of attention within the body, the focusing of awareness along the bodily axis toward the brain. As the breath, or life-force, rises in the body, attention ascends and leads to more and more subtle experiences. In the final stage of this process, the prana is guided into the topmost psychoenergetic center at the crown of the head. When prana and attention come to be fixed in that spot, the quality of consciousness changes radically, yielding the ecstatic state (samadhi).

But this is not the immediate result of pranayama. In the beginning, the regulation of the breath and life-force simply leads to emotional stability, deeper relaxation, inner clarity, and a growing ability to concentrate.

Sense-Withdrawal

The practice of posture and breath control leads to a progressive desensitization to external stimuli. More and more, the yogin comes alive in the inner environment of his mind. When consciousness is effectively sealed off from the environment, this is the state of sensory inhibition known as sense-withdrawal (pratyahara). The Sanskrit texts compare this process to a tortoise contracting its limbs. In the Mahabharata, sense-withdrawal is pertinently described thus:

> The Self cannot be perceived with the senses that, disunited, scatter to and fro and are difficult to restrain for those whose self is not prepared. (XII.194.58)

> Clinging thereto [i.e., to the highest reality], the sage should, through absorption, concentrate his mind to one point by "clenching" the host of the senses and sitting like a log. (XII.195.5)

> He should not perceive sound with his ear, not feel touch with his skin. He should not perceive form with his eyes and not taste tastes with his tongue. (XII.195.6)

> Also, the knower of Yoga should, through absorption, abstain from all smells. He should courageously reject these agitators of the group of five [senses]. (XII.195.7)

Even though the yogin practicing sensory inhibition is described as "sitting like a log," this does not mean he is in a coma. On the contrary, when the senses are shut down one by one, the mind generally becomes very active. This has been demonstrated in experiments on sensory deprivation, such as with the help of samadhi tanks invented by John C. Lilly. Here the subject is completely immersed in salt water in a dark, insulated container. Some subjects start to hallucinate after only a few minutes. In the case of the yogin, of course, the challenge is not to succumb to either hallucinations or sleep, but to hold the mind steady on the object of concentration.

Concentration

As a direct continuation of the process of sensory inhibition, concentration is the "holding of the mind in a motionless state," as the Tri-Shikhi-Brahmana-Upanishad (31) defines this advanced practice. Concentration, the fifth limb of the eightfold path, is the focusing of attention to a given point (desha), which may be a particular part of the body (such as a cakra) or an external object that is internalized (such as the image of a deity).

Patanjali's term for concentration is *dharana,* which stems from the root *dhri,* meaning "to hold." What is being held is one's attention, which is fixed on an internalized object. The underlying process is called ekagrata, which is composed of *eka* ("one, single") and *agrata* ("pointedness"). This one-pointedness, or focused attention, is a highly intensified form of the spurts of concentration that we experience, for instance, in intellectual work. But whereas ordinary concentration is mostly only a heady kind of state, accompanied by a great deal of local tension, yogic dharana is a whole-body experience free from muscular and other tension and therefore having an extraordinary dimension of psychic depth, where the creative inner work can unfold.

In the eleventh-century Katha-Sarit-Sagara ("River Basin of Stories"), a popular collection of tales by Somadeva, we find the following story that shows just how pointed concentration must be.

Vitastadatta was a merchant who had converted from Hinduism to Buddhism. His son, in utter disdain, persisted in calling him immoral and irreligious. Failing to correct his son's obnoxious behavior, Vitastadatta brought the matter before the king. The king promptly ordered the boy's execution at the end of a period of two months, entrusting him to his father's custody until then. Brooding on his fate, the lad could neither eat nor sleep. At the appointed time he was again brought to the royal palace. Seeing his terror, the king pointed out to him that all beings are as afraid of death as he was; therefore, what higher aspiration could there possibly be than practicing the Buddhist virtue of nonharming at all times, including showing respect to one's elders.

The boy, by now deeply repentant, desired to be put on the path to right knowledge. Recognizing his sincerity, the king decided to initiate him by means of a test. He had a vessel brought to him, filled with oil to the brim, and ordered the lad to carry it around the city without spilling a drop, or else he would be executed on the spot. Glad of this chance to win his life, the boy was determined to succeed. Undaunted, he looked neither right nor left, thinking only of the vessel in his hands. He returned at last to the king without having spilled a drop. Knowing that a festival was going on in the city, the king inquired whether the boy had seen anyone at all in the streets. The boy replied that he had neither heard nor seen anyone. The king seemed pleased and admonished him to pursue the supreme goal of liberation with the same single-mindedness and passion.

The practice of concentration is difficult. At the beginning of his book

Waking Up, psychologist Charles Tart challenges his readers to pay continuous attention to the second hand of a watch while simultaneously remaining aware of their breathing. Exceedingly few people can do this without soon veering off in their thoughts. Presumably, those who can maintain constant concentration for even such a relatively short span of time are skilled in meditation or a comparable practice.

Concentration is not only difficult; it is also attendant with perils, as is acknowledged in the Mahabharata:

> It is possible to stand on the sharpened edge of a knife, but it is difficult for an unprepared person to stand in the concentrations of Yoga.
>
> Miscarried concentrations, O friend, do not lead men to an auspicious goal, [but are] like a vessel at sea without a captain. (XII.300.54–55)

The Yoga-Sutra (I.30) enumerates nine obstacles that can arise in the attempt to pacify the inner world, including illness, doubt, and inattention. Yogic concentration is a high-energy state, and it is easy to see how the psychic energy mobilized in it can backfire on the unwary practitioner. As Shankara observed in his Viveka-Cudamani ("Crest Jewel of Discrimination"):

> When consciousness deviates even slightly from the goal and is directed outward, then it sinks, just as an accidentally dropped ball rolls down a flight of stairs. (325)

When consciousness "sinks," it returns to ordinary preoccupations but with a higher psychic charge that can cause the undisciplined practitioner great trouble. Often it galvanizes latent obsessions, notably those related to sexuality. The number of fallen yogins is legend. All esoteric traditions warn the neophyte that, once he or she takes the first step on the path, the only safe direction is forward.

Meditation

Prolonged and deepening concentration leads naturally to the state of meditative absorption, or dhyana, in which the internalized object or locus, such as the image of one's chosen deity, fills the entire space of consciousness. Just as one-pointedness of attention is the mechanism of concentration, "one-flowingness" (eka-tanata) is the underlying process of meditation. All arising ideas (pratyaya) gyrate around the object of concentration and are accompanied by a peaceful, calm emotional disposition. There is no loss of lucidity; on the contrary, the sense of wakefulness appears to be intensified, even though there is little or no awareness of the external environment.

In his highly original work *A Map of Mental States,* the British psychologist John H. Clark aptly characterized dhyana thus:

Meditation is a method by which a person concentrates more and more upon less and less. The aim is to empty the mind while, paradoxically, remaining alert.

Normally, if we empty our minds, as we do when we settle down to sleep—for instance, "counting sheep" to narrow our thoughts—we become lethargic and eventually go to sleep. The paradox of meditation is that it both empties the mind and, at the same time, encourages alertness.[9]

The initial purpose of yogic meditation is to intercept the flux of ordinary mental activity (vritti), which comprises the following five categories:

1. Pramana—knowledge derived from perception, inference, or authoritative testimony (such as the sacred scriptures)
2. Viparyaya—misconception, perceptual error
3. Vikalpa—conceptual knowledge, imagination
4. Nidra—sleep
5. Smriti—memory

The first two kinds of mental activity are disposed of by the practice of sense-withdrawal. The tendency toward conceptualization gradually diminishes as meditation deepens. Sleep, which is due to a preponderance of the tamas (inertia) constituent, is also overcome by maintaining a state of wakeful attentiveness in the practice of concentration and meditation. Memory, the source of the mechanically arising thought fragments or imagery that are so troubling to the beginner, is the last to be blocked out. It is still active in the lower ecstatic states, where it generates presented ideas (pratyaya) of the nature of spontaneous insights. Memory is fully transcended only in the highest type of ecstatic realization, which is known as asamprajnata-samadhi. In this sublime condition of temporary identification with the Self, the subliminal activators (samskara) responsible for the externalization of consciousness are uprooted. Memory can be said to have two aspects, a gross one that is effectively disabled through meditation, and a subtle one that is neutralized through the supraconscious ecstasy.

The process of restriction (nirodha) has three major levels:

1. Vritti-nirodha, the restriction of the five categories of gross mental activity (vritti) in meditation, mentioned above.
2. Pratyaya-nirodha, the restriction of the presented ideas (pratyaya) in the various types of conscious ecstasy (samprajnata-samadhi). Thus, the yogin must go beyond the spontaneously arising insights or thoughts (vitarka) in the ecstatic state of savitarka-samapatti, described in the next section, just as he must go beyond the feeling of bliss (ananda) in the ecstatic state of ananda-samapatti, which is also described below.
3. Samskara-nirodha, the restriction of the subliminal activators in the supraconscious ecstasy (asamprajnata-samadhi). In this elevated

state, the yogin disables the depth memory itself, whose traits constantly generate new psychomental activity.

Ecstasy

In the same way in which concentration, when sufficiently acute, leads to meditative absorption, the ecstatic state (samadhi) ensues when all the "whirls" (vritti) of the ordinary waking consciousness are fully restricted through the practice of meditation. Thus, concentration, meditation, and ecstasy are phases of a continuous process of mental unification; this process, when it unfolds in relation to the same internalized object, is called constraint (samyama) by Patanjali.

The ecstatic condition, as the culmination of a long and difficult process of mental discipline, is as elusive a phenomenon as it is crucial to a proper appraisal of Yoga. It has often been interpreted as a self-hypnotic trance, a relapse into unconsciousness, or even an artificially induced schizophrenic state. But these labels are all inadequate. What is seldom understood is, first, that samadhi comprises a great variety of states and, second, that those who have actually experienced this unified condition in its various forms unanimously confirm that mental lucidity is one of its most striking features. Yoga psychologists are well acquainted with pseudoecstatic states that can rightly be understood as relapses into unconsciousness (jadya).

Genuine samadhi, however, is always accompanied by suprawakefulness—a point that, for instance, C. G. Jung failed to appreciate, and his views are still being echoed by others. Even if we were to find the cultivation of the different samadhi states impractical or undesirable, we cannot deny that they are stations on a road that leads not to a diminution of consciousness or of the human being, but to a greater reality and good. The great significance of India's psychotechnology for our age lies precisely in that it has amassed evidence for the existence of a condition of being, namely the condition of Self-Identity or transcendental Being-Consciousness, about which modern science is ignorant and which is barely recognized in our Western spiritual heritage.

For this reason, we must be cautious about passing summary judgment on yogic states, ideas, and practices—unless we have tested them in the unbiased manner for which science prides itself. As Mircea Eliade, world-renowned authority on spirituality and mythology, warned in his groundbreaking work on Yoga:

> Denial of the reality of the yogic experience, or criticism of certain of its aspects, is inadmissable from a man who has no direct knowledge of its practice, for yogic states go beyond the condition that circumscribes us when we criticize them.[10]

Although it is possible to define samadhi formally, no amount of description can fully convey the nature of this extraordinary condition, for which there is no reference point in our everyday life. Its most momentous component is undoubtedly the experience of complete fusion between subject and object: The yogin's consciousness assumes the nature of the contemplated object. This identification is accompanied by acute wakefulness, a mood of bliss, or the sense of mere existence, depending on the level of ecstatic unification.

Patanjali has elaborated a phenomenology of samadhi states that is distilled from centuries of yogic experience. He distinguishes between two major species of samadhi, namely conscious ecstasy (samprajnata-samadhi) and

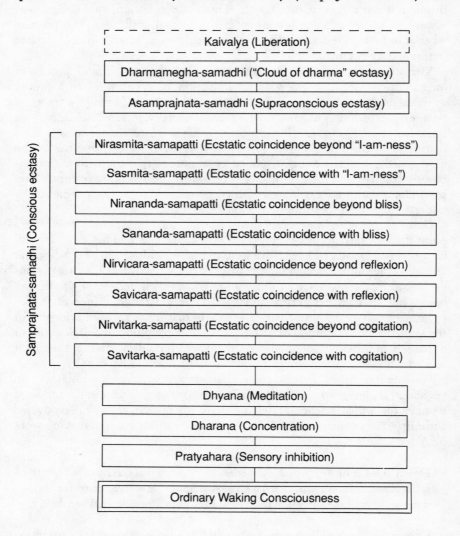

Types of ecstatic practice (samadhi) according to Patanjali's classical school of Yoga.

supraconscious ecstasy (asamprajnata-samadhi). These correspond to the Vedanta distinction between ecstasy tied to a particular form (savikalpa-samadhi) and formless ecstasy (nirvikalpa-samadhi) respectively.

Whereas supraconscious ecstasy is of a single type, conscious ecstasy has a variety of forms. These forms also bear the technical designation of "co-incidence" (samapatti), because subject and object coincide. The simplest form is vitarka-samapatti, which is ecstatic unification in regard to the coarse aspect of an object. For instance, if the object of contemplation is a particular deity—say, the blue form of four-armed Krishna—the yogin entering samadhi now becomes one with Krishna's image. That image is vividly experienced as a living reality, so that the yogin experiences himself as Krishna. His unified experience is interspersed with all kinds of spontaneous (nondiscursive) thoughts, but, unlike during meditation, these do not disrupt his ecstatic enjoyment. Upon the cessation of all ideation (vitarka), the yogin enters the supracogitative ecstasy (nirvitarka-samadhi).

The next higher or deeper level of ecstatic unification occurs when the yogin identifies with the subtle dimension of his object of contemplation. In our example, he would experience himself as Krishna on progressively less differentiated planes of existence, until there is only the irresoluble matrix of Nature left. This condition, again, has two forms, depending on the presence or absence of spontaneous thoughts. The first is known as reflexive ecstasy (savicara-samadhi), the second as suprareflexive ecstasy (nirvicara-samadhi).

According to Vacaspati Mishra's interpretation of the Yoga-Sutra as embodied in his ninth-century Tattva-Vaisharadi, there are four additional levels of subtle unitary experience: sa-ananda-samapatti ("coincidence with bliss"), sa-asmita-samapatti ("coincidence with I-am-ness"), nirananda-samapatti ("coincidence beyond bliss"), and nirasmita-samapatti ("coincidence beyond I-am-ness"). The first type consists in the experience of pervasive bliss. The second type is simply the overwhelming sense of being present, in our case as the very essence of Krishna. There is a sense of "I," or individuated existence, but no longer any role identity. The I is expanded infinitely. It is rather difficult to gain even an intuitive sense of the content of the third and the fourth types. We may question that the scholar Vacaspati Mishra actually experienced these additional types of ecstasy for himself or whether they were merely inferred by him. At any rate, Vijnana Bhikshu, who was a yoga practitioner, explicitly rejected the last two types of ecstasy.

All these types are forms of conscious ecstasy (samprajnata-samadhi). They are experiential states in which the ego-personality is partially transcended. From one perspective, they can even be regarded as means of obtaining knowledge about the universe through the capacity of the human consciousness for chameleon-like identification with the object of contemplation.

Radically different from these ecstatic states is the supraconscious ecstasy (asamprajnata-samadhi), which coincides with temporary Self-realization.

Here, for the duration of the experience, the yogin transcends the realm of Nature and identifies with his authentic being, the Self (purusha). This presupposes a total turnabout, or metanoia, in his consciousness, a complete transformation of the body-mind. It cannot be accomplished through sheer exertion of will. Rather, the yogin must empty and open himself to the higher Reality beyond the ego-personality. Since this is not something he can initiate at will, the moment of radical opening is often described, as we have seen, in terms of the intervention of grace.

Asamprajnata-samadhi is the only avenue to recover conscious awareness of the transcendental Self-Identity and its eternal freedom. In this supraconscious ecstasy, there is neither an object of contemplation nor a contemplating subject. To the ordinary mind it appears as a state of frightening voidness. When maintained over a sufficiently long period, the fire of this ecstasy gradually transmutes the unconscious, obliterating all the subliminal activators (samskara) that lead to renewed ego-conscious activity and the resultant karma.

At the peak of this ecstatic unification, the yogin reaches the point of no return. He becomes liberated. According to the dualistic model of Classical Yoga, this implies the dropping of the finite body-mind. The liberated being abides in perfect "aloneness" (kaivalya), which is a transmental state of sheer Presence and Pure Awareness. Some schools of Vedanta, which hold that the ultimate Reality is nondual, argue that liberation does not have to coincide with the death of the physical body. This is the ideal of liberation in life (jivan-mukti). Patanjali, however, does not appear to have subscribed to it. For him, the yogin's greatest good lies in severing himself completely from the round of Nature (prakriti) and abiding merely as the attributeless Self, one among many and, as we must assume, intersecting with all other Selves in eternal infinity. This is also the ideal of Classical Samkhya, whose philosophical approach is equally rationalistic.

It is difficult to imagine what such untarnished Selfhood would be like, even when one has had glimpses of ego-transcendence in meditation. What is clear is that, by definition, it is not an experience, because there is neither a subject nor an object left to give rise to the knowledge connection. But neither is it a state of unconsciousness. All realizers agree that it is an utterly desirable condition, worthy of our absolute commitment.

The laborious path of Yoga leads thus beyond itself. Yogic psychotechnology is merely a ladder that the spiritual practitioner climbs, only to cast it off in the last moment. Patanjali's formulations are useful only to the degree that they can guide us to that instant of recognizing our inherent freedom, which gives us the authority and power to see Reality in its nakedness and to go beyond all formulations, creeds, dogmas, models, theories, and points of view.

योग स्रानन्दकल्पनः

chapter 10

The Nondual
Approach to God:
Post-Classical Yoga

OVERVIEW

Everything is only the Absolute (brahman). There is no other. I am That. Verily, I am That. I am only That. I am only That. I am only the everlasting Absolute. (31)

I am only the Absolute, not the worldling (samsarin). I am only the Absolute. I have no mind. I am only the Absolute. I have no wisdom-faculty (buddhi). I am only the Absolute, and not the senses. (32)

I am only the Absolute. I am not the body. I am only the Absolute, not the "cow-pasture" [i.e., the field of cosmic existence]. I am only the Absolute. I am not the psyche (jiva). I am only the Absolute, not differentiated existence. (33)

I am only the Absolute. I am not unconscious. I am the Absolute. There is no death for me. I am only the Absolute, and not the life-force (prana). I am only the Absolute, higher than the highest. (34)

Everything is only the Absolute. The triple world is pure Consciousness, the pure Absolute. There is nothing but Bliss, supreme Bliss (parama-ananda). (42)[1]

The experience of ecstatic unity expressed in the above passage is at the heart of the Upanishadic tradition. The sages of the early Upanishads were the first to speak of this grand realization so explicitly and with unbridled enthusiasm. Their nondualist metaphysics was an attempt to find a rational explanation for what was a living experience for them. This realization of all-embracing unity (ekatva) is more difficult to accommodate in Patanjali's dualistic framework. However, it is not impossible to do so, because Patanjali still regards Nature

199

(prakriti) as the transcendental source of all manifest forms. Yet, for him, merging with the ground of the world is not equivalent to gaining liberation. As Patanjali sees it, there can be no ultimate salvation within the province of Nature. True liberation involves going beyond all of Nature's dimensions, including its transcendental basis (pradhana).

Only the realization of the transcendental Self (purusha) amounts to genuine everlasting freedom. This, however, is not a matter of union but of simple identity. Self-realization is the yogin's awakening to his authentic or essential being, which abides forever beyond the orbit of Nature, vast as it is.

Patanjali did not accept the Upanishadic or Vedantic equation of the transcendental Self (atman) with the transcendental Ground of Nature, called brahman. Even though his Yoga-Sutra was very influential, his dualistic metaphysics has always been considered an oddity within the fold of Hinduism. Most Yoga schools during his time and in subsequent periods espoused some form of nondualism as it had been taught since the early Upanishads. The Yoga teachings that succeeded Patanjali but did not adopt his dualistic metaphysics can be referred to collectively as Post-Classical Yoga.

The Post-Classical literature of Yoga is even more diversified and richer in content than the Pre-Classical. First of all, there are the yogic teachings of the so-called Yoga-Upanishads. These are scriptures from various epochs and geographical areas, which represent different points of view within the Yoga tradition. They will be discussed in more detail shortly. Then there are the yogic teachings found scattered in the vast Purana literature, again dating from around the time of Patanjali to the twelfth century A.D. The Puranas, as we will see, are popular encyclopedias that contain, among other things, brief treatments of Yoga and numerous fascinating stories about aspirants and masters of Yoga.

Another rich mine of Yoga teachings is the Samhitas ("Collections"), the religious works of the Vaishnavas, both of the north and south of the Indian peninsula. The same is true of the Agamas ("Traditions"), the religious writings of the Shaivas, and likewise the Tantras ("Looms") of the Shakti worshippers. These "sectarian" literatures have been barely researched, and their teachings are incredibly intricate. In presenting them, I can do no more than scratch the surface.

An important phase of Post-Classical Yoga, covering the period from approximately the seventh to seventeenth centuries A.D., is represented by the schools belonging to the tradition of body-culture (kaya-sadhana), such as the Siddha movement and Nathism. These include orientations like Hatha-Yoga that seek to accomplish Self- or God-realization by probing the spiritual potential of the human body. These schools will be discussed over several sections of this chapter, because of their significance with regard to the development of Hinduism and because of the growing attention they receive in the West.

A Post-Classical work that deserves to be singled out for special treatment is the tenth-century Yoga-Vasishtha. Its radical idealism has for centuries been an unfailing inspiration, particularly to Hindus of the Himalayan region. I will introduce this remarkable poetic creation in the final section of the present chapter.

We will start this treatment of Post-Classical Yoga with the more extreme sects of the ramified Shaiva tradition. Some of their practices are rather radical, inasmuch as they severely challenge conventional morality. They are considered to be "left-hand" schools because they champion the literal enactment of the ultimate truth of nonduality, while the "right-hand" schools, by and large, condone only the symbolic expression of that truth. The difference between these two approaches is best epitomized in their contrasting attitudes to sexuality. While the adherents of the right-hand schools generally see sexuality as a threat to spiritual growth, the followers of the left-hand schools of Shaivism employ sexuality for their spiritual transformation.

In India, as in many other parts of the world, the left side is associated with evil, and the right with good. The Sanskrit term *vama-acara* ("left conduct") has negative connotations in conventional contexts. It is used by the left-hand schools themselves, but not because they admit to being partial to evil. Rather, in their exploration of our spiritual potential, they acknowledge the existence of the dark or shadow aspects of the human personality and of life in general. More than that, they actively associate with that which the "normal" person fears, avoids, or represses. The reason for this eccentric approach is partly to reclaim the repressed aspects of human existence and partly to demonstrate that life can and should be lived, under all circumstances, from the point of view of the ultimate truth of nonduality: If there is only the One Being, then, to put it bluntly, It must also be the essence of genitals, death, and garbage.

THE LEFT-HAND FOLLOWERS OF SHIVA: "SKULL-BEARERS," "PHALLUS-WEARERS," AND OTHER ASCETICS

In their quest for ultimate security and happiness, the spiritual seekers of India have, as have those of other countries, at times ventured into territory that lies well outside the social establishment. There were and still are individuals and small groups whose practices look extreme, even bizarre, to the conventional mind.

Hindus have the reputation of being exceptionally tolerant in matters of religion, and indeed no culture on earth has produced so much variety in its religious practices and ideas as Hinduism. But even the ordinary Hindu looks askance at some of the manifestations of religious fervor and spiritual aspiration that make up the colorful tapestry of Hinduism. In this respect, he is no different from the well-groomed New York businessman of the 1980s who raises his brows when he passes a long-haired latter-day hippie playing guitar at a street corner. In both cases powerful biases are at work. It is important to remember this in the following discussion of some of the more unusual manifestations of Hindu spirituality.

In the Mahabharata epic (XII.337.59), five religious traditions are mentioned as being prominent: the followers of the sacrificial religion of the Vedas, Yoga, Samkhya, Pancaratra, and Pashupata. Here we are interested in the Pashupata tradition, which is a particular phase in the development of the religious community of Shaivism that identifies the Absolute with God Shiva.

The Pashupata Tradition

The Pashupatas actually formed a religious order; in all probability an ascetic named Lakulisha, who may have lived in the second century A.D., was its founder. We know of him only through legends. The name Lakulisha means literally "Lord of the Club" and is explained by the fact that the Pashupatas carried a club (lakula) as one of their sectarian insignia. Lakulisha, or Lakulin ("Club-Carrier"), was venerated as an incarnation of God Shiva himself.

According to the Karavana-Mahatmya, a relatively recent work, he was born into a brahmin family of what is now Gujarat. He was an extraordinary child, possessing all kinds of superhuman powers. However, Lakulin died in his seventh month. His grieving mother cast his tiny body into the river. A group of tortoises carried it to the holy site of Jaleshvara-Linga, where the life-force reentered his limbs. He was brought up as an ascetic and later became a renowned teacher. According to one set of legends, Lakulin died after a life of severe austerities, and Shiva entered his body to reanimate it so that the Pashupata doctrine could be disseminated in the world.

Lakulin is said to have had four principal disciples, and sometimes the name of Patanjali is added as a fifth. But this is doubtful, since nowhere in the Yoga-Sutra is there any suggestion of Patanjali condoning the extreme practices for which the Pashupata sect was notorious. The connection between Patanjali and Lakulin, however, is not without historical interest, because it strengthens the traditional claim that Patanjali belonged to the tradition of Shaivism.

Hindu iconography typically depicts Lakulin seated in the lotus posture, with a citron in his right hand and a club in his left, and his penis stiff with life-force. We may see in the club and citron the symbols of the male and female aspects of the Divine respectively, though undoubtedly they have other esoteric significances as well. The erect penis suggests not sexual licentiousness but mastery of the sexual drive and the conversion of semen into the mysterious ojas, or subtle force, that is an important part of the alchemical processes occurring in the body of the Yoga adept.

What was so controversial about the Pashupatas was their insistence on shocking the public with their eccentric behavior, such as babbling, making snorting sounds, imitating the walk of a cripple, pretending to suffer from tremor of the limbs, making foolish statements, and making sexual gestures in the presence of women. With these escapades they sought to court public disapproval, which would test their capacity for humility and self-transcending practice. In his commentary on the Pashupata-Sutra, Kaundinya observes:

> He should appear as though mad, like a pauper, his body covered with filth, letting his beard, nails, and hair grow long, without any bodily care. Hereby he cuts himself off from the estates (varna) and stages-of-life (ashrama), and the power of dispassion is produced. (III.1)

But there was a further purpose to this strange practice. The Pashupatas thought that by attracting censure, they absorbed the bad karma of others while transferring their own good karma to them, thereby enhancing their impulse toward total transcendence of the realm of good and bad. This curious practice is known as the pashupata-vrata, or "Pashupata vow."

As is evident from the Pashupata-Sutra, ascribed to Lakulisha, the earlier schools of this tradition were heavily ritualistic, and philosophy played only a secondary role. The ritual Yoga of the Pashupatas included many ecstatic practices, such as singing, dancing, and laughter. But these were only engaged in the unmanifest (avyakta) or concealed state, when the initiates were amongst themselves, whereas the above-mentioned eccentric behavior was displayed in the manifest (vyakta) or public state, when they removed all identifying sectarian marks and behaved like complete outcastes.

The Pashupatas were surprisingly successful, and their order grew rapidly in size and influence. By the sixth century, Pashupata temples were scattered throughout India. There are two possible explanations for the success of this sectarian movement. The first is that it offered a sense of belonging that was not based on the prevalent caste hierarchy. The second is that the movement promised active participation in simple religious rituals, as well as an emotion-based experience of the sacred.

The philosophical elaboration of the Pashupata sect began with Kaundinya, who composed his Panca-Artha-Bhashya ("Commentary on the Five Topics [of the Pashupata-Sutra]") sometime in the fifth century A.D. A further level of philosophical sophistication is present in the Gana-Karika, attributed to a certain Haradatta. It has a fine commentary called Ratna-Tika ("Jewel of Exposition"), by the famous tenth-century logician Bhasarvajna.

In brief, the Pashupatas are theists. The Lord (ishvara) is the creator, sustainer, and destroyer of the world. He comprises a manifest and an unmanifest aspect and is utterly independent of the world. He has unlimited power of knowledge (jnana-shakti) and unlimited power of action (kriya-shakti). One of the most controversial dogmas of the Pashupatas is the notion that the Lord's will is entirely independent of the law of karman. He can, theoretically, reward evildoers and punish the good. The consummate state of liberation, which is called the "end of suffering" (duhkha-anta), is entirely a gift of grace (prasada). This is explained as a state of undiminished attention (apramada) on Reality.

Prior to liberation is the accomplishment of the condition of yoga, which is defined as "the union of the self (atman) with the Lord." As is made clear in the Pashupata-Sutra (V.33) itself, this union is not a complete merging of the self with the ultimate Reality, as in nondualistic Vedanta, but a form of transcendental bonding, which Lakulisha gives the technical designation of *rudra-sayujya*, "alliance with Rudra," Rudra being Shiva. Here the yogin's body-mind is constantly informed by the Divine, and his practice consists in continual surrender to Shiva.

The liberated being shares in most of the transcendental capabilities of the Lord, such as freedom from fear and death and lordship over the universe. As in Classical Yoga, the relationship between the liberated beings and the Lord is a curious one: Although they are absolutely one with God, God is at the same time something more than those liberated beings, either individually or collectively. Whereas Patanjali rejected the deistic idea of the Lord as Creator, Lakulisha celebrated Shiva as Pashupati, the Lord of Beasts. The beasts (pashu) are none other than the fettered souls that, in birth after birth, are forever recycled in the great ecology of Nature—unless they experience the grace of Shiva.[2]

The Kalamukha Order

Lakulisha was also venerated by the Kalamukhas, a well-organized sect that developed out of the Pashupata tradition. None of their scriptures have survived, and we know of their beliefs and practices only from the writings of their critics. The Kalamukha order may have originated in Kashmir. It thrived, together with the Pashupata order, in the southeast of the peninsula between the eleventh and thirteenth centuries A.D. It appears that there may have been migration of Lakulisha adherents from north to south at the beginning of the eleventh century, perhaps because they had lost patronage in Kashmir.

The name *kalamukha*, meaning "black-faced," probably derives from the fact that these ascetics wore a striking black mark on the forehead, indicating their renunciation. They existed in two major divisions, known as the power assembly (shakti-parishad) and the lion assembly (simha-parishad), which had their own subdivisions. We may speculate that the former were in practice and theory oriented more toward the female or power aspect of the Divine, whereas the latter's orientation was more toward the male or Shiva aspect of the transcendental Reality.

The Kalamukhas were fond of learning and had a special relationship with the Nyaya school of thought, a traditional system of logic. Thus, according to one epigraphic record, Someshvara, a renowned teacher of the Kalamukha order, received in A.D. 1094 a generous donation from his township in recognition of his great yogic accomplishments and his equally great learning in the arts and sciences. As is clear from many other temple inscriptions, the

Kalamukhas laid great store by the careful observance of the moral virtues codified by Patanjali under the categories of moral observance (yama) and self-restraint (niyama). The epigraphic evidence does not bear out the widespread belief that the Kalamukhas practiced revolting and obscene rituals. It appears that they were commonly confused with another Shaiva order, the infamous Kapalikas, who definitely did not belong to mainstream Shaivism but were Tantric in character.

The Kapalikas

The early history of the Kapalikas ("Skull-Bearers"), also called Mahavratins ("Great-Vowed"), is unknown. They got their name from the strange custom of carrying around a human skull, which served as a ritual implement and an eating utensil. References to skull-bearing are found already in pre-Christian works, but it appears that the Kapalika order originated only toward the middle of the first millennium in the south of India. Certainly by the sixth century A.D. the Kapalikas were frequently referred to in the Sanskrit literature.

As in the case of the Kalamukhas, no Kapalika scriptures have come down to us, and the little we know of them stems largely from the opponents of this extreme form of asceticism, though we also have a few positive (or at least neutral) accounts. For the most part these descriptions seem accurate, since to this day the small group of surviving Kapalikas in Assam and Bengal engages in the practices for which they have been notorious for many centuries.

In his Harsha-Carita, a beautifully crafted but incomplete Sanskrit biography of the seventh-century king Harsha, the celebrated court poet Bana describes an encounter between King Pushpabhuti and the Kapalika adept Bhairava. The ascetic accepted the king into pupilage and soon asked him to participate in the kind of nocturnal rite for which the Kapalikas were famous. After anointing a corpse with red sandalwood, Bhairava, painted black and wearing only black garments and ornaments, seated himself on its chest. Then he lit a fire in the corpse's mouth and offered black sesame seeds into it, while reciting magical incantations. Suddenly the ground before them split open and a fierce-looking spirit entity emerged and attacked Bhairava, the king, and three other disciples who were present. Bhairava managed to disable the entity but refused to kill it and was later rewarded for his mercy by Goddess Lakshmi. At any rate, the ritual proved successful and Bhairava acquired the status of a vidya-dhara, possessor of wisdom.

That not all Kapalikas were such relatively benign individuals is brought home by another story, found in the Dasha-Kumara-Carita ("Biography of the Ten Princes") by the renowed seventh-century poet Dandin. According to this story, Mantragupta, one of the ten princes, overheard a husband and wife complain that they had to constantly do chores for their teacher, so that they had no time for each other. They called their guru a black magician (dagdha-siddha)—literally "burnt adept." Curious about it all, the prince surreptitiously followed them back to their teacher's hermitage.

Soon Mantragupta spotted the adept seated at a fire. He was smeared with ashes and wore a necklace of human bones, and his appearance was quite frightening. Then the prince heard the magician sternly order his hapless servants to sneak into the palace and abduct the king's daughter, which they did. The prince remained in hiding. Then, to his horror, he saw the magician swing his sword to decapitate the princess. Just in time, Mantragupta jumped forward, seized the sword, and beheaded the magician instead.

In Madhava's Shankara-Dig-Vijaya ("Shankara's World Conquest"), a fourteenth-century biography of Shankara, the great teacher of nondualist Vedanta, there is another worthwhile story. One day, so the story goes, a cruel-hearted Kapalika approached the venerable Shankara, praising him as a true adept who has realized the Self and begging him for mercy. Shankara listened to him openheartedly, but with sublime indifference. The Kapalika explained that he had been performing austerities for a hundred years to win Shiva's favor. He wanted to ascend into Shiva's heavenly domain with the physical body, and Shiva promised that he would fulfill this desire if the Kapalika were to offer him the head of a king or an all-knowing sage. Having failed to procure the head of a king, the Kapalika now asked for Shankara's head. He had gauged the great adept correctly, for Shankara agreed without a moment's hesitation. He fixed a time and place where the transaction could take place without the knowledge of Shankara's disciples, who would surely try to prevent the decapitation. At the appointed hour Shankara entered into the state of formless ecstasy (nirvikalpa-samadhi), patiently awaiting the sword blow across his neck.

The Kapalika approached him with eyes rolling wildly from alcohol intoxication. He raised his trident to lop off Shankara's head. In that moment, Padmapada, one of Shankara's main disciples, saw in his mind's eye what was about to happen. He uttered an invocation to his chosen deity, Nri-Simha, the Man-Lion incarnation of God Vishnu. Instantly the disciple assumed the god's leonine form and flew through the air to the secret hiding place. Just as the Kapalika swung his trident, Padmapada jumped on him and tore open his chest. Shankara returned to his ordinary consciousness and, seeing the mutilated body of the Kapalika and the blood-drenched shape of Nri-Simha before him, begged the god to withdraw his terrific aspect and manifest mercy instead. Thereupon Padmapada regained his ordinary consciousness and form and promptly prostrated himself at his teacher's feet.

There undoubtedly were villains and psychotics among the Kapalikas, but most were probably content with wearing skulls stolen from cemeteries where they practiced their strange magical rituals. And there were a few genuine masters, like the Buddhist adept Kanha of the eleventh century A.D. who calls himself a skull-bearer (kapalin). He speaks of mating with and then killing the licentious washerwoman (dombi), who here stands for the female aspect of the transcendental Reality. To murder the Shakti means to transcend her.

This contains a reference to the sexual practices of the Kapalikas. Though renunciates, they gathered every spring and autumn for a big orgiastic ceremony. In the course of the ceremony they performed the "five M's" for which Tantrism achieved notoriety: the consumption of liquor (madya), meat (mamsa), fish (matsya), and parched grain (mudra), which is thought to have aphrodisiacal properties, as well as the performance of ritual intercourse (maithuna) with specially prepared women.

The Kapalikas were, like the Pashupatas and Kalamukhas, worshippers of Shiva—but Shiva in his terrifying aspect as Bhairava. The purpose of all the Kapalika rites was to achieve communion with God, through which the practitioner acquired both superhuman powers (siddhi) and liberation. They offered human flesh in their ceremonies and have been accused—probably rightly—of performing human sacrifices. Human sacrifice (purusha-medha) was already known in ancient Vedic India, and over the centuries continued to be resorted to as a means of propitiating the Divine by kings and Tantra practitioners alike. In 1832 the British raj finally outlawed this custom.

From the perspective of the evolution of human consciousness, this gruesome Kapalika practice must be regarded as a terrible diminution of the growth in moral sensibility seen, for instance, in the Buddhist and Jaina virtues of nonviolence and compassion. From a yogic point of view, it was likewise a step back into unfortunate literalism, for the Upanishadic sages had already understood that sacrifice was a matter of the renunciation of the ego, not of animal slaughter or murder. By the fourteenth century the Kapalika order was virtually extinct, perhaps brought down by the cumulative karma of those who failed to grasp that Yoga consists in the metaphorical sacrifice of the self.

The Aghori Order

The Kapalikas were replaced by the Aghori order. The word derives from *aghora,* meaning "nonterrible," which is one of the names of God Shiva in his terrific aspect. Presumably, only the initiate who knows how to propitiate Shiva is not terrified by the God's Bhairava aspect. The Aghoris, who are both venerated and feared by the villagers of India to this day, aspire to obliterate all human-made distinctions in their way of life. Thus, they live in cremation grounds or on dunghills, drink liquor or urine as readily as water, and break all social conventions by eating meat and the flesh of human corpses.

Recently an outstanding book was published that documents the life and teachings of a modern Aghori master, Vimalananda (d. 1983), who said about himself: "Either I must be mad or everyone else is; there are no two ways about it."[3] The author of the book, who was a close disciple of Vimalananda, comments about his teacher's extremist approach:

Aghora is not indulgence; it is the forcible transformation of darkness into light, of the opacity of the limited individual personality into the luminescence of the Absolute. Renunciation disappears once you arrive at the Absolute because then nothing remains to renounce. An Aghori goes so deeply into darkness, into all things undreamable to ordinary mortals, that he comes out into light.[4]

The Lingayat Sect

Another Shaiva sect that achieved great popularity after the decline of the Kapalikas is the Lingayat cult, so called because its members worship Shiva in the form of a phallic symbol (linga), standing for the creative process in the Divine. They carry a miniature stone linga in a small box attached to a necklace. Twice a day, the faithful sit quietly in meditation with the linga in the left hand and perform various rituals. Six stages (sthala) of meditation are distinguished:

1. Bhakti, or love-devotion, as expressed in ritual worship at the temple or in the home.
2. Maha-isha, or great Lord, the phase of disciplining one's mind, with all the trials this entails.
3. Prasada, or grace, the peaceful stage in which the devotee recognizes the Divine working in and through everything.
4. Prana-linga, or phallus of the life-force: Certain of the Lord's grace, the devotee now begins to experience the Divine in the consecrated temple of his or her own body-mind.
5. Sharana, or "[going] for refuge," the phase in which the devotee becomes a "fool of God," where he no longer identifies with the body-mind but is also not yet completely at one with the Divine, but longs for Shiva as does a woman for her absent lover.
6. Aikya, or union with the Divine: Here worship is at an end because the devotee has *become* the Lord; the pilgrim has arrived at his destination and found that he was never apart from it.

The devout Lingayat aspires to see Shiva in everyone and everything. As Basava expressed it so beautifully in one of his poems:

The pot is a god. The winnowing
fan is a god. The stone in the
street is a god. The comb is a
god. The bowstring is also a
god. The bushel is a god and the spouted
cup is a god.

Gods, gods, there are so many
there's no place left
for a foot.

There is only
one god. He is our Lord
of the Meeting Rivers.[5]

The Lingayats are also known as Vira-Shaivas, "Heroic Followers of Shiva." This sect originated in the twelfth century A.D., through its adherents believe that the roots of their faith reach back into the hoary past and that the adept Basava ("Bull"), or Basavanna (A.D. 1106–1167), merely reorganized their tradition. The popularity of the Lingayats was largely due to the fact that they championed greater social equality—favoring, for instance, the removal of caste distinctions, the remarriage of widows, and late marriage. This more moderate sect affords a convenient bridge to Agamic Shaivism, another conservative religious movement, which I will discuss next.

THE POWER OF LOVE: THE SHIVA WORSHIPPERS OF THE NORTH AND THE SOUTH

By no means all devotees of God Shiva follow the perilous path of the Kapalikas and Aghoris discussed in the previous section. Indeed, most of them cultivate a far more moderate approach to God-realization, though it may well include such Tantric rites as sexual intercourse with a consecrated partner.

Both mainstream and left-hand Shaiva beliefs and practices are found codified in the vast Agama literature of the north and the south. We will look at the northern branch of Shaivism first because it appears to be marginally older.

The Agamas—the word means simply "tradition"—understand themselves as a restatement of the ancient wisdom of the Vedas and are therefore often called the fifth Veda. They purport to be for the spiritual seeker of the "dark age" (kali-yuga), who lacks the moral fiber and mental concentration necessary to pursue the path of liberation by the more traditional means. The same intent is expressed in the Tantras, which are Agama-like scriptures that have Shakti (the feminine counterpart of Shiva) as their metaphysical and practical focus. However, mainline brahmins, who accept the revelatory authority of the Vedas, reject both the Agamas and Tantras as false.

The Agama canon is traditionally said to comprise twenty-eight scriptures, but we have knowledge of many more. It is impossible to do justice to the complexity of their history or philosophy in the context of this volume. To simplify matters, we can say that the southern and northern schools of Shaivism found vindication in the Agamas for their own distinct positions. Southern Shaivism favors a qualified monism that in practice is dualistic, with Lord Shiva on one side and the devotee (bhakta) on the other. This is epitomized in the devotionalism of such great saints as Tiruvalluvar, Sundarar, and Manikavacakar. By contrast, northern Shaivism leans toward an idealist or a radically nondualist interpretation of reality, similar to Advaita Vedanta.

Northern Shaivism

In Kashmir, where the Shaiva tradition flourished, it is known as the triadic (trika) system because it acknowledges the interdependence of the following three aspects of the Divine: Shiva (the male pole), Shakti (the female pole), and Nara (the conditional personality seeking liberation). The trika tradition comprises the original doctrines of the Agamas with their preeminently dualistic orientation, the teachings of the Spanda or "Vibration" school, and the doctrines of the Pratyabhijna or "Recognition" school. At the beginning of the ninth century A.D., the Kashmiri adept Vasugupta "discovered" the Shiva-Sutra, which is a digest of the earlier Agama teachings that had the declared intention to bring to light the nondualistic approach of these doctrines. According to Kshemaraja, author of a tenth-century commentary on the Sutra, God Shiva appeared to Vasugupta in a dream and revealed to him the secret location in which the Shiva-Sutra could be found inscribed in rock. Upon waking, Vasugupta promptly went to the place shown to him in the dream and found the seventy-seven aphorisms revealed by Shiva.

Even though the word *yoga* is nowhere used in the Shiva-Sutra, this scripture is a unique treatise on Yoga. It distinguishes four levels of yogic means (upaya):

1. Anupaya ("nonmeans"): The practitioner realizes the Self spontaneously, without effort, as a result of the teacher's transmission of the teaching.
2. Shambhava-upaya ("Shambhu's means"; Shambhu is another name for Shiva) or iccha-upaya ("means of the will"): When the mind is perfectly still, the transcendental Shiva-Consciousness flashes forth spontaneously, without exertion on the part of the practitioner.
3. Shakta-upaya ("Shakti's means"): The shambhava-upaya calls for a degree of spiritual maturity that few possess. Most people find it impossible to go beyond conceptualization (vikalpa) and to simply rest in perceptual awareness. The very effort to outwit the conceptual mind merely tends to produce new conceptual content. Therefore, Vasugupta puts forward an alternative: to attach attention to what he calls pure (shuddha) concepts. By this he means such intuitions as the following: Our true identity is not the ego-personality but the transcendental Self, and the knowable universe is not external to us but a manifestation of our transcendental Power. In this way, we can remove the ingrained illusion of duality between subject and object.
4. Anava-upaya ("limited means"): The shakta-upaya seeks to trick the mind into a new way of looking at its own nature and the nature of the apparently external world. Vasugupta particularly recommends Mantra-Yoga for this process, since the dwelling of the mind on the

hidden meaning of such mantras as "I am Shiva" ultimately blots out the distinction between the mantra and the mind, and so forms a foundation for the revelation of Shiva-Consciousness. In the level of anava-upaya, the practitioner resorts to such common yogic practices as breath control, sense-withdrawal, concentration, and meditation. Ultimately, the practitioner has to transcend this level and discover the transcendental "I"-Consciousness through the more direct means of shakta-upaya and then shambhava-upaya.

The commentaries on the Shiva-Sutra contain invaluable materials on the technique of pranayama, which is more sophisticated than that expounded in the Yoga-Sutra. Especially interesting is the teaching that associates different forms of delight, or bliss (ananda), with the contemplation of the various types of life-force (prana) in the body. The doctrine of the ascent (uccara) of the life-force as subtle vibration is connected to complicated speculations about the mystical sound matrices (matrika) that are the root of all mantras. This and other forms of the anava discipline are found, for instance, in the Vijnana-Bhairava, a much-loved treatise composed probably in the seventh century A.D.

A further developmental stage of the tradition of northern Shaivism is present in the Spanda-Sutra and its commentarial literature. The Spanda-Sutra, also called Spanda-Karika, is generally ascribed to Vasugupta as well, though some traditions name his disciple Kallata as its composer. The technical term *spanda* is generally defined as "a sort of movement." It is not successive motion as we encounter it in space-time, but an instantaneous vibration in the transcendental Reality itself, which is the source of all manifest movement—perhaps what physicist David Bohm styles "holo-movement."

Spanda is the ecstatic throb of the Shiva-Consciousness. This notion is in striking contrast to the static interpretation of Selfhood in Classical Yoga, where the Self is merely an eternally disinterested watcher of events in the body-mind. This new dynamic concept was no doubt invented to account more adequately for the Self- or God-realization as experienced by the adepts of Shaiva Yoga.

The Pratyabhijna School

The third phase or camp of northern Shaivism is represented by the Pratyabhijna ("Recognition") school founded by Somananda (ninth century A.D.), a disciple of Vasugupta. The two key scriptures of this school are the Pratyabhijna-Sutra of Utpala, a pupil of Somananda, and the several commentaries of Abhinavagupta, a tenth-century adept who was also a remarkably prolific writer. Abhinavagupta composed some fifty works, including his Tantra-Aloka ("Light on Tantra"), a work of encyclopedic proportions on the philosophy and ritual of Agamic Shaivism. Madhuraja Yogin, a pupil of Abhinavagupta, left us this devotional portrait of his guru:

> His eyes are rolling with spiritual bliss. The center of his forehead is clearly marked with three lines, made with ashes. His luxuriant hair is tied with a garland of flowers. His beard is long, his body rosy. He is dressed in silk, white like the rays of the moon, and is seated in the heroic posture on a soft cushion placed on a throne of gold. He is attended by all his pupils, with two female devotee-messengers standing by his side.[6]

Local tradition has it that, after completing his final commentary on the Pratyabhijna system, Abhinavagupta, accompanied by 1200 disciples, entered the Bhairava cave near the Kashmiri village of Magam and was never seen again. He is remembered even today as a fully realized adept (siddha). Abhinavagupta and many of the other great masters of northern Shaivism are a wonderful illustration that mystical aspiration and philosophical acuity can be successfully combined.

One of the most popular manuals of the Pratyabhijna school is the Pratyabhijna-Hridaya ("Heart of Recognition"), written by Rajanaka Kshemaraja, a disciple of Abhinavagupta. It is evident from this and Abhinavagupta's own writings, as well as other related scriptures, that the Pratyabhijna practitioners were well acquainted with Yoga, not least Kundalini-Yoga. They are therefore important sources for our understanding of the early developmental phase of Hatha-Yoga.

The Pratyabhijna school gets its name from its principal doctrine that liberation is a matter of "recognizing," or remembering, that our true identity is not the limited body-mind but the infinite Reality of Shiva. In their analysis of existence, the Pratyabhijna masters arrived at the following thirty-six categories or principles (tattva):

1. Shiva, the ultimate Reality, which is pure Being-Consciousness.
2. Shakti, the Power aspect of the ultimate principle, which is not really separate from Shiva but merely appears so from the unenlightened point of view. Shakti is the transcendental source of the entire manifest and unmanifest cosmos. The yogin experiences Shakti as bliss (ananda).
3. Sada-Shiva ("Ever-Shiva"), or Sada-Akhya ("Ever-Named"), is the will aspect of the One Being. In the scale of yogic realizations, this elevated principle is the ecstatic experience of "I am this," where Consciousness encounters itself vaguely as an object.
4. Ishvara ("Lord") is a further progression of the psychocosmic evolution, where the objective or "this" (idam) side of the universal Consciousness is still more accentuated. The ecstatic experience on this level is now "This am I" rather than "I am this."
5. Sad-vidya ("Being-knowledge"), or Shuddha-vidya ("Pure

Knowledge"), is ecstatically experienced as a perfect balance between the subject ("I") and the objective ("this") aspect of universal Consciousness.

6. Maya ("Illusion") is the first of the so-called "impure" (ashuddha) principles, because it relativizes existence through the agency of its five functions, known as "jackets" (kancuka) because of their concealment of the truth that there is only the One Being-Consciousness, which is Shiva. These five functions are (7–11):

7. Kala[7] ("part"), which stands for secondary, or partial, creatorship.

8. Vidya ("knowledge"), which signifies limited knowledge as opposed to omniscience.

9. Raga ("passion"), which is desire for limited objects rather than universal bliss and satisfaction.

10. Kala[8] ("time"), which stands for the reduction of eternity to the temporal order, divisible into past, present, and future.

11. Niyati ("destiny"), which is the law of karma as opposed to the eternal freedom and independence of the Divine.

12. Purusha ("male") is the individuated being, the source of subjective experience, resulting from the activity of the maya-tattva. The purusha is here different from the purusha of Classical Yoga, which is utterly transcendental.

13. Prakriti ("nature") is the matrix of all objective aspects of manifestation. Unlike Classical Yoga and Samkhya, Kashmiri Shaivism proposes that every purusha has its own prakriti.

14.–36. The remaining principles are identical to the twenty-four principles known in the Samkhya tradition, namely the higher mind (I prefer to call it the wisdom-faculty) [buddhi], the "I-maker" (ahamkara), the lower mind (manas), the five cognitive organs (jnana-indriya), the five conative organs (karma-indriya), the five subtle elements (tanmatra), and the five coarse elements (bhuta).[9]

Yoga is understood as a gradual ascent to the transcendental Source, which involves the progressive penetration of the various layers of illusion created by the maya principle. While success on the spiritual path depends on the guidance of a realized master, ultimately it is the grace of Shiva that bestows liberation on the deserving practitioner.

The mysticism of northern Shaivism holds great attraction for the Westerner interested in India's wisdom, because it is well argued in rational language. In recent years, northern Shaiva teachings have been brought to Europe and America by the late Swami Muktananda, an adept of the Siddha tradition. He empowered numerous Westerners through the method of shakti-pata ("descent of the power"), either through his touch or his mere glance. Joseph Chilton Pearce reported the following incident:

A young heart surgeon from Florida, who was disturbed by the hard emotional attitude in his profession, met Muktananda during a meditation intensive. Muktananda grabbed him by the bridge of the nose and held on. In that instant, the young doctor experienced himself as a "body of blue energy." Then he had a visionary experience of his right arm clinging tightly to the branch of a tree. He felt his fingers being pried loose from the branch. Then something snapped inside him. He experienced himself entering Muktananda's head. In his words, "there I found myself in an immense vacuum—an infinite space. A wave of emotion swept up from my belly and I wept for fifteen minutes or more." Afterward, he felt "cleaned out" and peaceful. Pearce called this a "classical account of Shaktipat," which turned the young surgeon's life around, granting him the empathy for his patients he had been hoping for.[10]

Southern Shaivism

During the period between the seventh and ninth centuries A.D., Agamic Shaivism also gained momentum in the south. The Tamil-speaking Shaivas deny that their Agamas hailed from the north. Be that as it may, they produced a vast and beautiful literature whose doctrines are known as Shaiva-Siddhanta. The metaphysics of this tradition is, as already mentioned, a form of qualified nondualism: Shiva is the One Reality, and the insentient (acit) world of multiplicity is no illusion, but a product of Shiva's power (shakti). This is an important distinction from the northern tradition, which favors an illusionist interpretation of the world. However, in both traditions liberation is dependent on grace (prasada).

Rejecting the Vedas, the Tamil Shaivas have their own sacred corpus, the Tirumurai, also often referred to as the Tamil Veda. This collection of ancient hymns in praise of God Shiva was put together by Nambiandar Nambi, who lived toward the end of the eleventh century A.D. These hundreds of hymns are arranged into eleven chapters, of which the tenth is the best known: the famous Tirumantiram of the adept-bard Tirumular (seventh century A.D.). It consists of more than 3000 verses. Tirumular's teaching is a mixture of devotionalism, yogic technique, and gnosis (jnana).

We may see in Tirumular an early master of the Siddha tradition, which will be dealt with shortly. In one stanza (1463), he defines a siddha, or adept, as someone who has experienced the divine light and acquired power (shakti) through yogic ecstasy. For the historian of Yoga, the most important part of Tirumular's work is the third section, consisting of 333 verses, where he explains the eightfold limbs of the Yoga path (a la Patanjali) and the fruits of correct Yoga practice, including the eight great supernormal powers (mahasiddhi). He also introduces several Tantric practices, notably the khecarimudra, which is defined (verse 779) as the "simultaneous arresting of the movement of breath, mind, and semen." The Tirumantiram is as important to southern Shaiva Yoga as the Bhagavad-Gita is to the northern Vaishnava Yoga tradition.

Another eleventh-century work is Sekkirar's Peria-Purana, which tells the life stories of sixty-three prominent Shaiva saints. This work is as edifying to read as are the Christian hagiographies, providing we put ourselves in a spiritually receptive mood and are willing to ignore cultural differences, for the human heart speaks a universal language. This scripture is filled with samples from the poetic outpourings of the saints in which they glorify the Divine Lord, asking for nothing but to be devotees, forever absorbed in contemplating Him.

The Shaiva saints were ascetics of the heart, but in their external lives it would have been difficult to distinguish them from their neighbors. They were married, had children, had work to accomplish and properties to care for. But inwardly they had renounced everything and become humble servants of Lord Shiva, ennobling their entire culture. Thus, the age-old Shaiva community continued to keep the spirit of Bhakti-Yoga alive.

GOD IS LOVE: THE VISHNU WORSHIPPERS OF THE NORTH AND THE SOUTH

When the heart is open it bursts into song and poetry. The ecstatic literature of the Shiva worshippers, especially of the southern part of the Indian peninsula, is a lasting testimony to this fact. And so is the great devotional literature of the Vishnu community, to which we turn next. The Bhagavad-Gita ("Song of the Lord"), the most popular of all Yoga works, was an early blossom on the Vaishnava tree of wisdom. It inspired later generations to compose such incomparable devotional works as the poetry of the Alvars, the Bhagavata-Purana, and the Gita-Govinda, all of which will be introduced shortly. The Gita even served poets of other religious communities as a model for similar songs in praise of their own deities.

The sacred literature of the Vaishnava community is as vast and complex as that of the Shiva community, which I have touched on in the previous section. The early post-Christian centuries saw the creation of the Samhitas ("Collections"), which are the Vaishnava equivalent to the Shaiva Agamas and the Tantras of the Shakti worshippers.[11] The anonymous composers of these scriptures were familiar with Yoga practice, and their understanding of what this entails is roughly similar. The emphasis of their teachings, however, is not so much on achieving mystical states of inwardness as on ritual worship and a moral way of life, interspersed with philosophical considerations.

The Vishnu-Samhita (chapter XIII) introduces a sixfold Yoga (shad-anga-yoga), which it styles bhagavata-yoga. But many other works of the Vaishnava canon—which is traditionally held to comprise 108 Samhitas—recommend Patanjali's eightfold Yoga. However, they do not appear to add much to our understanding of Yoga, including Bhakti-Yoga. For the most part, they make for dry reading unless one happens to be a historian of religion.

The opposite is true of the devotional poems of the Alvars (or Arvars), who flourished in the eighth and ninth centuries A.D. The Alvars are a group of twelve southern adepts of Bhakti-Yoga, whose poetry is gathered in the Nalayira-Prabandha, which is given the same respect as the sacred Vedas of the brahmins. Their poems sparkle with passionate love for the Divine, and their archetypal symbolism touches us deeply even in translation. Most of the 4000 poems or hymns in this collection were composed by Tirumankaiy and Namm. The latter is the most popular of these saints. He is said to have been born absorbed in yogic ecstasy and to have crawled into a hollow tree trunk, where he remained in samadhi for sixteen years until his chief disciple arrived. The Alvars were steeped in Krishna mythology: Krishna, the youthful shepherd, a full incarnation of the Divine Vishnu, at play with the shepherdesses, the gopis.

> In the spiritual experiences of these Arvars we find a passionate yearning after God, the Lord and Lover. . . . The emphasis is mostly on the transcendent beauty and charm of God, and on the ardent longings of the devotee who plays the part of a female lover, for Krishna, the God. . . . The rapturous passions are like a whirlpool that eddies through the very eternity of the individual soul, and expresses itself sometimes in the pangs of separation and sometimes in the exhilaration of union. The Arvar, in his ecstatic delight, visualizes God everywhere, and in the very profundity of his attainment pines for more. He also experiences states of supreme intoxication, when he becomes semi-conscious, or unconscious with occasional breaks into the consciousness of yearning. . . . The Arvars were probably the pioneers in showing how love for God may be on terms of tender equality, softening down to the rapturous emotion of conjugal love.[12]

The Bhagavata-Purana

The theme of erotic spirituality is fully explored, if not exploited, in the Bhagavata-Purana, also known as the Shrimad-Bhagavata, which depicts the God-man Krishna as husband to 16,108 women, each of whom bore him tens sons and one daughter. The Bhagavata-Purana is a magnificent tenth-century work that has been called "the richest treasure hidden in the bosom of the liberated, the incomparable solace to the disturbed soul."[13] No other scripture, with the exception of the Bhagavad-Gita, has enjoyed such widespread popularity through the centuries. Numerous commentaries have been written on this work, which holds aloft the great ideal of love-devotion (bhakti) to the Lord (bhagavat).

Yoga is mentioned in many passages of the Bhagavata-Purana. In one place (XI.20.6), three approaches are distinguished, namely the path of wisdom for those who are weary of rituals, the path of action for those who are still inclined toward worldly and sacred activity, and the path of devotion for those who are fortunate enough to be neither weary of actions nor overly inclined to them but simply have faith in the Lord. The Bhagavata-Purana accepts Patanjali's eight limbs but rejects his dualistic philosophy. Also, the limbs are defined somewhat differently. This is most apparent in the delineation of the constituent practices of moral observance (yama) and self-discipline (niyama). Where Patanjali lists five practices for each set, the Bhagavata-Purana (XI.19.33ff.) has twelve. But always it is devotion that is recommended as the supreme means of reaching liberation. The adept Kapila, who is remembered as the founder of the Samkhya tradition and is identified with God Vishnu, puts it this way:

> When the mind is firmly fixed on Me by intense Bhakti-Yoga, it becomes still and steady. This is the only way for attaining the highest bliss in this world. (III.25.44)

On the path of devotion, concentration is always the fixing of attention upon the Divine Person, whereas meditation is the contemplation of the Lord's form, as depicted in iconography: with a four-armed, garlanded dark-blue body, a serene expression on his kind face, holding a conch, a disc, and a mace in his hands, wearing a crown on his head and the magical kaustubha jewel around his neck, and bearing the shri-vatsa ("blessed calf") mark on his chest. The dark-blue hue of Krishna's body is the result of his drinking the poisoned milk of the female demon Putana who suckled him. The implements in his hands are instruments of war, and their use destroys the enemy—the ego—and leads to liberation. The magical jewel was created during the churning of the world ocean at the beginning of time. The mark on Krishna's chest is one of the signs of his superior birth and of his principal vocation as a shepherd—a shepherd of cattle and of human souls.

Liberation is thought to be of different degrees, depending on the devotee's level of proximity to, or identification with, the Lord. At the lowest stage, the devotee dwells in the divine location—Vaikuntha Heaven—in the Lord's company. This is called salokya-mukti. When the devotee's power and glory equals that of the Lord, it is known as sarishti-mukti. When he is abiding in close proximity to the Lord, it is called samipya-mukti. The penultimate level of liberation is sarupya-mukti, where the devotee attains perfect conformity with the Lord. Finally, there is ekatva-mukti, or the "liberation of singleness," where the last trace of difference between the devotee and the Divine is lifted.

Of particular interest for the Yoga student are chapters 6–29 of the eleventh book (skandha) of the Bhagavata-Purana. This section is known as the Uddhava-Gita, after the sage Uddhava to whom the God-man Krishna expounds the Yoga of devotion. Here are some typical stanzas from this Song, which is sometimes referred to as Krishna's "last message":

> Just as fire that is ablaze with flames reduces wood to ashes, so devotion to Me, removes all sin, O Uddhava. (XI.14.19)

Neither through [conventional] Yoga nor Samkhya, nor righteousness (dharma), nor study, nor austerities, nor renunciation (tyaga) does he reach Me as [readily as he does through] devotion (bhakti), or the worship of Me. (XI.14.20)

I, the beloved Self of the virtuous, am realized through singular devotion, through faith. Devotion established in Me purifies even outcastes like the "dog-cookers" (shva-paka) from their [lowly] birth. (XI.14.21)

He whose speech is interrupted by sobs, whose heart (citta) melts, who unashamedly sometimes laments or laughs, or sings aloud or dances—[such a person] endowed with devotion to Me purifies the world. (XI.14.24)

Faith in the nectar-like stories about Me, constant proclamation of My [greatness], deep reverence (parinishtha) in worshipping [Me], and praising Me with hymns; (XI.19.20)

delight in service [to Me], making prostrations [before Me], rendering greater worship to My devotees, and considering all beings as Me; (XI.19.21)

doing bodily activities for My sake, to recite My qualities in sayings, offering the mind to Me, and banishing all desires; (XI.19.22)

renouncing things, pleasure, and enjoyment for My sake, [undertaking] whatever sacrifice, gifting, oblation, recitation, vow and penance for My sake; (XI.19.23)

—by such virtues, O Uddhava, self-surrendered people acquire love-devotion (bhakti) for Me. What other task remains for such a one? (XI.19.24)

Perhaps the most extraordinary teaching of the Bhagavata-Purana is the Yoga of hatred (samrambha-yoga), according to which a person who thoroughly hates the Divine can achieve God-Realization as readily as one who deeply loves the Lord. Sage Narada, a frequent spokesman for the Bhagavata religion, expresses it thus:

All human emotions are grounded in the erroneous conception of "I" and "mine." The Absolute, the universal Self, has neither "I"-sense nor emotions. (VII.1.23)

Hence one should unite [with God] through friendship or enmity, peaceableness or fear, attachment or love. [The Divine] sees no distinction whatsoever. (VII.1.25)

Narada goes on to mention Kamsa, who reached God through fear, and Shishupala, king of the Cedis, who reached God through hatred. In fact, Shishupala's hatred was cultivated over several incarnations. He was the demon Hiranyakashipu ("Gold-Cloth") who tortured his son Prahlada for his devotion to Vishnu and was disemboweled by the god, who assumed the form of the Man-Lion (nara-simha). In another birth Shishupala was the demon Ravana who was slain by Rama, an incarnation of Vishnu.

The idea that hatred can turn out to be a pathway to God, shocking as it is to conventional sensibilities, is a logical consequence of the ancient esoteric doctrine that we become whatever we meditate upon. Because of the intense hatred that Shishupala entertained toward Lord Vishnu, he thought about the Divine incessantly, and therefore ultimately became absorbed in it. This brings home the fact that the spiritual process is a matter of the play of attention.

The Gita-Govinda

While the Bhagavata-Purana, true to its Puranic character, deals with all kinds of theological, philosophical, and cosmological matters besides telling the story of Krishna's heroic life, the somewhat later Gita-Govinda ("Song of Govinda") is solely dedicated to celebrating Lord Krishna's love of his favorite shepherdess, Radha. The name Govinda is one of Krishna's many appellations. It means literally "cow-finder" and refers to the God-man's occupation as cowherd in the Vrindavana region. There is also an esoteric significance to the name, since the Sanskrit word *go* also stands for "wisdom." Thus, Govinda is the finder, or shepherd, of gnosis.

This Sanskrit poem by the twelfth-century Bengali writer Jayadeva is a profound allegory of the love between the personal God and the human self, which has strong erotic overtones. It is expressive of a new trend in the Vaishnava devotional movement, coinciding with its expansion to the north of the Indian peninsula. Suddenly great prominence was given to the figure of Radha as an embodiment of the feminine principle of the Divine. Confiding in a friend, Radha recounts her love adventure with Krishna thus:

> Secretly at night I went to his home in a concealed thicket where he remained in hiding. Anxiously I glanced in all directions, while he was laughing with an abundant longing for the delight (rati) [of sexual union]; O friend! Make the crusher of [the demon] Keshin love me passionately. I am enamored, entertaining desires of love! (III.11)

> I was shy at our first union. He was kind toward me, [showing] hundreds of ingenious flatteries. I spoke through sweet and gentle smiles. [Then] he unfastened the garment around my hips. (III.12)

> He laid me down on a bed of shoots. For a long time he rested on my breast, while I caressed and kissed him. Embracing me, he drank from my lower lip. (III.13)

> I closed my eyes from drowsiness. The hair on his cheeks bristled from my caresses. My whole body was sweating, and he was quite restless because of his great intoxication with passion. (III.14)

Radha pines for her lover, as the awakened heart yearns for God. The Gita-Govinda, reflecting the spirit of Tantrism, extensively uses sexual metaphors to convey the bodily passion that the devotee feels when he or she contemplates God. In its explicitness it surpasses the comparable literature of the bridal mystics of medieval Christendom.

The Bhakti-Yoga of the Vaishnava Preceptors

The ecstatic devotionalism of the Alvars attracted not only the illiterate masses, who were moved by the Alvars' strong sentiments of love, but also stimulated the intelligentsia to develop sophisticated philosophies revolving around the ideal of love (bhakti). The first of these learned Vishnu devotees was Nathamuni, who lived in the tenth century A.D. He is said to have often walked about naked, chanting the sacred name of God Vishnu. Some scholars identify him with Shri Natha, the author of several works, including the Yoga-Rahasya ("Secret Doctrine of Yoga"). Another important figure among the so-called "preceptors" (acarya) of Vaishnavism was Yamuna, grandson of Nathamuni. He wrote six works, of which the Siddhi-Traya ("Triad of Perfection") is the most significant. According to tradition, Yamuna, who described himself as a "vessel of a thousand sins," learned the eightfold Yoga from Kurukanatha, to whom Nathamuni had entrusted this teaching for the benefit of his grandson.

The most influential preceptor was unquestionably Ramanuja (A.D. 1017–1137). Yamuna, who had expressed a keen interest in meeting the brilliant Ramanuja, was dead by the time Ramanuja came to pay homage to him. Three of Yamuna's fingers were curiously twisted, and Ramanuja took this to be a final message to him. He understood it to mean that he should preach the Vaishnava doctrine of unconditional surrender, or prapatti, and write a commentary on the Brahma-Sutra, as well as many other works championing the Vaishnava faith as taught by the Alvars.

The visit to Yamuna occurred after Ramanuja had been asked to leave by his own teacher, Yadavaprakasha, a learned but irascible man. Ramanuja's discipleship had been stormy because he begged to differ from his guru in points of doctrine. Whereas Yadavaprakasha avowed a strictly nondualistic interpretation of the Vaishnava scriptures, Ramanuja was at heart a qualified nondualist, believing that the Divine is not a mere distinctionless One but comprises infinite differentiation. Ramanuja lived a long and eventful life, and his many works expounding the philosophy of Vishishta-Advaita formed the foundations of a comprehensive exegetical literature, which offered the most serious challenge to the radical nondualism of Shankara's school.

Ramanuja and his followers oppose Shankara's notion that the experienced world of multiplicity is unreal. They place no faith in the doctrines of maya ("illusion") and avidya ("ignorance"), by which the Shankara camp seeks to explain the fact that, even though there is only the Absolute, we actually experience distinctions. If there were such an agent as ignorance, the Ramanujites argue, it could not be located in the omniscient transcendental Reality. But if it is not located in the Absolute, it would form an alternative reality to it, which would completely undermine the idea of radical nondualism.

Ramanuja was an eager protagonist of Yoga, which he understood as Bhakti-Yoga. For him, the purpose of meditation is to generate love for the Divine Person. He was consequently rather critical of Patanjali's Yoga, which is not only dualistic but also aims at stilling the mind rather than turning the heart to God. Ramanuja was similarly wary of Jnana-Yoga, as taught by Shankara, because in the beginner it tends to lead to intellectualism and self-delusion. In preparation for meditation, or the contemplative remembrance of the Divine, one should instead engage in Karma-Yoga.

From Ramanuja's point of view, liberation is not the annihilation of the self but rather the removal of its limitations. The liberated being attains the "same form" as the Divine, though this does not imply the obliteration of all distinctions either. Rather, liberation is conceived as a kind of fellowship with and in the Divine Person—a condition of continuous love-devotion. But whereas the Divine Person is infinite and the absolute creator of the universe, the liberated devotee is finite and has no power of creation. For Ramanuja, liberation occurs only after death. Love is the means and the goal, and it can and should be cultivated throughout one's life on earth or in any of the higher realms of existence.

Yogic teachings also played a role in the schools of the other three great Vaishnava preceptors—the Vedantic dualist Madhva (A.D. 1238–1317), the theologian of duality-in-nonduality Nimbarka (mid-twelfth century A.D.), the pure nondualist Vallabha (A.D. 1479–1531), and the ecstatic Krishna Caitanya (A.D. 1486–1533), who argued that the true nature of Reality is imponderable.

These teachers and their numerous adherents all enlist the capacity for self-transcending love and surrender as the principal means of liberation. It is here that psychospiritual technology is the most artful and the least in danger of degenerating into gross manipulation of the body-mind. Of course, the path of the heart, or Bhakti-Yoga, has its own risks, such as rampant irrationalism and unbridled emotionalism. Yet it appears to be inherently more conducive to a balanced approach. The heart (hrid, hridaya) has from ancient times been acknowledged as a primary focus of the spiritual process. "The heart," says a modern sage, "is the cradle of love."[14] And it is at the heart that, according to many schools and traditions, the great awakening occurs.

THE YOGINS AND ASCETICS OF THE PURANAS

The Naked Ascetic

Once upon a time God Shiva, in the youthful guise of the skull-carrying naked ascetic Kalabhairava, was wandering in the Devadaru forest. He was accompanied by his spouse Sati and God Vishnu in human form. The forest was inhabited by many saints, seers, and sages, and their families. Wherever Kalabhairava went, the women became so infatuated with him that they ripped off their clothes, touched and embraced him, and followed him around. The young men were similarly affected by him. But the holy men were infuriated by the stranger's outrageous demeanor and his magical effect on their women and sons. They demanded that he cover his genitals and start doing real penance (tapas). Using their store of psychic power, gathered over decades of fierce austerities, they repeatedly cursed Kalabhairava. Yet their curses bounced back "like starlight falling upon the sun's brightness," without doing any damage whatsoever. Unthinking, they started to beat the naked ascetic with sticks, and he had to flee.

Then Kalabhairava and his entourage arrived at the hermitage of Sage Vashishtha, where he begged for alms. The sage's wife, Arundhati, approached the visitor with great reverence, wanting to feed him. But again Kalabhairava was driven away. The holy men shouted after him to tear out his penis so that it could not offend people any longer. Without hesitation, Kalabhairava tore out his genitals—and instantly vanished. Suddenly the entire world was plunged into darkness, and the earth quaked.

At last it dawned on the seers and sages that Kalabhairava was none other than God Shiva himself, and they were overcome with shame and terror. Upon the advice of Brahma, the first to emerge at the creation of the universe, they sought Shiva's forgiveness by worshipping his phallus (linga), the principle of creativity. In due course, Shiva returned to the forest and revealed to the penitent sages the secrets of the Yoga of the Lord of Beasts (pashupata-yoga).

This story, which is told in the Kurma-Purana (chapter II), is typical of the legendary materials with which the Purana literature abounds. These stories were intended for the ears of the rural folk, and they never failed to entertain and edify as well as to explain the sacred practices and ideas of those who had dedicated their lives to the pursuit of liberation or paranormal powers, as the case may be.

Yoga in the Puranic Encyclopedias

The Puranas are popular encyclopedias in the rambling style of the Mahabharata, though they are more structured. The word itself means "ancient" and here denotes an age-old narrative; it refers to the contents of these narratives, which deal with the origins of things—from genealogies of families to the "genealogy" of the universe itself. This type of literature dates back to Vedic times, when the Puranas were still memorized rather than written down. None of these early compositions have survived. Of the eighteen great Puranas that are extant today, the oldest, such as the Vayu-, the Matsya-, and the Vishnu-Purana, belong (in part at least) to the same period as the Bhagavad-

Gita. Most, however, were created in the post-Christian era, and some, like the Bhagavata-Purana, are medieval compositions. They are all said to have been authored by Sage Vyasa—a superhuman feat indeed.

These works seek to instruct the faithful and have been most influential in the education of the masses. They purport to deal, ideally, with five principal themes: Usually they start with a mythological account of the creation (sarga) of the world. This is followed by a treatment of the world's re-creation (pratisarga) after its destruction at the end of time. A third major topic is the genealogies (vamsha) of the gods and seers. Then there is a mythological account of the cosmic eras called manvantara ("Manu interim"). These are the great cycles of existence, each of which has its own Manu who, like the Hebrew Adam, gives birth to humankind. Lastly, the Puranas are supposed to deal with the genealogical histories (vamsha-anucarita) of the royal dynasties.

Few Puranas conform to this traditional ideal, and most contain much extraneous matter, including brief treatments of yogic teachings, which are usually found toward the end. The types of Yoga differ greatly, though they are all integrally connected with the worship of particular deities, primarily Vishnu and Shiva. Not surprisingly, therefore, most of these teachings have a ritual character, though some offer a more contemplative type of Yoga.

The Padma ("Lotus")-Purana, for instance, has an appendix to its last book, entitled "The Essence of Ritual Yoga" (Kriya-Yoga-Sara), which recommends that Vishnu should be worshipped not through meditation (dhyana) but through prayers and sacrificial rites. In contrast, the Vishnu-Purana, which deals with Yoga in its short sixth book, understands Yoga as the path of meditation. The Vayu ("Wind")-Purana, in its concluding chapters, introduces Yoga as a means of attaining "Shiva's city" (shiva-pura), which corresponds to the Vaishnava notion of Vaikuntha, Vishnu's heavenly domain.

The Ritual Yoga of the Markandeya-Purana

The Markandeya-Purana, which gets its name from Sage Markandeya, a central figure in this narrative, belongs to the early post-Christian centuries. It speaks of Yoga in chapters 36–43. The following passage from the fortieth chapter, where Sage Dattatreya instructs his disciple Alarka, conveys a sense of the ritualized nature of that yogic teaching:

> He should set his foot only after [the path in front of him] has been purified by the eye. He should drink only water filtered through cloth, only utter words purified by truth, and only think of what has been purified completely by the mind (buddhi). (4)

> The knower of Yoga should nowhere be a guest, and he should not participate in ancestor worship, sacrifices, pilgrimages to [the shrines of] deities and festivals. He also should not mix with the crowd for purposes of demonstration. (5)

The knower of Yoga should wander about begging [his daily sustenance] and live off what he finds in the refuse. [He should beg] at places where no smoke arises [from the hearth], where the coal is extinguished, and among all those who have already eaten, but also not continually among these three. (6)

Since the crowd despises and mocks him because of this, the yogin should, yoked [in Yoga], tread the path of the virtuous, [so that he might] not be tarnished. (7)

He should seek alms among the householders and the huts of mendicant monks: their mode of life is considered the foremost and best. (8)

The ascetic (yati) should furthermore also always stay [close to] the pious, self-controlled, and magnanimous householders versed in the Vedas. (9)

In addition [he should stay close to] the innocent and non-outcastes. Begging among the casteless is the lowest mode of life that he could wish. (10)

The begged food [may consist of] gruel, diluted buttermilk or milk, barley broth, fruit, roots, millet, corn, oil-cake, or groats. (11)

And these are pleasant eatables that support the yogin's [struggle for] perfection (siddhi). The sage should turn to them with devotedness and highest concentration (samadhi). (12)

After first having drunk water, he should collect himself silently. Then he should [offer] the first oblation to the [life-force] called prana. (13)

The second [oblation] should be to apana, the next to samana, the fourth to udana, and the fifth to vyana. (14)[15]

After having completed one oblation after the other, [all the while practicing] the restraint of the life-force (prana) [through controlled breathing], he may then enjoy the remainder to his heart's content. Taking again water and rinsing, he should touch his heart. (15)

Nonstealing, chastity, dispassion, absence of greed, and nonharming are the five most important vows of the mendicant (bhikshu). (16)

Absence of wrath, obedience toward the teacher, purity, moderation in eating, sustained study—these are the five well-known rules (niyama). (17)

Above all, [the yogin] should dedicate himself to knowledge that leads to the goal. The multiplicity of knowledge as it exists here [on earth] is an obstacle to Yoga. (18)

He who seized-by-thirst (trishita) dashes along [in the belief that he must] know this or that, will not even in a thousand eons obtain that which is to be known, [namely the ultimate Reality]. (19)

Abandoning society, curbing wrath, eating moderately, and controlling the senses, he should block the gates [of the body] by means of the wisdom-faculty (buddhi) and let the mind come to rest in meditation. (20)

That yogin who is yoked incessantly should always practice meditation in empty rooms, caves, and in the forest. (21)

Control of speech, control of action, and control of the mind—these are the three [masteries]. He who [practices] these restraints unfailingly is a mighty "three-restraint" ascetic. (22)

The Markandeya-Purana speaks in detail about the qualities of an individual suited for Yoga and also the environmental conditions necessary for success in its practice. The body is recognized as an important instrument on the spiritual path. This Purana offers an original measure for assessing yogic perfection: There should be no fear in the yogin toward other beings, and other beings should not fear him.

Yogins are subdivided according to the prevalence of one of the three primary constituents (guna) of Nature. They are also distinguished by their achievement on the path. Thus, at the pratibha ("understanding") stage, the yogin comprehends all the sacred scriptures and other branches of knowledge. At the shravana ("listening") stage, he understands the significance of the different realms of existence. At the daiva ("divine") stage, he perceives higher beings, such as the deities ("deva"). At the bhrama ("roaming") stage, the yogin's mind is fickle, impeding his progress.

Yogic Teachings in Other Puranas

The Linga ("Phallus")-Purana introduces yogic concepts at the outset, in chapters 7–9. Here the eightfold Yoga, as outlined by Patanjali, is said to arise from understanding (jnana), which is given by grace. The different limbs are described, and a long list of obstacles and omens is given. Chapter 88 is a review of this Pashupata-Yoga.

The Kurma ("Tortoise")-Purana, so called because of Vishnu's incarnation as a tortoise, contains many fascinating myths about Vishnu and Shiva. In its second part, we find two well-known Gita imitations—the Ishvara-Gita and the longer Vyasa-Gita.

The Agni ("Fire")-Purana, a massive but late work that is more encyclopedic in character than the other Puranas, contains extensive information about rituals, including mantra recitation, mudras (hand gestures), the construction of yantras (mystic diagrams similar to the circular mandalas), and pranayama (ritual breath control). Patanjali's eightfold Yoga is explained in chapters 352–358.

An important place is assigned to Yoga in the Garuda ("Eagle")-Purana, which dedicates three chapters (14, 49, and 118) to the eightfold path. Tapas is defined as sense-control rather than penance. Only two meditation postures are mentioned: the lotus and the bound lotus. Concentration, again, is said to be of the duration of eighteen cycles of breath control, whereas meditation is twice that long, and the unbroken chain of ten cycles of concentration leads to ecstasy (samadhi). This text also refers to Bhakti-Yoga and to Tantric Yoga.

Lastly, the voluminous Shiva-Purana deals with Yoga in different places. Thus, in chapter 17 of the first book, the Yoga of mantric recitation is introduced. It is said that 1,080,000,000 repetitions of the sacred mantra *om* lead to the mastery of "purified Yoga" (shuddha-yoga), which is synonymous with liberation. The text further explains that shiva-yogins are of three types: the kriya-yogin, who engages in sacred rites (kriya); the tapo-yogin, who pursues asceticism (tapas); and the japa-yogin, who observes the practices of the other two types and in addition constantly recites the holy five-syllabled mantra "Om, obeisance to Shiva" (om namah shivaya).

Yoga makes its appearance again in chapters 37–39 of the concluding book of the Shiva-Purana. Yoga is here defined as the restraint of all activities and mental concentration upon Shiva. Five types or degrees are distinguished:

1. Mantra-Yoga is the focusing of attention by means of the sacred five-syllabled invocation of Shiva.
2. Sparsha-Yoga ("Contact Yoga") is Mantra-Yoga coupled with the control of the life-force (pranayama).
3. Bhava-Yoga ("Yoga of Being") is a higher form of Mantra-Yoga, where contact with the mantra is lost and consciousness enters a subtle dimension of existence.
4. Abhava-Yoga ("Yoga of Nonbeing") is the meditation of the universe in its entirety, associated with the transcendence of object-related awareness.
5. Maha-Yoga ("Great Yoga") is the contemplation of Shiva without any restricting conditions.

The Puranas thus contain records of and references to a variety of yogic schools. Some of these schools follow Patanjali's model of the eightfold path, though occasionally they interpret the limbs differently from that great Yoga authority. But what distinguishes them most markedly from Patanjali's tradition is that they all propose a single ultimate principle, the Self or God.

Puranic Yoga has been little researched, though fortunately many of the Puranas are available in more or less reliable English translations. The fund of myths and legends preserved in these scriptures is a perennial inspiration to the Yoga student.

MIND ONLY: THE IDEALISM OF THE YOGA-VASISHTHA

> Whatever is in this [book], is also [to be found] in others, but what is not in it, will also not [be found] elsewhere. Hence the learned know this [work] as the treasury of the entire philosophical learning. (III.8.12)

Thus announces proudly the composor of the Yoga-Vasishtha-Ramayana, a philosophical work of nearly 30,000 stanzas, written in the finest poetic Sanskrit. The author, whom tradition fancifully identifies with Valmiki, the creator of the Ramayana epic, is poet, philosopher, psychologist, and yogin in one person. In the form of an imaginary dialogue between the ancient hero Ramacandra and his teacher Vashishtha,[16] Valmiki presents an abundance of ideas, stories, and experiences that show a rare depth and universality of outlook.

The original and now lost version of the Yoga-Vasishtha was probably composed in the eighth century A.D., and in the ninth century was fashioned into the still extant Laghu ("Smaller")-Yoga-Vasishtha by Gauda Abhinanda. The full version was created some time in the tenth century A.D. In its different forms, Valmiki's work has exercised considerable influence on Yoga and Vedanta theory and practice. It has been translated into a number of Indian vernaculars and has several commentaries and summaries. The modern saint Rama Tirtha called it "one of the greatest books, and the most wonderful according to me, ever written under the sun . . . which nobody on earth can read without realizing God-consciousness."[17]

The philosophy of the Yoga-Vasishtha is radically nondualist. The fundamental thesis of this scripture, reiterated innumerable times, is that there is only Consciousness (citta). It is omnipresent, omniscient, and formless. Sage Vashishtha also refers to it as the Absolute (brahman), stating that as the mind of a painter is filled with numerous images of a great variety of objects, so the pure Consciousness is suffused with the images of the multiple forms of Nature—an idea that we also encounter in the teaching of the Christian mystic Meister Eckehart. Vashishtha defines the Absolute as follows:

It is the Self (purusha) of volition (samkalpa), devoid of physical form such as earth [and the other material elements]. It is singular (kevala), Consciousness only, the essential cause of the existence of the triple universe.[18] (III.3.11)

Like the chest of a stone [sculpture], which is void inside and void outside, [the Absolute] is tranquil, lucid as the vault of the sky, neither to be seen nor beyond vision. (VI.53.24)

Just as there is butter in every [kind of] milk, similarly the Supreme abides in the bodies of all things. (VI.53.49)

Just as the lustre of all [kinds of] gems and treasures of the sea [shines] within and without, so I am in [all] bodies, abiding [in them, and yet] seemingly not abiding [in them]. (VI.53.50)

Just as space is inside and outside thousands of pots, so I abide as the Self in the bodies of the three worlds. (VI.53.51)

Just as a thread strung with a mass of hundreds of pearls [is concealed but nevertheless present], so does this invisible Self abide in the visible bodies [of all beings]. (VI.53.52)

That which is the universal Being (satta) in the multitude of things—from [the Creator-God] Brahma down to a blade of grass—know that to be the unborn Self. (VI.53.53)

The phenomenal world is but a reflection of that universal Mind. It *is* that Mind. It is merely on account of spiritual ignorance (avidya) that we fail to realize this truth. The world is neither real nor unreal. It is situated in Consciousness but appears to the unenlightened mind as something external. It is like a dream, or a bubble rising in the absolute Consciousness. Once it is understood that the world we perceive is "our" world, "our" creation, and that bondage and freedom are states of mind, the next step is to break down the habit of wrong conceptualization. The mind (manas) itself must be transcended.

The spiritual path outlined in the Yoga-Vasishtha is essentially Jnana-Yoga and has great similarity to the Buddhi-Yoga taught in the Bhagavad-Gita, where action and knowledge are blended harmoniously. Vashishtha disdains the kind of asceticism that is performed empty-minded or is attended with pain. The genuine yogin, according to him, is free from the push and pull of passionate attraction on the one side and hostile rejection on the other. Such a yogin looks at a lump of gold and a pile of rubbish with the same unperturbed mind.

According to Vashishtha, it is the human mind alone that creates the illusion of bondage or the reality of liberation. There is, therefore, no point in external renunciation. Rather, what is needed is a total inner reorientation. He calls this doctrine mental liberation (cetya-nirmuktata). Yoga is variously defined by him as "the restriction of the fluctuations of the mind," "nonemotionality" (avedana), and "separation from the effects of the poison of passion." In contrast with the teachings of the God-man Krishna, which emphasize our emotional capacities in the form of devotion (bhakti), Vashishtha stresses the cognitive side of our psychic life. However, he has little patience with those who are merely interested in intellectual gyrations without proper application in life. The knowledge he deems useful is wisdom, or real insight, that leads to illumination.

Thus, the author of the Yoga-Vasishtha seeks, in ever new ingenious phrases and metaphors, to evoke in his readers or listeners the conviction that they are absolutely in charge of their own destiny, if only they can see the trick the human mind is playing on them. Destiny (daiva) is a formidable force, but human effort (paurusha) is superior to it.

According to one passage (VI.13), Yoga consists of both Self-knowledge (atma-jnana) and the restriction of the life-force (prana-samrodha). The former is the path of meditative absorption; the latter approach may be identified with Kundalini-Yoga, involving the arousal of the latent consciousness-energy of the body.

The mind and the life-force are said to be most intimately associated. The stoppage of the one leads to the cessation of the other. By "mind" (manas), Vashishtha means the ego-consciousness, which projects its own world through the process of imaginative volition (samkalpa), propelled by the force of root desire (vasana). He compares the mind to a madman with a thousand hands who constantly beats himself, inflicting pain on his body. The mind is galvanized by the vibration (spanda, parispanda) of the life-force circulating in the body, while the life-force is impelled by primal desire (vasana). Control of the quivering of the life-force (prana) is the most direct means of quieting the mind and transcending the compelling force of desire. But Vashishtha also recommends concentration and meditation as superb aids for taking charge of the mind.

Vashishtha's Yoga comprises the following seven stages:[19]

1. Shubha-iccha ("desire for what is good"): A person becomes aware of his or her spiritual ignorance and state of suffering and begins to desire to know the truth through study of the traditional lore.
2. Vicarana ("consideration"): Through the deepening of study and contact with holy people, the practitioner's conduct improves and his or her desire for liberation is kindled.
3. Tanu-manasa ("refinement of thinking"), characterized by a growing sense of indifference to the things of the world.
4. Sattva-apatti ("attainment of being"): The practitioner becomes capable of getting in touch with pure Consciousness through meditation.
5. Asamsakti ("nonattachment"): By virtue of true illumination, the mature practitioner becomes perfectly indifferent to the world, which is recognized as being a mere production of the mind.
6. Pada-artha-abhavana ("non-imagining of external things"): The world is recognized to be unreal like a dream.
7. Turya-ga ("abiding in the Fourth"): The yogin transcends everything and remains perpetually in pure Consciousness, which is called the "Fourth" as in Upanishadic Vedanta, since it transcends the states of waking, sleeping, and dreaming.

The yogin who has realized the Fourth, or the Self, is liberated even while the body-mind continues to exist. This is the ideal of living liberation (jivan-mukti). Because he is no longer ensnared by the ego-illusion, he can be all things to all people, reflecting their own states of mind, but himself living in perpetual bliss.

Those whose body is not subdued by the antidote ["nonpoisonous powder"] to the "I," while they are acting or even slaying—they cannot [cure their malady of spiritual] indigestion. (VI.53.10)

[For him who is] defiled by the impure [idea of] "mineness" toward the body, Consciousness (cit) does not shine forth. Even though he may be wise and very learned, he is like an ill-bred person. (VI.53.11)

With all volition (samkalpa) cast off, an equable, tranquil-minded sage, performing [actions] with the self yoked through the Yoga of renunciation—thus cultivate a liberated mind. (VI.53.19)

> When all volition is tranquilized, the mass of desires (vasana) are pacified as well. The form [for which there is] no conception (bhavana) whatsoever, is known as the supreme Absolute. (VI.53.22)

> Application (udyoga) toward That, the mature-minded (krita-buddhi) know as wisdom and Yoga. "The Absolute is the whole world as well as the 'I' (aham)"—[this realization] is known as the offering to the Absolute. (VI.53.23)

Enlightenment is ego-transcendence in every moment, regardless of whether the body-mind is active or in a state of repose. Vashishtha relates the story of King Bhagiratha, who abandoned his kingdom in order to dedicate himself to spiritual life. After years of meditation at a remote place, Bhagiratha attained enlightenment. One day he happened to wander through his former kingdom, and when the people recognized him they begged him to accept the throne again, as his successor had just died. Because nothing can bind a Self-realized adept, Bhagiratha accepted and for many years ruled over his people, bringing justice and wisdom into their lives.

The Yoga-Vasishtha is a truly remarkable creation that has had a strong influence on the more literate community of Yoga and Vedanta practitioners of medieval India. It is a lasting monument to the wisdom of nondualism.

योग आनन्दकल्पनः

chapter 11
God, Visions, and Power: The Yoga-Upanishads

INTRODUCTION

"That art thou" (tat tvam asi). "I am the Absolute" (aham brahma asmi). "All this is the Absolute" (sarvam brahma asti). These are the three great maxims of the ancient Upanishadic sages. What they seek to communicate is that Reality is singular and that, therefore, we are in truth only that all-encompassing single Being, which is unsurpassably blissful and superconscious. The Upanishads call it by many names, but the most common designations are the Absolute (brahman) and the Self (atman). These maxims were more than pious affirmations. Throughout the more than 200 extant Upanishads, we find scattered testimonies to the fact that for their composers and transmitters the nondual Being-Consciousness-Bliss was a living reality, not merely an abstract hypothesis or a belief.

Patanjali's philosophical system was among the few schools within the Yoga tradition to break with the Vedantic metaphysics of nondualism and to boldly assert a plurality of transcendental Selves (purusha). This led to a great deal of controversy and debate, from which the proponents of nondualist Vedanta emerged as final victors. For the basic tenor of Hindu thought is distinctly nondualistic. As a result, Patanjali's compilation of Yoga aphorisms, though widely respected, came to be exploited more for its practical contents than its philosophy. Thus we find that many later Yoga authorities refer to his definitions of the different limbs of Yoga but virtually ignore his metaphysics, unless they criticize it.

This is also the situation in the so-called Yoga-Upanishads, which all promulgate a Vedantic type of Yoga. These are works modeled on the earlier Upanishads but belonging for the most part to the post-Patanjali era. They have not yet been critically edited or studied, and therefore their interrelation-

231

ships and dates are still uncertain. But they contain important expositions of the yogic path, and practitioners of Yoga can certainly benefit from a close reading of these works, which are all available in reasonably reliable translations.

In the following sections, I will provide brief summaries of the contents of twenty Yoga-Upanishads.[1] I will start with the five so-called Bindu ("Point")-Upanishads: the Amrita-Bindu, the Amrita-Nada-Bindu, the Tejo-Bindu, the Nada-Bindu, and the Dhyana-Bindu, which make use of mantras as a means of focusing and ultimately transcending the mind. Sound also plays an important role in the teachings of the Hamsa, the Brahma-Vidya, the Mahavakya, and the Pashu-Pata-Brahma. These works are followed by the Advaya-Taraka and the Mandala-Brahmana, which expound a Yoga of light phenomena. The short but unusual Kshurika-Upanishad epitomizes the essence of all forms of Yoga. The concluding category comprises those Upanishads that tend to be more comprehensive and textbook-like treatments of Kundalini-Yoga, namely the Yoga-Kundali, Darshana, the Yoga-Shikha, the Yoga-Tattva, the Yoga-Cudamani, the Varaha, the Tri-Shikhi-Brahmana, and the Shandilya-Upanishad.

SOUNDING OUT THE ABSOLUTE

> The world is sound. It sounds in pulsars and planetary orbits, in the spin of electrons, in the quanta of atoms and the structure of molecules, in the microcosm and in the macrocosm. It also sounds in the sphere between these extremes, in the world in which we live.[2]

This is how Joachim-Ernst Berendt, a well-known German producer of radio programs and musicologist, begins one chapter in his remarkable book *Nada Brahman*. His excursion into the mystery of what he calls primal sound, the transcendental sound that gives rise to all manifestation, shows that religiospiritual traditions around the world have explored sound as part of their quest for the transmutation of consciousness.

In India, undoubtedly the oldest and most sacred power-word (mantra) is the syllable *om*, symbolizing the Absolute. It is pronounced with a strongly nasalized or hummed *m*, which is indicated in Sanskrit by a dot (called bindu, "seed-point") under the letter *m*. Whereas the syllable *om* by itself is said to represent the creative or manifest dimension of the Divine, the echo, or bindu, of the sound *m* is thought to represent the Divine in its unmanifest dimension. Shyam Sundar Goswami, a modern practitioner of Laya-Yoga ("Yoga of [Mental] Absorption"), explained the esoteric significance of the bindu as follows:

> Bindu is a state in which power is at maximum concentration. When mental consciousness is in the bindu state, diversified mental powers are collected and

highly concentrated as mental dynamism. . . . Bindu—the power point—is a natural and indispensable condition associated with power in its operation. Bindu occurs both in the mental and material fields. The atom is the bindu of matter; the nucleus the bindu of a protoplasmic cell; and samadhi consciousness the bindu of the mind.[3]

Thus, the bindu is latent concentrated power—whether it be of consciousness or of sound or of Nature itself. The five Bindu-Upanishads build upon the age-old Vedic speculations around this sacred sound. They espouse a form of Mantra-Yoga.

Amrita-Bindu-Upanishad

The Amrita-Bindu ("Immortal Point")-Upanishad, also known as the Brahma-Bindu, is a short work of only twenty-two stanzas. It makes a distinction between the practice of the tonal (svara) syllable *om* and the higher practice of the nontonal or unsounded (asvara) syllable. They are also respectively referred to as lettered (kshara) and nonlettered (akshara) aspects of this great mantra. By meditating upon the latter aspect, the spiritual practitioner is assured of finding peace of mind. To this end, he or she is also advised to dispense with all book knowledge, just as one winnows the husk from the grain. The ultimate realization of this Mantra-Yoga is identification with the Absolute in the form of Vasudeva ("All-God").

Amrita-Nada-Bindu-Upanishad

With a total of thirty-eight stanzas, the Amrita-Nada-Bindu ("Immortal Sound-Point")-Upanishad is only slightly longer than the Amrita-Bindu. But it makes several interesting disclosures about Mantra-Yoga. First of all, it treats mantra meditation as part of a sixfold (shad-anga) Yoga, consisting of sense-withdrawal, meditation, breath control, concentration, inspection (tarka),[4] and ecstasy—in that order.

Breath control (pranayama) is defined as the triple recitation of the gayatri-mantra with a single breath. I have already introduced this famous Vedic mantra (see the third section of Chapter 5), which includes the sacred syllable *om*. The regulation of the breath in this manner causes a switch in consciousness, whereby attention becomes more and more focused. This enables the yogin to contemplate the transcendental Self in the practice of concentration (dharana), which consists in merging the desire-filled mind with the Self. One full cycle of pranayama, as described above, is known as a measure (matra). Concentration is said to be seven or eight such measures long, whereas the condition of union (yoga)—that is, ecstatic realization (samadhi)—is reckoned to be twelve such measures.

Of interest is the doctrine of the "seven gates" (sapta-dvara) that can lead the yogin to liberation. These are respectively called "heart gate" (hrid-dvara), "wind gate" (vayu-dvara), "head gate" (murdha-dvara), "liberation gate" (moksha-dvara), "cavity" (bila), "hollow" (sushira), and "circle" (mandala). They refer to different anatomical structures, though the author does not divulge anything about them. The last four are probably all esoteric loci in the head. These technical terms hint at the fact that the composer of this Upanishad was steeped in esoteric lore that was far more sophisticated than his own composition. The yogin who diligently follows this Yoga, sketched with such tantalizing brevity, is promised liberation (kaivalya) in the sixth month.

Nada-Bindu-Upanishad

The Nada-Bindu ("Sound-Point")-Upanishad comprises fifty-six stanzas. It starts with an exposition of the esoteric meaning of the sacred syllable *om*, which is said to consist of three and a half "measures" (matra—namely the sounds *a, u, m,* and the half-measure (ardha-matra) that is the nasalized echo of *m,* elsewhere referred to as the point (bindu). This mantra is called the vairaja-pranava, "resplendent humming." In one place (9–16), twelve such measures are spoken of, as well as the states of consciousness correlated with them.

There is also a passage describing the practice of the inner sound (nada), which can be located in the right ear during meditative absorption. Through repeated practice this sound can become so prominent that all external sounds are drowned by it. It also gives rise to a variety of other inner sounds, resembling those produced by the ocean, a waterfall, a kettledrum, a bell, a flute, and so on. The inwardly perceived sound becomes increasingly subtle, until the mind becomes so completely one with it that the individual forgets himself or herself. The mind undergoing this process is compared to a bee that is only interested in the nectar of a flower, not the scent that attracted it. The end-state is one of total mental repose, perfect indifference to worldly existence. The yogin who has achieved this sublime state is described as being a videha-mukta, one who has reached disembodied liberation.

Dhyana-Bindu-Upanishad

The Dhyana-Bindu ("Meditation-Point")-Upanishad, having 106 verses, expands on the mystical speculations of the Nada-Bindu. Employing an old Upanishadic metaphor, it likens the syllable *om* to a bow, with oneself as the arrow and the Absolute as the target. The individual who truly realizes the import of this metaphor is liberated even while being embodied. Meditation on the "lotus of the heart"—that is, the esoteric center at the heart—is recommended, and prescriptions for its visualization are given.

From verse 41 on, which lists the limbs of a sixfold Yoga, the text changes gear and reads like a Hatha-Yoga work. Thus, we find a description of other principal psychoenergetic centers (cakra) of the body, including the "bulb" (kanda) in the lower abdomen where the 72,000 currents or ducts (nadi) of the life-force are said to originate. This is followed by a discussion of the ten types of life-force animating the body and how the life-force relates to the dynamics of the psyche (jiva).

The psyche, it is stated, continually recites what is called the hamsa ("swan")-mantra. The sound *ham* is associated with inhalation, the sound *sa* with exhalation. The sequence *hamsa-hamsa-hamsa* can also be heard as *so'ham-so'ham-so'ham*, which has the esoteric meaning of "I am He"; that is to say, "I am the Divine." Thus, the body itself is constantly affirming its own true Essence. This spontaneous recitation, effected by the automatic breathing process, is known as the ajapa-gayatri, or the "gayatri of nonrecitation." The yogins of yore calculated that we normally inhale and exhale around 21,600 times in the course of a day. The yogin's task is to aid this natural process through controlling the breath and thus the mind.

This six-limbed Yoga is clearly a form of Kundalini-Yoga. The "serpent power" (kundalini-shakti) is sought to be awakened by a variety of means, including "locks" (bandha) applied to the anal and abdominal muscles and the throat, and such practices as the famous "space-walking seal" (khecari-mudra) and the "great seal" (maha-mudra), which are both explained in Chapter 13 on Hatha-Yoga. Again, the goal of this Yoga is the state of "aloneness" (kaivalya), or liberation. The term is borrowed from Patanjali, but here it means merging with the Divine rather than perfect separation from Nature.

Tejo-Bindu-Upanishad

The Tejo-Bindu ("Radiance-Point")-Upanishad has six chapters with a total of 465 verses. Chapters II–IV and chapters V–VI appear to have once been two independent texts. Only the first chapter and the beginning of the fifth somewhat justify the title of this Upanishad, while the remaining sections are expositions of Vedanta nondualism and have nothing to do with the practice of Mantra-Yoga.

The reader is exhorted to meditate on the "swan" (hamsa), by which is here meant the transcendental Self beyond the three states of consciousness (waking, dreaming, and sleeping). The anonymous composer of this work puts forward a fifteen-limbed (panca-dasha-anga) Yoga, consisting of the following constituents:

1. Restraint (yama), which is defined as the "restraint of the senses by means of the knowledge that everything is Absolute" (I.17).
2. Self-discipline (niyama), which stands for "application to the

innate [Self] and dissociation from what is alien" (I.18); what is "alien" is everything that is perceived to be other than the Self.

3. Renunciation (tyaga), which is explained as the "abandonment of the phenomenal world as a result of beholding the true superconscious Self" (I.19).

4. Silence (mauna), which is not so much ritual silence as the quieting of mind and mouth in virtue of the awe felt when the transcendental Self appears on the horizon of the meditative consciousness.

5. Place (desha), which is esoterically explained as "that by which this [world] is eternally pervaded" (I.23)—that is, the Space of Consciousness.

6. Time (kala), which is likewise explained in mystical rather than conventional terms.

7. Posture (asana), which is further stipulated as the "adept posture" (siddha-asana).

8. "Root-lock" (mula-bandha), a Hatha-Yoga practice that is here given a new, occult significance, for the author interprets it as "the root of the world" (I.27).

9. Bodily balance (deha-samya), which is here explained as a merging with the Absolute. The conventional interpretation of this term, as the practice of standing like a tree, is explicitly rejected.

10. Steadiness of vision (drik-sthiti), which is seeing the world as the Absolute rather than the common yogic practice of fixing one's sight on the spot between the eyebrows, where the "third eye" is situated.

11. Breath control (prana-samyama), which is defined as "the restriction of all fluctuations [of consciousness]" (I.31).

12. Withdrawal (pratyahara), which is understood here not as sensory withdrawal but as the mental state of locating the Self in the objects of the world.

13. Concentration (dharana), which is explained as the mental state of having the vision of the Absolute wheresoever the mind may wander.

14. Contemplation of the Self (atma-dhyana), which yields supreme bliss.

15. Ecstasy (samadhi), which is defined as "the complete forgetting of the fluctuations [of consciousness], by [assuming] repeatedly the form of the Absolute, the unchanging fluctuation [of transcendental Consciousness]" (I.37).

The Tejo-Bindu (I.42) makes the further point that the ecstatic state entails the realization of the Absolute as fullness (purnatva), whereas the experience of emptiness (shunyata) is considered an obstacle on the path. This is a dig against the Mahayana Buddhists, who speak of the ultimate Reality as the Void.

The subsequent chapters are more formulaic, giving us hundreds of variations on the great theme of nondualism—"I am the Absolute." In chapter IV the ideal of living liberation (jivan-mukti) is referred to. The Self-realized adept, who experiences his perfect identity with the Divine while being embodied, is called a jivan-mukta. By contrast, the videha-mukta is described as having abandoned even the knowledge of being identical with the Absolute.

This group of Upanishads shows the high level of sophistication of yogic psychotechnology and metaphysical speculation that the Yoga tradition gained in the centuries after Patanjali.

SOUND, BREATH, AND TRANSCENDENCE

Unless we are consciously trying to muffle the sound of our breath, we are ordinarily quite unaware of it. However, as soon as we begin to meditate, we become awkwardly conscious of the sound produced by the two bellows in our chest. For beginners this can even be a disturbing experience. Yet for the yogin this rhythmic sound is music to his ears because he can fasten his attention on it, until the mind itself is transcended and he enters the soundless domain of the transcendental Reality.

The yogin regards the breath, which is technically known as hamsa ("swan"), as being a manifestation of the transcendental Life, or Self, which is also referred to as hamsa. As we have seen in the preceding section, the two syllables of the word—*ham* and *sa*—stand for the ingoing and outgoing breaths, as well as the ascending and descending currents of the life-force. They contain a great secret, for the continuous sound of the breath conveys the message "I am He, I am He, I am He." In other words, the breath is a constant reminder of the absolute truth that we are identical to the great Life of the cosmos, the Absolute, or transcendental Self.

Hamsa-Upanishad

This creative idea is at the core of the teaching of the Hamsa-Upanishad, a short work of twenty-one verses. Those who are incapable of contemplating the Self directly are advised to resort to the craft of silent hamsa recitation, which is the conscious observation of the spontaneous "prayer" of the breath. In this way, the text states, all kinds of internal sounds (nada) are generated. Ten levels are distinguished, and the practitioner is asked to cultivate only the tenth and most subtle level of the internal sound, which resembles that of a thundercloud. It leads to identification with the Self, the realization of Sada-Shiva, the "Eternal Shiva," who is the resplendent, peaceful Ground of all existence.

Brahma-Vidya-Upanishad

A more elaborate treatment of this Hamsa-Yoga is found in the Brahma-Vidya ("Knowledge of the Absolute")-Upanishad, a work of 111 stanzas. The practice of hamsa recitation and meditation is recommended for householders and forest anchorites as well as mendicant yogins. It is said to lead to spiritual perfection and paranormal powers. This form of Hamsa-Yoga is combined with practices designed to awaken the serpent power and to conduct it to the highest esoteric center at the crown of the head.

Mahavakya-Upanishad

Like the Tejo-Bindu, the Mahavakya ("Great Saying")-Upanishad, a tract of twelve verses, speaks of the goal of the yogic process as fullness. This condition, it states, is not merely ecstasy (samadhi), yogic perfection, or the dissolution of the mind. It is, rather, perfect identity (aikya) with the Absolute.

Pashu-Pata-Upanishad

The Pashu-Pata ("Lord of Beasts")-Brahma-Upanishad is a Shaiva work of seventy-eight verses distributed over two chapters. It gets its name from God Pashupati, who is none other than Shiva, the Lord of the "beasts," or souls, in bondage. This scripture builds on the sacrificial symbolism of the brahmins and introduces the practice of the hamsa-mantra as a form of internal or mental sacrifice. This process is also called nada-anusamdhana, "application to the [inner] sound." It is connected with an esoteric notion according to which there are ninety-six "solar beams" in the heart. These are rays, or links, originating in the transcendental Self through which It can be creative in the human body-mind. "This occult fact about the Absolute is not disclosed anywhere else," states the text (I.25). It is further stated that liberation is possible only for the yogin who is able to meditate on the identity of the hamsa as sound and the hamsa as the transcendental Self.

On the philosophical question of how the singular transcendental Reality can give rise to the world of multiplicity, the anonymous composer suggests silence as the wisest attitude to be assumed. Because of his radical nondualist philosophy, he can even declare that liberation is sought only by those who feel themselves bound. For the same reason, dietary restrictions do not apply to the liberated sage, for, as the ancient Taittiriya-Upanishad teaches, he is always food and the consumer of food: The transcendental Self is forever devouring itself in the form of the multiple objects of the phenomenal world.

PHOTISTIC YOGA

More than sound, mysticism is universally associated with experiences of light. In fact, the transcendental Reality is frequently described as utter brilliance and as such is compared to the sun. Liberation is also widely referred to as enlightenment or illumination.

> The enlightened are bathed in light. Likewise they irradiate light, which is represented by the aura that surrounds the heads of saints and *bodhisattvas* in Christian and Buddhist art. There is a subtle form of light that strikes the inward eye and suffuses the body. Enlightenment is no metaphorical term.[5]

One of the most memorable passages in the Bhagavad-Gita is Arjuna's description of his vision of Lord Krishna as the ultimate Being. Awed by Krishna's self-revelation to him, Arjuna exclaims:

> Without beginning, middle, or end, of infinite vigor, with infinite arms, and with the sun and the moon for your eyes: thus I behold you, your mouth a flaming offering-consumer burning up this entire [world] with your brilliance. (XI.19)

> Tell me who you of dread-inspiring Form are. Salutations be to you! O Foremost God, have mercy! I wish to know you [as you were] at first [in your human form], for I do not comprehend your Creativity. (XI.31)[6]

Prince Arjuna, who at the time of his vision had not yet undergone the full yogic process, was ill-prepared for this encounter with the God-man Krishna in his transcendental nature. He begged Krishna to restore his ordinary consciousness so that he could once again behold Krishna's familiar human body. It is always fear—the fear of losing oneself—that prevents the ultimate event of enlightenment even in those who are advanced on the spiritual path. Thus, in the Tibetan Book of the Dead, the person preparing for the great transitional process of death is instructed not to be afraid of the Clear Light that he or she will perceive in the after-death state.

Experiences of inner light occur well before the yogin has reached the point of spiritual maturity where the confrontation with the transcendental Light takes place, for which the only viable response is self-surrender. These experiences, known as photisms, can be looked upon as dress rehearsals for the encounter with the Light of lights. They can be quite spectacular internal fireworks, though more often they are simpler experiences of localized or sometimes diffused nonphysical light or lights. The experience of the "blue pearl" (nila-bindu), frequently talked about by the late Swami Muktananda, is such a preliminary manifestation.

Just as Mantra-Yoga or Nada-Yoga makes use of the vibrations of sound to internalize and transcend the ordinary consciousness, Taraka-Yoga avails itself of the higher vibrations of both white and colored light. Moreover, it includes aspects of the practice of the inner sound (nada).

The word *taraka* means literally "deliverer." It denotes the ultimate Reality, which is the true liberating agency. The term is found already in the Yoga-Sutra (III.54), where it refers to the liberating wisdom (jnana), which results from continuous discernment (viveka) between the transcendental Subject and the objective world, including the mind. It appears that this Yoga was fairly widespread in India during the medieval period, and it may have exercised considerable influence on Chinese Taoism.

Advaya-Taraka-Upanishad

Taraka-Yoga is dealt with in the Advaya-Taraka ("Nondual Deliverer")-Upanishad. This compact text of only nineteen passages happens to be among the most cohesive works of the Upanishadic genre. The "nondual deliverer" is the transcendental Consciousness, which reveals itself to the yogin in a "multitude of fires"—similar to the way Paul of Tarsus was visited by a blinding light on the road to Damascus in an experience that changed his entire life.

The Advaya-Taraka begins as follows:

> Presently we would like to expound the secret doctrine of the nondual Deliverer for the ascetic (yati) who has subdued the senses and is filled with the six virtues, namely quiescence and the rest. (1)

The six virtues praised in Vedantic circles are quiescence (shama), restraint (dama) of the senses, cessation (uparati) of desire or worldly activity, endurance (titiksha), collectedness (samadhana), and faith (shraddha).

> Always realizing "I am of the nature of Consciousness (cit)," with eyes completely shut or else with eyes somewhat open, by looking inward, above the eyebrows—he, beholding the Absolute, the Supreme, in the form of a multitude of fires of Being-Consciousness-Bliss, assumes that appearance [of luminosity]. (2)

> [This secret doctrine is known as] Taraka-[Yoga] because [it enables the yogin] to overcome (samtarayati) the great dread of the cycle of conception, birth, life and death. Realizing the psyche (jiva) and the Lord (ishvara) to be illusory, and abandoning all differentiation as "not this, not that" (neti-neti)—that which remains is the nondual Absolute. (3)

The photistic manifestations are seen as a means of reaching the unmanifest supreme Light. They are significant only as signs along the way.

This Upanishad appears to have served as model for the more elaborate Mandala-Brahmana-Upanishad. Unlike the latter scripture, the Advaya-Taraka makes no attempt to integrate the Yoga of light phenomena with Hatha-Yoga techniques.

Mandala-Brahmana-Upanishad

The Mandala ("Circle")-Brahmana-Upanishad comprises ninety-two verses distributed over five chapters. The teachings are attributed to Yajnavalkya, who propounds an eightfold Yoga, giving some unusual definitions of each limb. Restraint (yama), the first limb, is said to encompass the following four practices:

1. Mastery over heat and cold as well as food and sleep at all times
2. Peace (shanti)
3. Steadiness (nishcalatva) of the mind
4. Restraint of the senses in regard to objects

Self-discipline (niyama), the second limb, consists of the following nine practices:

1. Devotion to the teacher (guru-bhakti)
2. Adherence to the path to truth
3. Enjoyment of the Real (vastu) as it is glimpsed in pleasurable experiences
4. Contentment
5. Nonattachment (nihsangata)
6. Living in solitude (ekanta-vasa)
7. Cessation of mental activity
8. Nonattachment toward the fruit of one's actions
9. Dispassion (vairagya), which presumably stands for the renunciation of all desires

"Postural restraint" (asana-niyama), the third constituent of the eightfold path, is defined as any comfortable posture that can be maintained over a longer period of time. Breath control (pranayama), again, is divided into inhalation (puraka), retention (kumbhaka), and exhalation (recaka); these are said to be of the duration of sixteen, sixty-four, and thirty-two "measures" respectively. In other words, the breathing cycle has the well-known yogic rhythm 1:4:2.

Sensory withdrawal (pratyahara) is explained as restraining the mind from going out toward the sense-objects, while concentration, the sixth limb, is defined as stabilizing one's consciousness in the transcendental Consciousness (caitanya). Modifying Patanjali's definition, Yajnavalkya explains meditation (dhyana), the penultimate aspect of the eightfold path, as the "single flow" (eka-tanata) of attention toward the transcendental Consciousness, which is hidden in all beings. Finally, ecstasy (samadhi) is the state of forgetfulness (vismriti) in meditation, when the notion of "I" drops away and there is only the absolute Being-Consciousness-Bliss.

That blissful Reality manifests as different light phenomena, which can be seen within and without. As in the Advaya-Taraka-Upanishad, the former experiences are known as visions of the inner sign (antar-lakshya-darshana), the latter as visions of the outer sign (bahya-lakshya-darshana). These photistic phenomena are associated with the idea of "radiance-space" (akasha). This is not physical, three-dimensional space, but the expanse of the life-force and consciousness itself as it can be experienced in deep meditation. Five types of radiance-space are distinguished, which appear to be different levels of luminous experience. First is the radiance-space (akasha) existing both within and without, which is "exquisitely dark." Perhaps this corresponds to the experience of the "space of consciousness" at the beginning of meditation. The second level is superior radiance-space (para-akasha), which is said to be as bright as the conflagration when the cosmos is destroyed at the end of time. Next comes the great radiance-space (maha-akasha), which is radiant beyond measure. The fourth is sunlike radiance-space (surya-akasha). The fifth is supreme radiance-space (parama-akasha), which is all-pervading and unsurpassably blissful; its luminosity is quite indescribable.

We can only guess at the experiential significance of these luminous spaces. They are clearly supraphysical and only vaguely analogous to the "ether" once thought by physicists to be the medium for the propagation of light. It is easier for meditators than for nonmeditators to appreciate what these potent radiance-spaces might be.

This Upanishad, moreover, makes a distinction between two types of photistic experience. First is the "deliverer with form" (murti-taraka), which is within the range of the senses and consists in manifestations of light in the space between the eyebrows. The second type is the "formless deliverer" (amurti-taraka), which is the transcendental Light itself.

The ultimate condition aspired to in this Yoga is called the transmental state (amanaskata), or no-mindedness (unmani), or yogic sleep (yoga-nidra). The unmani state is the product of prolonged absorption in the formless ecstasy (nirvikalpa-samadhi). This leads to the dissolution of the mind, whereupon the transcendental Reality shines forth in its solitary majesty.

> The yogins immersed in the Ocean of Bliss become that [Absolute]. (II.4.3)

> Compared to that [ultimate Bliss], Indra and the other [deities] are only minimally blissful. Thus, he who has attained that Bliss is a supreme yogin. (II.4.4)

The yogin who has reached this lofty state is called a supreme swan (parama-hamsa) and an avadhuta, one who has cast off everything. "Even an ignorant person serving such a one," declares Yajnavalkya confidently, "is liberated" (V.9).

CUTTING THROUGH THE KNOTS OF ORDINARY AWARENESS

The Indian rope trick is a collective hallucination in which the bystanders witness the following: A fakir throws one end of a rope into the air. Instead of falling back on the ground, it stiffens and stands on its own. A boy climbs up the rope, followed by the fakir himself, carrying a dagger in his mouth. Both disappear. Suddenly, the boy's severed limbs fall from the sky, seemingly out of nowhere. The fakir reappears and reassembles the youth. When his head is placed back on the neck, the boy seemingly comes alive, with a broad smile.

The rope trick, though usually performed for public entertainment, has deep symbolic significance. The dismemberment is a symbolic enactment of the very essence of spiritual life, which is the death of the "old Adam" and the birth of the "new man."

This same motif is present in the Kshurika ("Knife")-Upanishad. This is a short work with an interesting angle on concentration, which describes well the core of all yogic activity: The yogin severs all the bonds that fasten him to conditioned existence, starting with "bioenergetic" blockages, or obstructions in the flow of the life-force in the body, and proceeding to faulty attitudes and ideas. Like a sharp blade, the Yoga described in this Upanishad cuts through all binding conditions and frees the spirit, which soars like a bird to the Absolute.

Of special interest is the concept of bodily vital-points (marman), which appear to be places of trapped life-energy. By a technique strikingly similar to contemporary bodywork, the yogin releases the dammed-up life-force and then applies it to stimulate the energy flow along the bodily axis (sushumna), guiding it gradually to the secret center in the head.

The following is a rendering of the whole text.

I will disclose the [doctrine of] the "dagger," the concentration [of attention] for perfection in Yoga, having attained which the Yoga-yoked will not be born again. (1)

That [teaching] is the essence and the goal of the Vedas, as has been declared by Svayambhu. (2)

Svayambhu, the "Self-Existent," is the Creator-God, whether he be called Brahma, Vishnu, or Shiva.

Settling in a quiet place, there assumed a [suitable] posture, confining the mind in the heart as a tortoise retracts its limbs—by means of the Yoga of twelve measures (matra) and the pranava [i.e., the syllable om] very gradually . . . (3)

. . . one should, all [bodily] openings blocked [by means of the fingers], fill up [with life-force] one's whole body (atman) from the chest to the head and from the hips to the nape, with slightly raised chest. (4)[7]

Thereon one should hold fast the life-forces (prana) moving through the nostril. Having achieved prolonged breath (ayata-prana), one should gradually exhale the breath (ucchvasa). (5)[8]

Having made oneself steady and firm, [one should practice breath control] by using the thumb [to close one nostril at a time] [and then draw the life-force in] through the ankles and also the calves, "three-by-three." (6)[9]

Then [one should draw the life-force in] through the knees and thighs, the penis, and the anus, "three-by-three." [Lastly], one should cause it to flow and rest in the area of the navel, [having drawn the life-force up from] the seat of the anus. (7)

There [at the lowest center of the body] is the sushumna channel, surrounded by ten [main] channels (nadi): the red, the yellow, and the black, the copper-colored, and the flame-colored ones, . . . (8)

. . . [which are] very fine and tenuous. One should cause the breath to flow to the white channel [of the sushumna]. Thereupon one should guide the life-forces as a spider [ascends] along its thread. (9)

Thence [the yogin reaches] that resplendent red lotus, the great seat of the heart, which is called the "dahara lotus" in the Vedanta [scriptures]. (10)

Having broken it open, he proceeds to the throat, and it is said that one should fill that channel [with the life-force]. The mind's supreme mystery, exceedingly spotless wisdom: (11)

The vital-point (marman) situated on the top of the foot can indeed be contemplated as having that character[?]. By means of the sharp blade of the mind, constantly devoted to [the practice of] Yoga, . . . (12)

. . . [one should bring about] the cutting of the vital-point of the calves, which is said to be "Indra's thunderbolt." He should cut through that [vital-point] with the powerful Yoga of meditation, through concentration. (13)

Practicing the four [types of meditation on external and internal as well as coarse and subtle objects], he should, by means of Yoga, unhesitatingly cut through the vital-point situated in the middle of the thighs, [thereby] freeing the life-force [in that place]. (14)

Thence the yogin should gather [the life-force and lead it] to the throat, [where] a multitude of channels [exists]. There, one among and above a hundred channels, is the supreme stable . . . (15)

. . . sushumna, far hidden, pure, embodying the Absolute. Ida stands to the left and pingala to the right [of the sushumna channel]. (16)[10]

Between these two is the supreme abode. He who knows it, knows the Vedas. Taitila, among the seventy-two thousand secondary channels, . . . (17)

. . . is cut off by means of the Yoga of meditation, [that is to say,] by the untainted, powerful blade of Yoga with its flaming energy. [However,] the solitary sushumna is not cut off. (18)

At that moment, the yogin can see the Taitila, which is like a jasmine flower. For, the sage should cut, in this very existence, the one hundred channels, because they are the cause [of future births]. (19)

Thus, one should dissociate from auspicious and inauspicious conditions [associated with] these channels. Those who have realized this achieve freedom from rebirth. (20)

With the mind conquered through asceticism, established in a wilderness, unattached, conversant with the limbs of Yoga, desireless, [practicing] step by step: [thus should the yogin approach liberation]. (21)

As a swan (hamsa), having cut through the fetters, flies straight up into the sky—similarly the psyche (jiva), having severed its bonds, always crosses over [the ocean of] existence (samsara). (22)

As a lamp, at the moment of [the flame's] extinction, having burnt up [its fuel], ceases to function—thus the yogin, having burnt out all karma, ceases to exist [as an individual separate from all other beings]. (23)

Having cut through the bonds by means of the blade of the measure (matra) [of meditation], well-sharpened through breath control and whetted on the stone of renunciation, the Yoga-adept is no [longer] fettered. (24)

BODILY TRANSMUTATION: THE UPANISHADS OF HATHA-YOGA

Sound, light, and breath: These are important tools for the yogin. They belong to the oldest and best-tried elements of India's psychotechnology. Their possibilities for psychospiritual transformation have been explored over the centuries by tens of thousands of practitioners. The Sanskrit and vernacular works on Yoga are, therefore, distillates of an immense wealth of factual information, though in many cases we still need to find the right key for unlocking their secrets. The spirit of experimentation on which modern science prides itself is intrinsic to Yoga as well. The yogins have always been fearless adventurers in the vast and mostly still unmapped territory of the human body-mind.

But at no time has this experimental mood been more prominent than during those centuries that saw the birth and rise of Tantrism—the period between the sixth or seventh and the fourteenth centuries A.D. It was during that span of time that the Indian "athletes of the spirit" intensively explored the hidden potential of the human body. Their curiosity, daring, and persistence led to the creation of what came to be called Hatha-Yoga, the "Yoga of the Force." The "force" is the esoteric serpent power (kundalini-shakti) celebrated in the Tantras. This is the universal life-force locked up in the human body, where it is said to be responsible for both bondage and liberation, depending on whether it is functioning unconsciously or consciously. The goal of the hatha-yogin is to bring the kundalini-shakti under his conscious control, inasmuch as this is possible.

We have encountered that formidable biospiritual energy in several of the Yoga-Upanishads discussed above, where it is mentioned in passing. The remaining texts of the Yoga-Upanishads all focus on Hatha-Yoga and therefore on techniques that are designed to awaken and harness the kundalini energy to the point where it can safely be conducted to the primary biospiritual center at the crown of the head, resulting in the blissful state of ecstatic merging with the Divine. The following Upanishads are all products of the twelfth to fourteenth centuries A.D. I will outline their contents only briefly here, because I do not want to anticipate too much of Chapters 12 and 13, which deal with the body-positive traditions of Tantrism and Hatha-Yoga.

Yoga-Kundaly-Upanishad[11]

The Yoga-Kundali, consisting of three chapters with a total of 171 stanzas, launches straight into an explanation of the serpent power, which it calls kundali and kundalini, both meaning the "coiled one," referring to the latency of this force. It mentions different types of breath control and the three "locks" (bandha)—at the base of the spine, the abdomen, and the throat—by which the life-force is restrained within the body. Its anonymous author preaches the ideal of disembodied liberation (videha-mukti), which is attained when the serpent power reaches the topmost center, where it unites with the transcendental male force of Shiva.

The second chapter deals with the highly esoteric practice of the "space-walking seal" (khecari-mudra), which, it is emphasized, must be learned from one's teacher. It is performed by using the tongue to block off the cavity behind the palate—a somewhat complicated maneuver that requires the elongation of the tongue. The third chapter consists of speculations about esoteric matters and hints at certain higher yogic processes.

Yoga-Tattva-Upanishad

The Yoga-Tattva ("Principles of Yoga")-Upanishad, a Vaishnava work of 142 verses, distinguishes and succinctly defines four types of Yoga: Mantra-Yoga, Laya-Yoga, Hatha-Yoga, and Raja-Yoga. This is a fairly systematic text that offers useful definitions of the constituent practices of Hatha-Yoga, including the obstacles on the path and also the paranormal attainments that the yogin may come to enjoy. It proposes a combination of gnosis (jnana) and yogic technology, with Hatha-Yoga preparing the practitioner for the demands of Raja-Yoga, which calls for both renunciation and discernment. Again the goal is "aloneness" (kaivalya), which is explained as disembodied liberation (videha-mukti).

Yoga-Shikha-Upanishad

With a total of 390 verses, the Yoga-Shikha ("Crest of Yoga") is the most comprehensive of the Yoga-Upanishads. It consists of six chapters, of which the concluding one appears to have been an independent tract at one time. This Shaiva work, like the Tantras, is said to be for spiritual seekers facing the difficulties inherent in the "dark age" (kali-yuga). Similar to the Yoga-Tattva, it propounds a teaching that combines gnosis or wisdom with yogic practice. Again and again the reader is reminded of the importance of transforming the body so that it becomes truly a "temple of Shiva."

> By means of the fire [of Yoga], [the yogin] should stimulate (ranjayet) the body made up of the seven constituents (dhatu) [i.e., the bodily humors—wind, bile, gall, blood, etc.]. (I.56a)

> All his diseases are cured. How much more so cuts, gashes, and so on. He acquires an embodied shape that is of the form of the supreme radiance-space (parama-akasha). (I.57)

The Yoga adept is not only Self-realized but his transmuted body is invested with all kinds of paranormal powers (siddhi), which are taken to be a sure sign of his spiritual attainment. "One should regard the man lacking powers as bound," declares the anonymous author (I.160). This does not invalidate the generally accepted attitude that the egoic use of these powers is detrimental to the yogin's spiritual welfare.

The second chapter deals with Mantra-Yoga, declaring that the inner sound (nada) is the highest mantra. In the third chapter, some of the metaphysical aspects of Mantra-Yoga are introduced. Sound is said to have several dimensions of subtlety, starting with the sound-transcending ultimate Reality and its lower or manifest form, the so-called shabda- ("sound") brahman. Subsequent stages in the progressive manifestation of sound are:

1. Para ("transcendental"), which is the "seed"-sound, or bindu
2. Pashyanti ("visible"), which is sound at a level that is inaudible but visible in yogic introspection
3. Madhyama ("middling"), which can be heard resounding "like a thunderclap" in the heart during deep meditation
4. Vaikhari ("harsh"), which is the sound (svara) created by vibrating air

The fourth chapter of the Yoga-Shikha-Upanishad is dedicated to expounding the Vedantic doctrine of the unreality of the world and the body, which are nothing apart from the single, all-encompassing Self (atman). In the fifth chapter, we learn about some of the main features of esoteric anatomy, such as the channels (nadi) and the centers (cakra). The concluding chapter covers somewhat similar ground but focuses on the central channel known as the sushumna-nadi, described as the "foremost place of pilgrimage" (VI.45). It is in or along this axial channel of the body that the yogin must force the awakened serpent power to the head.

Varaha-Upanishad

The Varaha ("Boar")-Upanishad, which is a late Vaishnava composition, has 263 verses distributed over five chapters. It begins with an enumeration of the categories (tattva) of existence. Vishnu, as the Boar (one of his incarnations), is said to be beyond all categories. Those who take refuge in him become liberated even while alive in the body.

The second and third chapters are a discourse on Vedanta metaphysics, which culminates in the recommendation to contemplate Vishnu in the manner of Bhakti-Yoga. Devotion to the Lord is regarded as the true means of liberation. But Kundalini-Yoga is also advised.

The fourth chapter explains the seven stages of wisdom, which are also mentioned in the Yoga-Vasishtha (see the final section of Chapter 10). The nature and life of the yogin who is embodied yet liberated is described. The Upanishad speaks of two approaches—that of the bird, as followed by the sage Shuka, and that of the ant, as followed by the sage Vamadeva. The former course leads to instant liberation (sadyo-mukti), whereas the latter orientation results in gradual liberation (krama-mukti).

The fifth chapter, which originally was probably an independent treatise that came to be appended to the Varaha-Upanishad, is a longer treatment of Hatha-Yoga. Its author recognizes only three types of Yoga—Laya-, Hatha-, and Mantra-Yoga, which should all be mastered. This compound Yoga has eight limbs, which match those specified by Patanjali. Its goal is enlightenment in this lifetime.

Shandilya-Upanishad

The same eightfold Yoga is taught in the Shandilya-Upanishad, which is a slightly shorter work than the Varaha-Upanishad and has a mixture of metric and prose passages. It covers much the same ground as the other texts dealing specifically with Hatha-Yoga concepts and techniques, but again insists on the complementarity of self-knowledge (jnana) and Yoga. A considerable amount of space is devoted to the channels (nadi). Their purification is seen as preparation for the higher practices of concentration and meditation, by which the vibrations (spanda) of the mind are brought under control. The text includes interesting descriptions of methods that the yogin is asked to use in order to control and manipulate the life-force (prana) in the body. Also a long list of paranormal powers is given. The last two of the three chapters of this Upanishad appear to have been appended. The teachings are ascribed to the sage Shandilya, after whom this work is named.

Tri-Shikhi-Brahmana-Upanishad

The Tri-Shikhi ("Triple Tuft")-Brahmana-Upanishad is similar to the Shandilya-Upanishad both in style and content, though it is about half as long. It gets its title from the unnamed brahmin wearing three tufts of hair who received the teachings given in this work directly from God Shiva. The Upanishad starts with an exposition of Vedanta metaphysics and then recommends a combination of Jnana-Yoga and Karma-Yoga (or Kriya-Yoga) for the seeker after liberation. It interprets the latter as strict attention to the observances laid down in the scriptures, which presumably means the works of Hatha-Yoga, for the rest of this Vaishnava Upanishad covers much the same ground as the above-mentioned works.

Darshana-Upanishad

The Darshana ("Vision")-Upanishad, which runs to over thirty pages in translation, presents itself as the teachings of Lord Dattatreya to the sage Samkriti. The limbs of the eightfold path are defined, and in general the approach of this text is refreshingly systematic. Nevertheless, this late scripture does not add substantially to our knowledge of Hatha-Yoga.

Yoga-Cudamany-Upanishad[12]

The last work to be examined here is the Yoga-Cudamany ("Crest-Jewel of Yoga")-Upanishad. It teaches a sixfold Yoga but fails to describe the higher stages of yogic practice. The reason for this is that it is a text fragment, the earlier portion of the Goraksha-Paddhati, which is an important Hatha-Yoga manual.

This concludes our survey of the psychotechnology of the Yoga-Upanishads. Their revealed teachings offer a convenient transition to the more detailed discussion of Tantra and Hatha-Yoga in the remaining two chapters.

योग आनन्दकल्पनः

chapter 12
The Esotericism of Medieval Tantra Yoga

BODILY PLEASURE AND SPIRITUAL BLISS: THE ADVENT OF TANTRISM

The quest for immortality and freedom is fundamental to human civilization. We see it expressed as much in the pyramids of Egypt and the cathedrals of medieval Europe as in the modern medical search for the fountain of youth and the race to the stars, as well as in the search for lasting peace between nations. But nowhere has that quest become so obvious a motive of aspiration as in India. Already the Vedic seers were preoccupied with discovering the immortal domain that is the homeland of the gods, beyond all grief and even beyond the delightful realms of the ancestral spirits. Later, the Upanishadic sages made the revolutionary discovery that immortality is not part of the topography of the hereafter but is the essential Ground of all existence. Consequently, they taught, we only need to realize our inmost nature in order to enjoy the Self, or Identity, of all beings—here and now.

The sages believed that the immortal Self (atman) could never be known, because it is not an object, but that it could be *realized*. That realization consists in a radical shift of our identity-consciousness, of who we experience ourselves to be. Whereas the ordinary mortal thinks of himself or herself as a specific, limited body-mind, the Self-realized being no longer identifies himself or herself as a skin-bound individual but as the timeless quintessence of all beings and things.

The way to that realization, the ancient sages believed, lies in the difficult path of renunciation and asceticism. They maintained that the splendor of the transcendental Reality reveals itself only to those who turn their attention away from the affairs of the world and instead, by exercising conscientious control over body and mind, focus it like a laser beam upon the ultimate concern of Self-realization. In the last analysis, to *become* the Absolute

250

(brahman), one has to transcend the human condition and human conditioning. One must desist from investing one's energies in the usual preoccupations through which people reinforce the illusion of being separate entities.

While the Upanishadic ideal of living liberation (jivan-mukti), of enjoying the Bliss of the Self while still in the human body, was an important step in the evolution of India's spirituality, it did not entirely overcome dualistic thinking. This idea raised the following question: If there is only the one Self, why should such a struggle be involved in realizing it? In other words, why do we have to think of the world, and thus the body-mind, as an enemy that has to be overcome? To put it still more concretely: Why do we have to abandon pleasure in order to realize bliss?

The New Approach of Tantrism

A new answer, and a new style of spirituality, was proposed by the masters of Tantrism, who made their appearance around the middle of the first millennium A.D. Their teachings are embodied in the Tantras, which are works similar to the Shaiva Agamas and the Vaishnava Samhitas but dedicated to the feminine psychocosmic principle, Shakti.[1] Hindu tradition speaks of there being sixty-four Tantras, but the actual number of these works is much higher. In addition, the Buddhists have their own Tantras.

Only a few of the most important texts of this genre of Hindu literature have been translated into European languages. Noteworthy are the Mahanirvana-, the Kularnava-, and the Tantra-Tattva-Tantra. The scope of topics discussed is considerable. They deal with the creation and history of the world, the names and functions of a great variety of male and female deities and other higher beings, the forms of ritual worship (especially of goddesses), magic, sorcery, and divination, as well as esoteric "physiology" (the mapping of the subtle or psychic body), the awakening of the mysterious serpent power (kundalini-shakti), techniques of bodily and mental purification, the nature of enlightenment, and (not least) sacred sexuality.

The revolutionary philosophy of Tantrism is best captured in the definition of the term *tantra* as given in the old Buddhist Guhya-Samaja-Tantra, which explains that "Tantra is continuity." The word is derived from the root *tan*, meaning "to extend, stretch." It is generally interpreted as "that which extends understanding" (tanyate vistaryate jnanam anena). But the concept of continuity expresses the nature of Tantrism far better, because this pan-Indian tradition seeks, in a variety of ways, to overcome the dualism between the ultimate Reality (Self) and the conditional reality (ego) by insisting on the continuity between the process of the world and the process of liberation or enlightenment.

The great Tantric formula, which is fundamental also to Mahayana Buddhism, is "samsara equals nirvana." That is to say, the conditional or phenomenal world is coessential with the transcendental Being-

Consciousness-Bliss. Therefore, enlightenment is not a matter of leaving the world or of killing one's natural impulses. Rather, it is a matter of envisioning the lower reality as contained in and coalescing with the higher reality, and allowing the higher reality to transform the lower. Thus, the keynote of Tantrism is integration—the integration of the self with the Self, of bodily existence with the spiritual Reality.

Orientalist and art historian Ananda Coomaraswamy made this pertinent observation:

> The last achievement of all thought is a recognition of the identity of spirit and matter, subject and object; and this reunion is the marriage of Heaven and Hell, the reaching out of a contracted universe towards its freedom, in response to the love of Eternity for the productions of time. There is then no sacred or profane, spiritual or sensual, but everything that lives is pure and void. This very world of birth and death is also the great Abyss.[2]

It is important to realize that the Tantric revolution was not the product of mere philosophical speculation. Though connected with an immense architecture of old and new concepts and doctrines, Tantra is intensely practical. It is, above all, a "practice of realization," or what is called sadhana. Thus, the spirit of Yoga is central to it. Historically, Tantrism can be understood as a dialectical response to the often abstract approach of Advaita Vedanta, which was and still is the dominant philosophy of the Hindu elite. Tantrism was a grass-roots movement, and many, if not most, of its early protagonists hailed from the castes at the bottom of the social pyramid in India, corresponding to the lower working class in our society. They were responding to a widely felt need for a more practical orientation that would integrate the lofty metaphysical ideals of nondualism with down-to-earth procedures for living a sanctified life without necessarily abandoning one's belief in the local deities and the age-old rituals for worshipping them.

So the Tantras are marked by an astonishing synthesis between theory and practice based on a vibrant eclecticism with a strong penchant for ritualism. The teachings of Tantrism were designed to serve the spiritual needs of the "dark age" (kali-yuga) that is thought to have commenced with the death of Lord Krishna after the great battle related in the Mahabharata epic. The psychotechnology described—or, more often than not, only hinted at—in the Tantras was invented for those who, like ourselves, are barely able to channel their aspirations to the Divine and are easily distracted by their conventional ideas and expectations.

In keeping with the basic nondualist orientation of Tantrism, the adepts of this movement introduced a battery of means that hitherto had been excluded from the spiritual repertoire of mainstream Hinduism, notably Goddess worship and sexuality. The tantrikas, or practitioners of Tantra, rejected the purist attitude of the Hindu and Buddhist orthodoxy and instead sought to bring the spiritual quest down to earth, into bodily existence. It was the introduction of sexuality that understandably caused the greatest opposition in conventional Hindu and Buddhist circles; the Tantric practitioners were accused of indulging in hedonism under the mantle of spirituality. In some cases, accusations of debauchery were no doubt justified, but such cases were the exception rather than the rule. Today Tantrism is held in low esteem in India, and left-hand Tantric gatherings (involving sexual rites) are actively suppressed by the Indian government.

Had it not been for Sir John Woodroffe (alias Arthur Avalon), a British judge of the Calcutta High Court who studied the Tantras with native Bengali scholars, we might still share that general prejudice. More than seven decades ago, Woodroffe boldly disregarded the hostile attitude toward Tantrism. In a number of pioneering studies he paved the way for a better understanding and appreciation of this many-faceted movement. In many respects, his writings are still unsurpassed, as is their tolerance.

The sexual revolution of the 1960s and 1970s has, among other things, put Tantrism on the map of our contemporary Western culture. Yet Tantrism remains widely misunderstood. Its sexual practices, which are enacted literally only in the left-hand schools but are understood symbolically by the right-hand tantrikas, are merely one aspect of Tantra Yoga.

Moreover, it is true that today we are perhaps not as easily shocked by the more controversial features of Tantrism, yet the Tantric masters, especially those teaching in the crazy-wisdom mode, can still manage to test even our more enlightened attitudes. They are spiritual radicals, and notwithstanding our sexual revolution, I believe that most people still carry in their heads a rather idealized image of how a spiritual teacher is supposed to behave. We still tend to think of sexuality and spirituality as incompatible and hence take great offense at gurus who are sexually active.

For instance, how would we relate to the fourteenth-century adept Chandidas if he were alive today? A brahmin, Chandidas managed to outrage his contemparies because he fell in love with a young girl, Rami, whom he had seen washing clothes at a riverbank. Their eyes met, and he became enchanted by her to the point of neglecting his priestly duties. He was rebuked, and when he continued to openly dedicate love songs to her he was deprived of his offices at the local temple and was "excommunicated." (Since Hinduism has no organized church, excommunication is strictly speaking not possible. A person can only be denied his caste rights.)

Chandidas' brother finally negotiated an official hearing, during which the adept was given the opportunity to publicly renounce his obsession and be forgiven for his folly. When the maiden heard about this, she went to the hearing. On seeing her, Chandidas forgot the promises he had made to his family and adoringly approached Rami with folded hands. What Chandidas' judges and revilers failed to see was that for him that young girl had become an embodiment of the Divine Mother. His love was for the Goddess in human form. It was an emotion of worship, triggered by a beautiful maiden.

The liberalism of the Tantric masters is of course not unique in the history of religion. Sexuality has been a part of the ritual dimension of many traditions outside India—notably China—where it has likewise led to occasional excesses and frequent accusations of debauchery. Orgiastic excesses were more likely where ritual praxis became separated from lofty metaphysics and associated with magical intentions. A good example of this is found in recent history in the homespun occultism of Aleister Crowley, who encouraged his followers to engage in homosexuality, premarital and extramarital intercourse, and bestiality.

Goddess Worship

The Tantric adepts reclaimed for the spiritual process all those aspects of existence that the mainline traditions excluded by way of renunciation—sexuality, the body, and the physical universe at large. In Jungian terms, we can see this as a concerted attempt at reinstating the anima, the feminine psychic principle.[3] That this interpretation is correct is borne out by the fact that the unifying element of all schools of Tantrism is precisely the attention they pay to the feminine principle, called shakti ("power") in Hinduism and depicted in iconography by such goddesses as Kali, Durga, Parvati, Sita, Radha, and hundreds of other deities.

Often the feminine principle is simply referred to as devi ("shining one")—the Goddess. The Goddess is, above all, the Mother of the universe, the Spouse of the Divine Male, whether he is invoked as Shiva, Vishnu, Brahma, Krishna, or simply Mahadeva ("Great God"). In the Ananda-Lahari ("Wave of Bliss"), a poem ascribed to Shankara, we find this verse:

> He who contemplates You, O Mother, together with Vashini and the other [attendant female dieties], who are lustrous like the moon-gem, he becomes a maker of great poems, with lovely metaphors, of speech [inspired] by Savitri, and of words that are as sweet as the fragrance of the lotus-mouth of that Goddess. (17)

Devi is not only the creatrix and sustainer, whose beauty is beyond imagination; she is also the terrible Force that blots out the universe when the appointed time has come. In the human body-mind, Devi is individuated as the "coiled power" (kundalini-shakti), whose awakening is the very basis of Tantra Yoga. We will hear more about this shortly.

But Shakti, or Devi, is nothing without the masculine pole of existence. Shiva and his eternal spouse are commonly portrayed in ecstatic embrace—what the Tibetans call Mother-Father (yab-yum). They belong together. On the transcendental plane, they are forever enjoying each other in blissful union. Their transcendental marriage is the archetype for the empirical correlation between body and mind, consciousness and matter, and male and female. "Shiva without Shakti," states a well-known Tantric dictum, "is dead." That is to say, Shiva remains uncreative.

But the same holds true of Shakti on her own, as is emphasized in the Buddhist Tantras, which invest the masculine rather than the feminine principle with dynamism. In Hindu Tantrism, at any rate, Shiva represents the primordial Condition in its unqualified aspect, as pure Consciousness or Light. Shakti represents that same Reality in its dynamic motion, its perennial "holo-movement," to use David Bohm's quantum-physical phrase.

Shakti is the Life-Force, the driving force behind all change and evolution. She is the universal Energy of Consciousness. Thus, Tantric metaphysics conceives of reality as a bipolar process. Creation is simply the effect of the preeminence of the feminine or Shakti pole, whereas transcendence is associated with the predominance of the masculine or Shiva pole.

The Tantric Antiritualist School

Tantrism is a movement comprehensive enough to contain its own antithesis. Thus, the pronounced ritualism characteristic of most Tantric schools is, for example, overcome and even criticized in the schools of the Buddhist Sahajayana, the "Vehicle of Spontaneity." The adepts of this school take the doctrine of the identity between the conditional world and the ultimate Reality as literally as possible. They prescribe neither a path nor a goal. For, from the viewpoint of spontaneity (sahaja), we are never truly separated from Reality. Our birth, the whole adventure of our life, and our death occur against the eternal backdrop of Reality. We are like fish who do not know they are swimming in water and are continuously sustained by it.

The term *sahaja* means literally "born together," which refers to the fact that the empirical reality and the transcendental Reality are coessential. The word has come to connote spontaneity, as the natural approach to existence, prior to interfering thought constructs about Reality. The sahaja-yogin lives from the point of view of enlightenment, of Reality.

When we breathe, it is the Divine that breathes as us. When we think, it is the Divine that thinks as us. When we love and hate, it is the Divine that loves and hates as us. Yet we are forever in search of a higher Reality, and this very quest merely reinforces our illusion of being separated from that Reality. The adepts of the Sahaja school, therefore, refused to put forward any program of liberation. As the ninth-century adept Lohipada says in one of his songs (doha):

Of what consequence are all the processes of meditation? In spite of them you have to die in weal and woe. Take leave of all the elaborate practices of yogic control (bandha) and false hope for the deceptive supernatural gifts, and accept the side of voidness to be your own.[4]

Or as Sarahapada, a great master of the eighth century A.D., declares in his Royal Song:

> There's nothing to be negated, nothing to be Affirmed or grasped; for It can never be conceived. By the fragmentations of the intellect are the deluded Fettered; undivided and pure remains spontaneity.[5]

The songs of the adept Kanhapada, who lived in the twelfth century A.D., contain similar pronouncements. He admonished practitioners to follow the example of the Tantric female consorts who sell their looms and woven baskets to join the Tantric circles. Looms and baskets have been interpreted allegorically as standing for thought constructs and superstitious ideas respectively. The follower of the path of spontaneity must give up the mental habit of experiencing Reality from within the cage of his or her particular mind-set. This includes the renunciation of magical or wishful thinking, which was as ripe among tantrikas as it was and is among most spiritual traditions.

If the practice-oriented (ritualistic) schools of Tantrism were a reaction to the abstractionist trend in Advaita Vedanta, the Sahajayana can perhaps be regarded as a critique of the extreme ritualism of mainstream Tantrism. But the sahajiyas, or sahaya-yogins, criticized scholarship as vigorously as they censured religious formalism. With unsurpassed single-mindedness, they lived and preached the truth of nondualism.

Strictly speaking, their no-path cannot be characterized as psychotechnology. Rather, Sahajayana understands itself as the negation of all techne or "skilfull means." It is unquestionably the epitome of the Tantric movement. However, the principle of sahaja, or spontaneity, is inherent in all Tantric teachings. After all, the purpose of even the most humble rite is to help the practitioner transcend all the artificial divisions made by the unenlightened mind and to restore the integrity between transcendence and immanence, between bliss and pleasure.

THE HIDDEN REALITY

It is a fundamental premise of all esoteric schools of thought that the world we perceive through our ordinary senses is only a minute slice of a much larger reality and that there are many more subtle planes of existence. Today we can understand this idea in terms of the metaphor of spectral wave bands, or frequencies of vibration. The distinct levels of existence proposed by traditional esotericism may be viewed as different aspects of the same cosmos vibrating at different rates. Thus, the psyche and mind, which exist on the subtle plane, are thought to vibrate many times faster than the material objects of the gross plane of space-time. The subtle dimension or dimensions of reality form a fifth axis to the four axes of ordinary space and time, namely length, breadth, height, and duration.

We can perhaps better understand these invisible higher dimensions of existence by referring to the new world-view formulated by quantum physicists. Quantum physics operates comfortably with the notion of electrons and other atomic particles, and yet no one has ever seen any of them directly. The British physicist Harold Schilling proposed that we should look upon reality as "a cybernetic network of circuits . . . more like a delicate fabric than an edifice of brick and mortar."[6] But it is a network that has interior depth. In fact, when we look at the inner hierarchy of reality we perceive, as Schilling put it, "depth *within* depth *within* depth"—an ultimately unfathomable, mysterious well of existence.

As we have seen in Chapter 9, which dealt with Patanjali's philosophy, Yoga metaphysics also subscribes to the view that there is an inner dimension to the universe: The objects we see have an invisible depth. That depth is progressively disclosed to the yogin in his sustained effort to internalize his awareness. He experiences subtle regions and nonmaterial entities, of which modern science knows next to nothing, though thanatologists (death researchers) encounter similar ideas in the reports of subjects who have undergone a near-death experience.

The hidden dimension of macrocosmic existence, of the universe at large, has its precise parallel in the microcosm of the human body-mind. The depth structures of the body share in the depth structures of its larger environment. All esoteric traditions assume that there is, a correspondence between inner and outer reality, and we also encounter the same idea in Jung's notion of synchronicity, which is really an attempt to explain the fact that there is, as he saw it, an occasional surprising coincidence between external events and psychic conditions. For instance, we may recount to a friend a dream we had about a rare butterfly, and just as we are describing the butterfly, our friend presents us with a gift. When we open the package, we find a book whose cover has a picture of the same type of butterfly.

The Subtle Body

The earliest explicit model of the inner hierarchy is that of the five "sheaths" (kosha)—a doctrine expounded, as we have seen, in the ancient Taittiriya-Upanishad. This model is generally accepted by the schools of Vedanta and other nondualist traditions, like Tantrism. At any rate, it is widely held in and outside India that the physical body has a subtle counterpart made not of gross matter but of a finer substance or energy. The "anatomy" and "physiology" of that supraphysical double—the so-called astral body or subtle body (sukshma-sharira)—has been the subject of intense yogic investigation, particularly in the traditions of Hatha-Yoga and Tantrism.

The Tantric literature is filled with descriptions of the centers (cakra) and currents (nadi) that are the basic structures of the subtle body. We will examine this in more detail shortly. Modern physicians typically dismiss these "organs" as entirely fictional, the products of an overheated imagination or an inadequate knowledge of anatomy. Others have suggested that they are "maps" for concentration and meditation, or that the cakras are created in consciousness through visualization. This point of view is apparently expressed even in some Tantric works, the Ananda-Lahari among them. In general, however, the organs of the subtle vehicle are thought to be as real as those of the physical body. Hence they are visible to clairvoyant sight.

But far more than the physical heart, lungs, or liver, the cakras and nadis are subject to great variation. They may be more or less active and more or less well defined. These differences reflect a person's psychospiritual condition. This explains, in part at least, why the enumerations and descriptions of the cakras given in different texts do not always tally. Another reason for these textual variations is that the descriptions are indeed intended to be models for the yogin. They are idealized versions of the structure of the subtle body, which are meant to guide the yogin's visualization and contemplation. Thus, the depiction of the cakras as lotuses whose petals are inscribed with Sanskrit letters is clearly an idealization, not an empirical observation. But it is an idealization based on actual perception: The activated cakras are, as the Sanskrit word suggests, wheels of energy, with radiant spokes that lend themselves to representation as lotus petals.

The Life-Force (Prana)

The form of energy composing the cakras and currents in the subtle body is unknown to science. The Hindus call it prana, which means literally "life"—that is, "life-force." The Chinese call it *chi*, the Polynesians *mana*, the Amerindians *orenda*, and the ancient Germans *od*. It is an all-pervasive "organic" energy. In modern times, psychiatrist Wilhelm Reich attempted to resuscitate this notion in his concept of the orgone, but he met with hostility from the scientific establishment. More recently, Russian parapsychologists have introduced the notion of bioplasma, which is explained as a radiant energy field interpenetrating physical organisms.

While Western science is still struggling to find explanations for such phenomena as acupuncture meridians, kundalini awakenings, and Kirlian photography, the yogins continue to explore and enjoy the pyrotechnics of the subtle body, as they have done for hundreds of generations. Some of their ideas have already fertilized current pioneering research in bioenergy, and I believe it is a matter of time before the emergent scientific paradigm will generate a comprehensive model of bioenergic fields that can also help us understand and vindicate some of the stranger practices of Hatha-Yoga.

According to the authorities of Yoga, the universal life-force is focalized in the individual subtle body, where it branches out into five primary and five secondary energy flows, each with its own specialized function. The five primary energy flows are as follows:

1. Prana ("breath")—draws the life-force into the body (chiefly through the act of inhalation); it is generally thought to be located in the upper half of the trunk, especially in the heart region but also in the head.
2. Apana ("out-breath")—expels the life-force (mainly through the act of exhalation); it is associated with the navel and the abdomen but also the anal and genital areas.
3. Vyana ("through-breath")—distributes and circulates the life-force (chiefly through the action of the heart and lungs); it is always present even when the activity of prana and apana is for some reason suspended; it is widely agreed to pervade the entire body.
4. Samana ("co-breath")—is responsible for the assimilation of nutrients; it is located in the digestive system.
5. Udana ("up-breath")—is primarily responsible for speech but also for belching (which has traditionally been looked upon as a positive sign that the food or drink is being digested properly); it is specifically connected with the throat.

Different scriptures explain these five energies somewhat differently and give different locations for them. The above version is the most common.

The five auxiliary bioenergetic functions are:

1. Naga ("serpent")—causes vomiting or belching
2. Kurma ("tortoise")—effects the closing and opening of the eyelids
3. Krikara (sound the stomach makes when one is hungry)—causes hunger
4. Deva-datta ("god-given")—effects yawning or sleep
5. Dhanamjaya ("conqueror of wealth")—is responsible for the disintegration of the dead organism

Again, there is no unanimity about the precise functions of these subsidiary energies.

The two most important species of the life-force are obviously prana and apana, which underlie the breathing process. Their incessant activity is seen as the principal cause of the restlessness of the mind, and their stoppage is the main purpose of breath control (pranayama). I will say more about this in Chapter 13 ("Yoga as Spiritual Alchemy") in connection with the Hatha-Yoga path of realization.

The Circuits (Nadi) of the Subtle Body

Rather like electricity, the life-force (prana) condensed in the subtle body travels along pathways, called nadi in Sanskrit. The word means "duct," but the nadis must not be mistaken for tubular structures. They are energy currents, distinguishable flow patterns within the luminous energy field that is the subtle body. The classical drawings of the network of nadis fail to convey the living, vibrant radiance of the supraphysical vehicle; to the trained eye, it looks like a shimmering, shifting mass of light with foci of different color and, sometimes, dark areas suggesting physical weaknesses, perhaps even disease.

Commonly, the Yoga scriptures mention that there are 72,000 nadis in all. Some speak of as many as 300,000. Several of the Yoga-Upanishads name nineteen and give their respective locations, but the names and positions do not always match. The following diagram shows the arrangement of the thirteen principal nadis according to the Darshana-Upanishad (IV.14ff.). The view is from above, looking down into the body.

All the nadis originate at the "bulb" (kanda), a structure shaped "like a hen's egg." According to some texts, the kanda is two fingers above the anus and two fingers below the penis, while others locate it in the region of the navel.

The Three Principal Circuits: Sushumna, Ida, and Pingala

Three chief pathways are universally recognized in the yogic literature. The central or axial pathway, which runs along the spine, is known as the sushumna-nadi, which means "the current that is most gracious." It is also called brahma-nadi, because it is the trajectory of the ascending kundalini-shakti, the awakened serpent power leading to liberation in the Absolute (brahman).

Some works speak of a channel within the sushumna, which they call vajra ("thunderbolt")-nadi, and within that channel another still subtler one known as the citrini ("shining")-nadi. This last term conveys the idea that within this innermost conduit or flow, the yogin locates the radiance of Consciousnes (cit) itself.

To the left of the axial current lies the ida-nadi, and to the right lies the pingala-nadi. The former gets its name from being "pale," the latter from being "reddish." They are respectively symbolized by the cool moon and the hot sun. These pathways wind around the sushumna, forming a helical stairway. They meet at each of the six lower cakras and terminate at the center situated behind and between the eyebrows. Only the sushumna extends all the way from the bottom cakra to the crown center.

The Tantric yogin's principal challenge is to stabilize the flow of bioenergy in the central pathway. So long as the life-force oscillates up and down the ida and pingala, attention is externalized; that is, the yogin's consciousness is dominated by the forces of "moon" and "sun." By forcing the life-energy (prana) along the axial channel, the yogin stimulates the dormant kundalini energy until it rushes upward like a volcanic eruption, flooding the crown center and thereby leading to the desired condition of blissful ecstasy (samadhi). The esoteric explanation of the word *hatha* is the union of "sun"

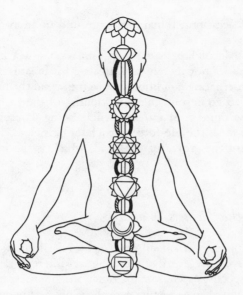

The seven "wheels" or cakras of the subtle body.

and "moon"—that is, the convergence of the life-force that ordinarily travels along the ida and pingala pathways.

I have mentioned the kundalini on a number of occasions, and I will say more about it shortly. Here it is important to point out that the life-force (prana), which is responsible for the functioning of the body-mind, and the kundalini-shakti are both aspects of the Divine Power, or Shakti. If we compare the life-force to electricity, the kundalini can be likened to a high-voltage electric charge. Or if we regard the life-force as a pleasant breeze, the kundalini is comparable to a hurricane.

Once the kundalini power is unleashed in the body, it produces far-reaching changes in our physical and mental being. If properly managed, this incredible power can, as the adepts of Tantra and Hatha-Yoga promise us, refashion our body-mind into a divine vehicle, a transubstantiated form capable of incredible feats.

Knowledge of the functioning of the ida- and pingala-nadis is deemed elementary in Hatha-Yoga. On the physical level, their activity governs the responses of the sympathetic and parasympathetic nervous systems respectively. Thus, through controlled breathing in which the life-force is guided along the pingala-nadi, the yogin can speed up his heart rate and metabolism and improve the functioning of his eyes and ears. On the other side, through controlled breathing in which the life-force is conducted along the ida-nadi, the yogin can greatly reduce his metabolism. This practice can be pushed to the point where the expert yogin can, as has been conclusively demonstrated on a number of occasions, remain underground in an airtight container for hours, even days.

But the rationale of breath control (pranayama) is a different one: The authentic yogin does not merely seek to stop his breath and heart rates and bring about a hybernating condition, but to transcend the human condition as such. He wants to go beyond the conditioning of the body-mind and break through into the domain of transcendental Being-Consciousness-Bliss. For this, he needs to focus the life-force like a laser beam and channel it along the spinal axis toward the crown of the head, which is the location of a major esoteric center.

The Seven Psychic Centers (Cakra)

There are seven major cakras in all, arranged vertically along the axial channel. These are pools of life-energy, vibrating at different rates. Each cakra is associated with specific psychosomatic functions, but these energy whirls must not be confused with the nerve plexuses of the physical body (with which they are, however, correlated). From the base up, the sequence of cakras is as follows:

1. Muladhara ("root-support")—Situated at the perineum, this center, also called adhara ("support"), is associated with the earth element, the sense of smell, the lower limbs, the Sanskrit mantra *lam*, and the elephant (symbol of strength). The presiding deities are Brahma (the Creator God) and the Goddess Dakini. It is generally depicted as a deep red four-petaled lotus, and it is the seat of the dormant kundalini-shakti and the issue-place of the sushumna-nadi.

2. Svadhishthana ("own-base")—Located at the genitals, this cakra is associated with the water element, the sense of taste, the hands, the mantra *vam*, and an aquatic monster resembling a crocodile (symbol of fertility). The presiding deities are Vishnu and the Goddess Rakini. This center is depicted as a crimson six-petaled lotus.

3. Manipura ("jewel-city")—Situated at the navel and also called nabhi-cakra ("navel wheel"), this center is associated with the fire element, the visual sense, the anus, the mantra *ram*, and the ram (symbol of fiery energy). The presiding deities are Rudra and the Goddess Lakini. This center is portrayed as a bright yellow lotus of ten petals.

4. Anahata ("unstruck")—This center is located at the heart and hence is also widely known as the hrit-padma ("heart lotus"), a blue lotus of twelve petals. The designation *anahata-cakra* derives from the esoteric fact that it is at the heart that the transcendental "sound" (nada)—Pythagoras' music of the spheres—which is "unstruck"—

that is, not produced by mechanical means—can be heard. The heart lotus is associated with the air element, the sense of touch, the penis, the mantra *yam*, and a black antelope (symbol of swiftness). The presiding deities are Isha and the Goddess Kakini.

5. Vishuddha or vishuddhi ("pure")—Situated at the throat, this cakra, which is depicted as a smoky-violet sixteen-petaled lotus, is associated with the ether element, the auditory sense, the mouth and the skin, the mantra *ham*, and a snow-white elephant (symbol of pure strength). The presiding deities are the androgynous God Ardhanarishvara (Shiva/Parvati) and the Goddess Shakini. It is at this center that the secret soma secretion is tasted; the soma drips from the lalana-cakra, a minor structure located behind the vishuddhi-cakra. The production of this nectar of immortality is stimulated, above all, through the practice of khecari-mudra ("space-walking seal"), which is described in Chapter 13 ("Yoga as Spiritual Alchemy").

6. Ajna ("command")—Located in the brain midway between the eyes, this center is also known as the third eye. It is so named because it is through this center that the disciple receives telepathic communications from the teacher. For this reason it is also called guru-cakra. This center is associated with the manas, that aspect of the mind concerned with the processing of sensory input. The ajna-cakra is also connected with the sense of individuality (ahamkara) and with the mantra *om*. The presiding deities are Paramashiva and the Goddess Hakini. The ajna center is depicted as a pale gray or white two-petaled lotus. It contains a symbolic representation of the phallus placed within a downward-pointing triangle (the whole signifying the polarity of Shiva and Shakti).

7. Sahasrara ("thousand-petaled")—Situated at the crown of the head, this cakra is so called because of the myriad of luminous filaments that compose it. Strictly speaking, it is not part of the cakra system at all but a body-transcending locus where Consciousness appears to be connected to the human form. This idea is indicated by the luminous linga, Shiva's symbol, placed in the middle of this lotus.

The symbolic elements connected with each cakra serve the yogin to build up complex visualizations that hold his mind steady and lead to various paranormal powers (siddhi) as well as ecstasy. In modern manuals of Hatha-Yoga, the seven cakras are also frequently associated with different psychomental functions. The lowest cakra is said to be connected with fear, the cakra in the genital region with sorrow, the navel center with anger, and the heart cakra with love. Kundalini-yogins are careful to raise the serpent power at least to the heart center, because the activation of the lower cakras can have undesirable effects on instinctual life. The center at the throat is sometimes associated with life-positive or life-negative attitudes, the ajna-cakra or "third eye" with the mood of doubt or basic trust in life, whereas the sahasrara-cakra at the crown of the head may be related to our feeling connected or separated from Reality.

Some schools of thought speak of cakras beyond the sahasrara, corresponding to different levels of transcendental realization. Thus, the Shaiva Agamas refer to the dvadasha-anta, a locus that is situated, as the name suggests, "twelve digits" above the crown. This idea was undoubtedly conceived as a result of certain advanced yogic experiences and can only really be understood by duplicating those experiences.

The same holds true of the rare concept of the "conduit of immortality" (amrita-nadi) spoken of by Ramana Maharshi, the sage of Tiruvannamalai in south India, and more recently by the Western adept Da Free John. The latter described this secret channel as the matrix of the sushumna-nadi. It manifests only upon full enlightenment, or sahaja-samadhi, when it creates a link between the ascending sushumna-nadi and the subtle center at the heart. Da Free John writes:

> It is as if a line of Light were plumbed between the deep center of the upper coil (midbrain to crown) and the deep center of the lower coil (below and behind the navel). Not only the sahasrar, but the whole body becomes full of Light or Radiant Bliss. This entire Fullness is the *reflection* of the Heart [i.e., the transcendental Self]. *All* of it is Amrita Nadi.[7]

The Knots (Granthi) and Vital Points (Marman)

The classical literature on Hatha-Yoga speaks of knots (granthi), or bioenergetic constrictions, that effectively prevent the ascent of the life-force and then the kundalini-shakti along the spinal axis. The first knot, which is called rudra-granthi, is at the base center; the vishnu-granthi is in the navel region; the brahma-granthi is at the throat. These knots must be pierced by the life-force so that the kundalini can travel unhindered to the crown center.

Some of the later works on Hatha-Yoga, moreover, recognize the existence of minor focal points of life-energy, called marman. These are bioenergetic blockages that must be removed by means of concentration and guided breath—as taught in the Kshurika-Upanishad, for instance.

Serpent Power (Kundalini-Shakti)

The most significant aspect of the subtle body is the psychospiritual force known as the kundalini-shakti. What is this mysterious presence in the human body? Metaphysically speaking, the kundalini is a microcosmic manifestation of the primordial Energy, or Shakti. It is the universal Power as it is connected with the finite body-mind. This is sometimes misinterpreted as meaning mere "Force," and is then conveniently contrasted with the principle of love. But, as Sir John Woodroffe noted long ago, Shakti is Power, or cosmic Capacity, and as such is Bliss (ananda), Supraconsciousness (cit), and Love (prema).[8] Some authorities call it Divine Intelligence.

So, in some sense, the phrase "kundalini energy" is a misnomer, because we tend to regard energy as a neutral physical force. The term *shakti*, by contrast, connotes something far more positive and creative. Above all, shakti is supraconscious. Nevertheless, it is convenient to use such English equivalents as "power" and "energy" rather than retain the word *shakti*.

The word *kundalini* means "she who is coiled" and refers to the fact that the kundalini (or kundali) is envisioned as a sleeping serpent curled three and a half times around a phallus (linga) in the lowest bioenergy center of the human body. That serpent blocks the central pathway with its mouth at the place of the first knot. This symbolism simply suggests that the kundalini is normally in a state of dormancy or latency.

As I have mentioned, in the human body, the primordial Energy is polarized into potential energy (i.e., the undifferentiated kundalini-shakti) and dynamic energy (i.e., the differentiated prana or prana-shakti). By regulating the flow of prana, the potential energy can be mobilized, which results in the well-known phenomenon of kundalini arousal. Thus, the prana is used to stir the dormant kundalini energy into action. The situation is analogous to bombarding the atomic nucleus with high-energy particles, which destabilizes the atom and leads to a release of tremendous energy.

Through controlled breathing, in which the life-energy (prana) is withdrawn from the left and right nadis and forced into the central pathway, the "sleeping princess" is awakened. Often this process is explained as one of heating the kundalini; it can be compared to the explosion of a conventional bomb in order to trigger a nuclear reaction. That this comparison is not too far fetched is evident from Gopi Krishna's description of the moment of kundalini awakening, which, subjectively at least, amounts to a phenomenal burst of energy:

> Suddenly, with a roar like that of a waterfall, I felt a stream of liquid light entering my brain through the spinal cord.
>
> Entirely unprepared for such a development, I was completely taken by surprise; but regaining self-control instantaneously, I remained sitting in the same posture, keeping my mind on the point of concentration. The illumination grew brighter and brighter, the roaring louder, I experienced a rocking sensation and then felt myself slipping out of my body, entirely enveloped in a halo of light.[9]

In Gopi Krishna's case, this experience was quite unexpected and uncontrolled. But the goal of Tantra Yoga and Hatha-Yoga is to induce this event under controlled conditions, so that the practitioner does not have to suffer the kind of disastrous side effects that Gopi Krishna and a good many other meditators as well as nonmeditators have had to endure, often for prolonged periods. The symptoms of an unintentionally and wrongly aroused kundalini can be severe—from splitting headaches to psychotic episodes.

The traditional model states that when the dormant kundalini-shakti is awakened, it shoots up to the crown center, where the blissful meltdown between Shakti and Shiva occurs. Implicit in this is the idea that the kundalini is completely dynamized, and that the body of the yogin is now sustained by the "nectar" that flows from the union of the two poles of Reality. Western students of Kundalini-Yoga find this model difficult to accept and have proffered other solutions, which are informed by the laws of physics.

A good contender is the model that compares the body to a bipolar magnet. Intense concentration and breath control lead to an oversaturation, which causes an inductive process in the static pole (i.e., the muladhara-cakra). The life-energy begins to stream from that cakra. The energy released is equivalent to the energy impacting on it, yet of an opposite kind, and the energy does not deplete itself.

The curious physical phenomena associated with the kundalini awakening, such as sensations of intense heat, light, sound, pressure, and even pain, must not be confused with the kundalini itself. Hence the American psychiatrist Lee Sannella has dubbed these phenomena collectively "physio-kundalini."[10] This aspect of the kundalini can be understood in neurophysiological terms, and the model developed by Isaac Bentov and used by Sannella is the most sophisticated available. Bentov looks at the kundalini process from a mechanical point of view that regards the body as containing standing electromagnetic wave systems, especially in the skull and heart. These wave systems are thought to trigger the brain into producing the sort of visionary, auditory, and other sensory experiences typical of kundalini awakenings. Undoubtedly, most psychic and mystical phenomena have a physiological basis. But beyond such physiological manifestations of the kundalini lies the mysterious realm of the kundalini as Consciousness-Bliss.

The kundalini experience is presumably as old as humanity's encounter with the spiritual dimension, though the special significance of that experience was not recognized until the dawn of Tantrism. Kundalini-Yoga is the mature product of a long history of psychospiritual experimentation, and it presupposed the discovery of the body as a manifestation or "temple" of the Divine.

More than anyone else, it was the Kashmiri pundit Gopi Krishna who democratized the kundalini phenomenon. Firstly, he made it widely known in the modern world and promoted its scientific investigation. Secondly, he saw in it the engine behind our entire psychospiritual evolution. On the one hand, Gopi Krishna was adamant that the kundalini is a *spiritual* reality, and on the other hand, he passionately advocated it as *the* biological mechanism that is responsible for sainthood, genius, and insanity alike. As he put it:

What my own experience has clearly revealed is the amazing fact that though guided by a Super-Intelligence, invisible but at the same time unmistakably seen conducting the whole operation, the phenomenon of Kundalini is entirely biological in nature.[11]

This states the problem in a nutshell. The kundalini cannot be both a spiritual reality and entirely biological, as we would normally understand the term *biological*. Of course, from a Tantric point of view, which holds that immanence and transcendence are coessential, any strict distinction between matter and spirit makes little sense. But for this elevated point of view to be relevant, it must be our lived truth. So long as we are not de facto enlightened but experience ourselves as individuated beings, we must concede the usefulness of making practical distinctions.

Even though Gopi Krishna's work has contributed greatly toward a phenomenology of the kundalini experience, there is a real need for further research and, not least, conceptual clarification.

The quest to awaken the sleeping goddess kundalini, as we have seen, is at the heart of Tantrism. I will turn next to the Tantric path itself, which has as its sole objective to arouse the hidden Goddess and induce her to embrace and melt with the equally hidden God, Shiva, residing at the solitary peak of Mount Meru, in the microcosm of the human body.

TANTRIC RITUAL PRACTICE

The Purification of the Elements (Bhuta-Shuddhi)

Before the prince in the well-known legend could kiss the sleeping princess, he had to combat monsters and cut a path to the castle. Similarly, before the wedding of Shiva and Shakti can occur in the human body-mind, the yogin must clear away all kinds of obstructions. The path of realization (sadhana) is, therefore, often couched in terms of purification (shodhana). In fact, the very process of kundalini arousal is understood as the progressive purification of the constituent elements (bhuta) of the body—earth, water, fire, air, and ether. It is known as bhuta-shuddhi.

As the kundalini is conducted upward along the axial channel (sushumna-nadi), it gradually "dissolves" the dominant element of each somatic region or cakra. Thus, by the time it reaches the sixth or ajna-cakra, the kundalini has successively dissolved the five elements. What this means in practice is that the withdrawal of the life-force from the body produces a state of coldness and insensitivity in the trunk and limbs. The kundalini's further progression to the crown or sahasrara-cakra signals the dissolution of the mind (manas) in the state of formless ecstasy or nirvikalpa-samadhi, which completely shuts down the yogin's individuated awareness of his environment, including his own body. His awareness-identity now rests in the All-Identity of the transcendental Self, which is indescribably blissful.

On a lower level, bhuta-shuddhi is a ritual that is performed as a preliminary practice to the worship of one's chosen deity or deities in the context of the Tantric lifestyle. It is the symbolic dissolution of the elements of the body. The process, described in the Mahanirvana-Tantra (V.93ff.), involves visualizing the process of elemental creation in reverse order. Thus the yogin pictures the lowest element, earth, associated with the cakra at the base of the spine, as dissolving into the water element at the second cakra, and that as dissolving into the fire element at the navel center, and so on, until he reaches the crown center. At that point, his body is thought to be purified.

This ritual is to be followed by a series of other practices by which the body is converted step by step into a temple, or sacred mound, ready to receive the great Being. Thus, through the practice of "life installation" (jiva-nyasa), the yogin assimilates the life-force of his chosen female deity. This is done by empowering certain body parts through touch and infusing them with the life of the god or goddess of the yogin's choice. Another form of installation is matrika-nyasa, which installs the fifty sounds of the Sanskrit alphabet in the yogin's body. The matrices or "little mothers" (matrika), as the Sanskrit alphabetic sounds are called, are thought of as the offspring of the primordial sound (shabda) of the Absolute. The body parts of the chosen deity are imagined as consisting of letters of the alphabet, which are visualized in the respective areas of the yogin's body.

Other similar rites include the installation of the seers (rishi-nyasa); the installation of the six limbs (shad-anga-nyasa), which is performed by placing the hands on six different bodily parts and empowering them; and the installation of the hands, which is the same kind of exercise but performed on the finger and palms of the hands only. Interspersed between the rites are complex visualization practices (dhyana), usually of the deity and his or her abode.

All this is combined with a great deal of mantra recitation, regulated breathing, and intense concentration. I have already spoken of mantras in connection with Mantra-Yoga. Mantras are also the principal tool of the Tantric practitioner.

Mantra Practice

Under the aegis of Tantrism, mantra practice became a sophisticated art. The Tantric scriptures are also known as treatises on mantra (mantra-shastra), because their favorite subject matter is the "science of mantras" (mantra-vidya). And the Tantric Buddhism of Tibet is known as the Mantrayana. The word *mantra* itself is esoterically explained as derived from the words *manana* ("thinking,") and *trana*, ("liberation"). In other words, a mantra is a potent form of thought, an instrument of conscious intention.

> Because the *mantra* is an expression of a more evolved consciousness, it offers a unique link with that higher level. For this reason, it not only makes the path to higher consciousness clearer by replacing interfering thoughts, its gradual incorporation pulls consciousness toward that state.[12]

Broadly speaking, mantras are sounds charged with numinous power. As Agehananda Bharati, a monk of the Dashanami order who has Tantric leanings, observed in his outstanding book on Tantrism, there are three possible purposes of mantras.[13] They can be used to appease the forces of the universe to ward off unpleasant experiences and foster pleasant ones; to acquire things by magical means; and to identify with an aspect of reality (such as a specific deity) or with Reality itself.

As the Tantras emphasize, mantras are not arbitrary inventions. They are revealed to yogic adepts in heightened states of awareness, and their effectiveness depends entirely on proper initiation (diksha). According to the esoteric traditions of India, the mere repetition of the mantra *om*, for instance, will have no spiritualizing effect unless its recitation is empowered by a qualified teacher. As the Kularnava-Tantra (XI) declares, there are countless mantras, which only distract the mind. For a mantra to bear fruit it must have been received through the teacher's grace. The recitation of a mantra that has been overheard or acquired by deceit or accident is considered to lead only to personal misfortune.

The recitation (japa) of mantras can be done aloud (vaikhari), whispered (upamshu), or mentally (manasika), which is deemed the best because it is the most potent. They should be carefully enunciated and never sloppily performed. A fourth way of benefiting from a mantra is by writing it out, which is known as written recitation (likhita-japa). Whichever form of japa is chosen, only conscientious and intensely conscious practice can awaken a mantra's potency and lead to success. Each mantra is associated with a specific state of consciousness (caitanya), and recitation is thought to be successful when that consciousness is actualized. Without its actualization, a mantra is mere sound that has no transformative power.

From another point of view, however, a mantra is the manifestation of the Absolute as sound (shabda-brahman). The eternal unmanifest sound is the root principle of all manifest sounds—a concept similar to the Greek idea of the logos, as found in the opening passage of the Old Testament. Shabda is the kinetic aspect of the Absolute. In its purely transcendental state, the Absolute is thought of as static and uncreative; it is through its aspect of sound, or vibration, that it generates the finite realms of existence, such as our space-time universe.

Like the world of forms, sound proceeds from the Absolute in a series of distinct stages. Tantrism proposes a four-phase model:

1. Supreme speech (para-vac)—sound as pure potentiality
2. Visible speech (pashyanti-vac)—sound as mental image
3. Intermediate speech (madhyama-vac)—sound as thought
4. Manifest speech (vaikhari-vac)—audible sound

For generations in the East, mantras have been employed not only in sacred contexts but have served widely as magical spells for profane ends, including occasional black magic. However, their nuclear significance is as a means of internalizing and intensifying awareness to the point of transcendence of all contents of consciousness. It is impossible to do justice to this far-ranging and recondite subject here, and I refer the reader to the works of Sir John Woodroffe for an abundance of technical details.

In addition to mantras, there are two other important elements of Tantric practice, namely hand gestures (mudra) and geometric representations of the levels and energies of the psychocosmos, which are known as devices (yantra).

Symbolic Gestures (Mudra)

The word *mudra* is derived from the root *mud*, "to gladden, delight." The reason given for this meaning is that mudras bring delight (muda) to the deities and cause the dissolution (drava) of the mind. But the term *mudra* denotes "seal," and it is employed in Tantric contexts because the hand gestures (or, in Hatha-Yoga, the bodily postures) "seal" the body. They are means of controlling the energy in the body. They are also symbolic representations of inner states. Anyone who is in the least sensitive to the body's energies can easily verify that by folding the hands, a change of mood is effected: We begin to feel more mentally collected. With a little experience, the different inner states associated with the mudras become clearly discernible.

There are said to be 108 hand gestures—108 being a favorite sacred number among Hindus. In reality there are many more, though according to the Mahanirva-Tantra (XI), fifty-five are the most common in use. The origin of the gestures used in the Tantric rituals is obscure. They probably go back to Vedic times, where the sacrificial ceremonies involved the meticulous handling of implements such as the ladle during the pouring of the soma libations. The Japanese tea ceremony is a good example of the intensely conscious conduct called for in such rituals. Another, later source of inspiration was Indian dance, which knows a great repertoire of mudras, though the possibility that the Tantric mudra ritual cross-fertilized the Indian kathakali dance cannot be excluded.

The most important hand gestures are the jnana-mudra ("wisdom seal"); vishnu-mudra ("seal of Vishnu"), which is commonly used during breath

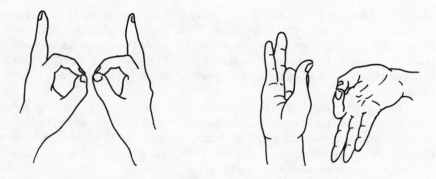

Two principal hand gestures or mudras employed in the Tantric ritual.

control; and cin-mudra ("consciousness seal"). They are depicted in the illustration above.

Geometric Meditation Devices (Yantra)

A yantra is a thumbnail sketch of the levels and energies of the universe and thus the human body (as a microcosmic replica of the macrocosmos). A yantra may be drawn on paper, wood, cloth, or any other material, or in sand if nothing else is available. Three-dimensional models made of clay or metal are also known.

A yantra has a function similar to that of the mandala ("circle") as used in Tibetan Tantrism. Mandalas, however, tend to be more pictorial and are based on a circular arrangement of the constituent elements.

A yantra typically consists of a square surround, circles, lotus petals,

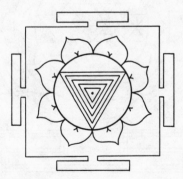

The kali-yantra, symbolizing the body of Goddess Kali.

triangles, and at the center the "point" (bindu). Each component has a more or less elaborate symbolism attached to it. Thus, the upward-pointing triangle denotes the masculine or Shiva pole of reality, while the downward-pointing triangle represents the feminine or Shakti pole. The point in the middle is the creative matrix of the universe, the gateway to the transcendental Reality itself.

In the higher stages of Tantic practice, the yantra must be completely internalized; that is, the yogin must construct its complex geometrical pattern mentally through visualization. The yantra is erected either from the innermost point outward—in accordance with the process of macrocosmic evolution—or from the outermost circumference toward the center—in alignment with the microcosmic process of meditative involution.

After having elaborately constructed the yantra internally, the yogin proceeds to dissolve it again. Since he is, in consciousness, identical with the structure of the yantra, its dissolution necessarily implies his own extinction as an experiencing subject. In other words, if successful at this advanced practice, the yogin transcends his conditioned mind and is catapulted into pure Being-Consciousness-Bliss, where the distinction between subject and object does not exist.

Tantrism employs a great number of yantras. In Chapter 20 of the Mantra-Mahodadhi ("Great Ocean of Mantras") twenty-nine yantras are

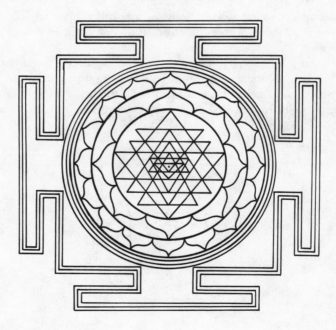

The famous shri-yantra of Tantrism.

described. The most celebrated is undoubtedly the shri-yantra, or shri-cakra, depicted above. The name *shri* refers to Lakshmi, the goddess of fortune. This yantra is composed of nine juxtaposed triangles arranged in such a way that together they produce a total of forty-three smaller triangles. Four of the nine primary triangles point upward, representing the male cosmic energy (Shiva); five point downward, symbolizing the female power (Shakti). These triangles are surrounded by an eight-petaled lotus symbolizing the deity Vishnu, who stands for the all-pervading ascending tendency in the universe. The next lotus, with sixteen petals, represents the attainment of the desired object, particularly the yogin's power over his mind and senses. Enclosing this lotus are four concentric lines that are symbolically connected with the two lotuses. The triple line surround is called "earth-city" (bhu-pura), which designates the consecrated place that may be the entire universe or, by way of analogy, the human body.

The Ritual of the "Five M's"

The term *mudra*, mentioned above, is applied to another practice of Tantrism. It refers to one of the elements of the central Tantric ritual of the "five M's" (panca-makara). These practices, which in Sanskrit all have names beginning with the letter *m*, are the following:

1. Madya, wine
2. Matsya, fish
3. Mamsa, meat
4. Mudra, parched grain
5. Maithuna, sexual intercourse

These five are understood metaphorically in right-hand schools and per-formed literally in left-hand schools. According to the Kularnava-Tantra (IV), wine is used in the left-hand ritual as a cathartic agent, cleansing the mind from the worries and concerns of everyday life. The object, however, is not drunkenness, which induces stupor rather than clarity. Similarly, the con-sumption of fish and meat, which are as strictly forbidden to the ordinary Hindu as is wine, has the sole purpose of achieving an altered state of awareness. Parched grain (mudra), like the other three ingredients mentioned, is supposed to act as an aphrodisiac—again an awareness-altering substance.

Not mentioned among the "five M's" but also prominent in Tantric rites are narcotic drugs (aushadhi). Commenting on the widespread use of awareness- or mood-altering drugs, Swami Satyananda of Bihar made the observation that, to this day, India's holy men take drugs such as ganja (cannabis) and datura (jimsonweed), while bhang (a preparation made from marijuana) is universally used during the Shivaratri festival, in which the marriage of Shiva and Parvati is celebrated. However, the Swami did not fail to remind us that drugs "allow us to taste the beyond but do not make us masters of the transcendental."[14]

The practitioner of the left-hand path (vama-marga) knows he is breaking profound social taboos, and his only justification for his conduct is that his goal is not sensual gratification but self-transcendence in the context of bodily existence. The philosophy of Tantrism is summarized in the following words from the Mahacina-Acara-Krama-Tantra:

> The yogin cannot be a sensualist (bhogin), and the sensualist is not one endowed with Yoga. Hence the kaula whose essence is Yoga and sensuality is held to be superior to everyone.[15]

Ritual Sex (Maithuna)

The Tantras make it clear that to be successful in the dangerous left-hand approach, the practitioner must not suffer from doubt, fear, or lust. He must be a "hero" (vira). This is especially important in the execution of the fifth practice, sexual congress (maithuna).

The female partner in this rite must be duly consecrated through ritual bathing and other ceremonies of purification, and she must be a spiritual practitioner herself. The yogin must see in her not a person of the opposite sex but the Goddess or Shakti, just as he must experience himself as Shiva. The ideal female partner should be lovely and quite uninhibited. Any woman qualifies except the yogin's mother. However, in an appendix to the Yoga-Karnika ("Ear-Ornament of Yoga"), a work of the eighteenth century, we find Shiva himself give the following instruction:

> One should place one's penis into the vagina of one's mother and one's slippers on one's father's head, while fondling [or licking] one's sister's breasts and kissing her fair seat. He who does this, O great Goddess, reaches the Abode of Extinction. He who worships, day and night, an actress, a female skull-bearer, a prostitute, a low-caste woman, a washerman's wife—he verily [becomes identical with] the blessed Sada-Shiva.

More likely than not, even extreme left-hand tantrikas would interpret the opening sentence metaphorically. Tantrism has a fully developed "twilight language" (sandha-bhasha), or secret symbolic language, which can be very misleading to the uninitiated.

In left-hand Tantrism, the term *mudra* also refers to the female partner in the "metasexual" ritual. She is also called *vama*, meaning both "woman" and "left"; hence the "left conduct" (vama-cara) or left-hand path. The maithuna rite, which incidentally has Vedic antecedents, often bears the technical designation yoni-puja, "worship of the vulva." This is meant to suggest that the rite is a sacred procedure. In fact, it can be an exceedingly complex affair,

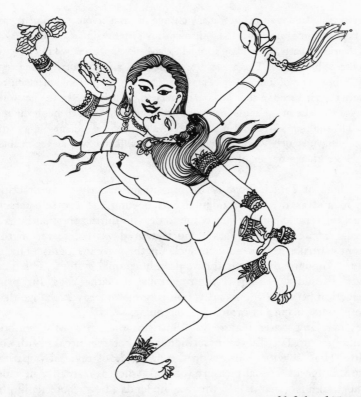

Ritual intercourse (maithuna) is an important part of left-hand Tantrism.

consisting of hours of painstaking ceremonial preparation and then an equally formal period of actual intercourse. Ordinarily, this ritual is performed among a circle (cakra) of initiates, with the teacher present. There is of course pleasure and delight, since the whole point of the ritual is to generate bliss (ananda) through bodily means. But there should be no self-indulgence, no egoic exploitation of the experience. The partners embrace as male and female deities, not ordinary mortals.

It is incumbent on the yogin to prevent the discharge of his semen at all cost. Semen (bindu, retas) is considered a most precious product of the life-force and must be conserved. The significance of coitus reservatus is that the semen is transmuted into a finer substance, called ojas, that nourishes the higher centers of the body, thereby facilitating the difficult ordeal of psychosomatic transformation attempted in Tantrism. From ancient times a spiritual practitioner who is adept at this inner alchemy has been known as urdhva-retas, "one whose semen flows upward." This can be experienced as a literal event, as is clear from Gopi Krishna's description:

There was no doubt an extraordinary change in my nervous equipment, and a new type of force was now racing through my system connected unmistakably with the sexual parts, which also seemed to have developed a new kind of activity not perceptible before. The nerves lining the parts and the surrounding region were all in a state of intense ferment, as if forced by an invisible mechanism to produce the vital seed in abnormal abundance to be sucked up by the network of nerves at the base of the spine for transmission into the brain through the spinal cord. The sublimated seed formed an intergral part of the radiant energy which was causing me such bewilderment and about which I was as yet unable to speculate with any degree of assurance.[16]

The climax of Tantric Yoga is not orgasm but ecstasy—the practitioner's abiding in and as the transcendental Self beyond the ego-self-personality. However, the female partner *may* come to orgasm during the maithuna ritual. Her sexual excitement produces a much-desired vaginal secretion that the competent tantrika knows how to suck up through his penis. The female ejaculate is thought to enrich the yogin's hormonal system. This practice, called vajroli-mudra, belongs to the repertoire of Hatha-Yoga. But primarily the interaction between yogin and yogini is one of energy exchange that goes far beyond what occurs in ordinary intercourse.

More than any other feature of Tantrism, the "five M's" embody its antinomian spirit: The Tantric practitioner deliberately breaks with conventional life. His behavior is based on the principle of reversal (viparita). He seems to indulge in sensual pleasure (bhoga), whereas in reality he cultivates transcendental bliss (ananda). In this way he lends a new, esoteric significance to his seemingly mundane actions. In Hatha-Yoga, it is the headstand that best symbolizes this principle of reversal.

The Tantric procedures are intended to construct a new reality for the yogin—a sacred reality analogous to the transcendental Reality: The yogin's body becomes the body of the chosen deity (ishta-devata). It is as that deity that the yogin approaches the transcendence of all forms, until he is one with the supreme Deity, or Godhead, which is sheer Being.

योग स्रानन्दकल्पनः

chapter 13

Yoga as
Spiritual Alchemy:
Hatha-Yoga

THE ENLIGHTENMENT OF THE BODY:
THE ORIGINS OF HATHA-YOGA
AMONG THE SIDDHAS AND NATHAS

The human body-mind is not what it appears to be: a limited, mobile digestive tube. We only need to relax or meditate to discover that this popular materialistic stereotype is untrue. For it is then that we begin to discover the energy dimension of the body and the deep space of consciousness. As the hard boundaries that we normally draw around ourselves dissolve, we feel more alive and enter a world of greater experiential intensity. Relaxation and meditation replace our ordinary body image with an experience of ourselves as a fluid process that is connected with the larger, vibrant whole. In this experience, the boundaries of the ego lose their rigidity.

Quantum physics tells us that everything is interconnected, and that the idea that "I" am a separate physical entity is an illusion. It tells us, moreover, that the so-called objective world is a hallucination, a projection of that imaginary point of subjectivity within us. We are slow in acknowledging the profound practical implications of the quantum-physical view, obviously because it requires us to make far-reaching and demanding changes in the way we think of ourselves and our universe.

The quantum-physical perspective is not as new as we would like to believe. It underlies the entire Tantric tradition, notably the schools of Hatha-Yoga, which are an offshoot of Tantrism. The image of the "dance of Shiva" best captures this orientation: Shiva, as Nata-Raja ("Lord of Dance") is forever dancing out the rhythms of the universe—the cycles of creation and destruction. He is the master weaver of space and time. This classical Hindu image has fascinated a number of quantum physicists. The first to draw

277

attention to it was Fritjof Capra in his justly famous book *The Tao of Physics*:

> The ideas of rhythm and dance naturally come to mind when one tries to imagine the flow of energy going through the patterns that make up the particle world. Modern physics has shown us that movement and rhythm are essential properties of matter; that all matter, whether here on earth or in outer space, is involved in a continual cosmic dance.
>
> The Eastern mystics have a dynamic view of the universe similar to that of modern physics, and consequently it is not surprising that they, too, have used the image of the dance to convey their intuition of nature.[1]

It was the adepts of Tantrism who pioneered this dynamic view of the universe, and it was also they who inaugurated a new attitude toward the human body and bodily existence in general. In pre-Tantric times the body was typically looked upon, in Gnostic fashion, as a source of defilement, the enemy of the spirit. This attitude prompted the anonymous author of the Maitrayaniya-Upanishad to compose the following litany:

> Venerable, in this ill-smelling, unsubstantial body [which is nothing but] a conglomerate of bone, skin, sinew, muscle, marrow, flesh, semen, blood, mucus, tears, rheum, feces, urine, wind, bile, and phlegm—what good is the enjoyment of desires? In this body, which is afflicted with desire, anger, greed, delusion, fear, despondency, envy, separation from the desirable, union with the undesirable, hunger, thirst, senility, death, disease, sorrow, and the like—what good is the enjoyment of desires? (I.3)

We may find the pessimistic tone of this passage strange and exaggerated, and yet it expresses our own culture's materialistic point of view very well. So long as we consider the body as a walking alimentary canal, there is little solace in the pursuit of pleasure, since any pleasure the body can afford us is inevitably limited in intensity and duration and usually purchased at great cost. Besides, the pursuit of pleasure certainly cannot save us from death.

The Tantric revolution led away from the model of the body as an "inflated bladder of skin."[2] "In tantrism," observed historian of religion Mircea Eliade, "the human body acquires an importance it had never before attained in the spiritual history of India."[3] This new attitude is pithily expressed in the Kularnava-Tantra, an important Hindu Tantric work, thus:

> Without the body, how can the [highest] human goal be realized? Therefore, having acquired a bodily abode, one should perform meritorious (punya) actions. (I.18)
>
> Among the 840,000 types of embodied beings, the knowledge of Reality cannot be acquired except through a human [body]. (I.14)

What the Tantric masters aspired to was to create a transubstantiated body, which they called adamantine (vajra) or divine (daiva)—a body not made of flesh but of immortal substance, of Light. Instead of regarding the body as a meat tube doomed to fall prey to sickness and death, they viewed it as a dwelling-place of the Divine and as the caldron for accomplishing spiritual perfection. For them, enlightenment was a whole-body event. As the Yoga-Shikha-Upanishad puts it:

He whose body (pinda) is unborn and deathless is liberated in life (jivan-mukta).—Cattle, cocks, worms, and the like verily meet with their death.

How can they attain liberation by shedding the body, O Padmaja?—The life-force [of the yogin] does not extend outward [but is focused in the axial channel]. How then can the shedding of the body [occur]?

The liberation that is attainable by the shedding of the body—is that liberation not worthless? Just as rock salt [is dissolved] in water, so the Absolute (brahmatva) extends to the body [of the enlightened yogin].

When he reaches the [condition of] non-otherness (ananyata), he is said to be liberated. [But others continue to] distinguish different bodies and organs.

The Absolute has attained embodiment (dehatva), even as water becomes a bubble. (I.161–165a)

The embodiment of an enlightened master is not limited to the physical organism with which he appears to be specifically associated. His body is really the Body of all, and therefore he can assume any form at will—a feat that is attributed to many ancient and contemporary adepts. This transubstantiated body is also styled ativahika-deha, "superconductive body." This omnipresent, luminous vehicle is endowed with the great paranormal powers (siddhi) acknowledged in all the scriptures of Yoga and Tantra. In the Yoga-Bija, possibly composed in the seventeenth or eighteenth century, we find the following stanzas:

The fire of Yoga gradually bakes the body composed of the seven constituents [such as bone, marrow, blood, etc.].

Even the deities cannot acquire the exceedingly powerful yogic body. [The yogin] is freed from bodily bonds, endowed with various powers (shakti), and is supreme.

The [yogin's] body is like the ether, even purer than the ether. His body is more subtle than the subtlest [objects], coarser than any coarse [objects], more insensitive [to pain, etc.] than the [most] insensitive (jada).

The [body of] the lord of yogins conforms to his will. It is self-sufficient, autonomous, and immortal. He entertains himself with play wheresoever in the three realms [i.e., on earth, in the midregion, and in the celestial worlds].

The yogin is possessed of unthinkable powers. He who has conquered the senses can, by his own will, assume various shapes and make them vanish again. (50b–54)

Thus, the adept is not merely an enlightened being but a magical theurgist who is on a par with the Creator-God. There are few Yoga and Tantra scriptures that do not make reference to this occult aspect of the yogic way of life. Patanjali, for instance, dedicates an entire chapter of his Yoga-Sutra to the paranormal powers, which he calls manifestations (vibhuti). Their more common designation is attainments or perfections (siddhi).

While the spiritual masters of India recognize a vast range of such paranormal powers, most traditions distinguish eight "superpowers" (maha-siddhi), whose possession is taken as a sign of liberation or enlightenment:

1. Animan ("miniaturization"), the ability to make oneself infinitely small.
2. Mahiman ("magnification"), the ability to make oneself infinitely large.
3. Laghiman ("levitation"), the ability to defy the law of gravity.
4. Prapti ("extension"), the ability to "touch the moon with one's fingertips."
5. Prakamya ("[irresistible] will"), the ability to defy the properties of the material elements, such as the capacity to move through earth as if it were water.
6. Vashitva ("mastery"), dominion over material Nature as a whole.
7. Ishitritva ("lordship"), supremacy over Nature to the point where the adept has the power of creating and destroying whole universes.
8. Kama-avasayitva ("fulfillment of desires"), the power of determining events according to one's desires, such as converting poison into nectar.

What are we to make of these abilities? Are they merely the product of a lively fantasy triggered by too much solitary introspection? Or are they manifestations of a psychic dimension of reality that science still needs to discover? Over the centuries, all kinds of anecdotal reports have come down to us of the uncommon powers of yogins and strange phenomena witnessed in their company. While there is ample evidence today of the yogins' incredible control over bodily and mental functions that had long been thought to be outside the reach of personal will, their claims to paranormal abilities have so far been only scantily researched. However, the cumulative weight of the findings of parapsychological research on nonyogic subjects increasingly lends credence to at least some of the claims made in yogic circles.

The Siddha Movement

The ideal of the adamantine body was at the core of a ramifying cultural movement, comparable perhaps to the body-awareness movement of the 1970s and 1980s. This was the Siddha cult, which flourished between the eighth and twelfth centuries and which completed the great pan-Indian synthesis of the spiritual teachings of Hinduism, Buddhism, alchemy, and popular magic.

The designation *siddha* means "accomplished" or "perfected." It refers to the Tantric adept who has attained enlightenment as the ultimate perfection (siddhi) and also possesses diverse paranormal powers (siddhi). The southern adept Tirumular defined a siddha (cittar in the Tamil language) as someone who has realized, through yogic ecstasy, the transcendental Light and Power (shakti). The siddha is a spiritual alchemist who works on and transmutes impure matter, the human body-mind, into pure gold, the immortal spiritual essence. However, he is also said to be capable of the literal transmutation of matter, and the renowned Czech indologist Kamil V. Zvelebil recalled a baffling demonstration of this power by one of his siddha informants.[4] The yogic process peculiar to this Tantric tradition, which straddled Hinduism and Buddhism, is known as kaya-sadhana, "body cultivation." It was the cradle of Hatha-Yoga.

The most important schools of the Siddha movement were those of the Nathas and the Maheshvaras. The former had their home in the north of the peninsula, especially Bengal. The latter had their provenance in the south. The Buddhist Tantras speak of a pantheon of eighty-four great adepts, or maha-siddhas, many of whom are even today revered as demigods. They were "mostly rustic folk without much liking for and no pretence to learning."[5] The Tibetan sources, relying on Sanskrit works that are no longer available, furnish us with biographical sketches of these adepts. While the bulk of the material is entirely legendary, there is good reason to assume that the personages behind these wonderfully imaginative stories were historical. For some of them, we even have extant literary works and mystical songs.

According to the Tibetan tradition, the first and foremost adept of the eighty-four siddhas was Lui-pa, whom some scholars identify with Matsyendra(natha), the famous teacher of the still more famous Goraksha(natha). Innumerable legends and songs tell of the magical and spiritual accomplishments of these two great masters. I will shortly relate some of them. Another remarkable siddha was the Buddhist Nagarjuna, the teacher of Tilopa, who initiated Naropa, who was the guru of Marpa, who, in turn, instructed the illustrious yogin-poet Milarepa. In the opening chapter of the Hatha-Yoga-Pradipika, one of the standard manuals on this type of Yoga, we find a list of maha-siddhas that overlaps with the Tibetan catalog of names.

The Tamil tradition of southern India remembers eighteen siddhas; some were of Chinese and Singhalese origin, and one is said to have hailed from Egypt. The number eighteen is as symbolic as the number eighty-four of the north, suggesting completeness. Among the southern siddhas, it was particularly Akattiyar (Sanskrit: Agastya), Tirumular, and Civavakkiyar whose teachings and magical feats have captivated the imagination of the people.

It appears that the southern branch of the diffuse Siddha movement tended to be more radical in its rejection of ritualism and other establishment values than its northern counterpart.[6] One of Civavakkiyar's poems reads:

Why, you fool,
do you utter *mantras,*
murmuring them, whispering,
going around the fixed stone
as if it were god,
putting garlands of flowers around it?
Will the fixed stone speak—
as if the Lord were within?
Will the cooking vessel,
or the wooden ladle,
know the taste of curry?[7]

But this rejection of popular forms of worship often amounting to idolatry can be found also among the siddhas of the north, notably the followers of the Buddhist Sahajiya tradition of spontaneity, as well as the Bauls of Bengal, who to this day roam the countryside singing their initiatory songs. Of course, the siddhas did not dismiss devotional feelings as such.

We can nonetheless detect a certain mechanistic trend among some members of the Natha school who place magical rituals and Hatha-Yoga practices above ego-transcendence, leaving little room for the cultivation of devotion. Where the acquisition of power is given priority over self-transcendence, it is easy enough to succumb to ego-inflation and a stony heart. Or, to put it differently, when the kundalini produces its characteristic kaleidoscope of fascinating inner phenomena, we are apt to forget that the kundalini is, ultimately, the Goddess and that the inner display is Her play. Like modern scientific technology, Indian psychotechnology is not without its perils. When the supreme value of self-transcendence is lost from sight, any technology runs the danger of becoming the servant of merely egoic purposes.

It was none other than Jnanadeva, the great adept of Maharashtra, who criticized those hatha-yogins who, "day and night measure the wind with upstretched arms" but sadly lack the slightest degree of devotion. They should, he oracled, expect only sorrow and tribulations in their path. Jnanadeva (A.D. 1271–1293), who voluntarily abandoned his body at the age of twenty-two, had been initiated into Hatha-Yoga by his elder brother Nivrittinatha. His Jnaneshvari, composed in melodious Marathi, is one of the most illumined independent commentaries on the Bhagavad-Gita. It represents a successful attempt to combine the Hatha-Yoga teachings Jnanadeva received from his family with the way of the heart taught by Lord Krishna of yore. It is difficult to read this work, which is available in a good English translation, without being deeply touched by its wisdom and lyrical beauty. By the time of Jnanadeva, Hatha-Yoga could already look back on a history of some 300 years.

Matsyendra, Goraksha, and Other Nathas

This brings us to the founder of the tradition of Hatha-Yoga himself, Goraksha(natha) (Hindi: Gorakhnath), and his teacher Matsyendra(natha). Matsyendra, who probably lived in the early part of the tenth century A.D., was a chief representative, if not the originator, of what is known as Nathism. Shiva himself is considered the source of the Natha lineage and is invoked as Adinatha, "Primordial Lord." The term *natha* simply means "lord" and refers to a yogic adept who enjoys both liberation (mukti) and supernatural power (siddhi). The nathas are locally thought of as immortal beings, who roam the Himalayan region. Matsyendra himself is venerated as the guardian deity of Nepal, in the form of the transcendental bodhisattva Avalokiteshvara.

Other prominent adepts of Nathism are Jalandhari, better known as Hadisiddha (a co-disciple of Matsyendra); Bhartri (son of King Bhoja and disciple of Jalandhari); Kanhu (disciple of Jalandhari); King Gopicandra (disciple of Kanhu); Prince Caurangi (whose stepmother abandoned him in the forest after cutting off his hands and feet; disciple of Matsyendra); as well as Carpata and Gahini (chief disciples of Goraksha). Numerous legends are told

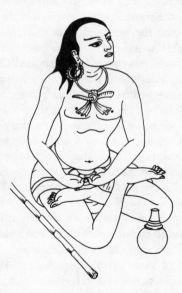

Gorakshanatha, founder of the Kanpatha sect of Hatha-Yoga.

about these personages. Many concern Gopicandra and are gathered in a popular epic that is still recited from Bengal in the northeast to the Punjab in the northwest of the peninsula.

According to legend, Gopicandra was born as a direct result of Shiva's grace, for there was no son written in his royal mother's destiny. The queen was told that her newborn son was a disciple of the adept Jalandhari and would have to be returned to that teacher after Gopicandra had ruled over his kingdom for twelve years. She was also told that if Gopicandra were to submit to his guru at the appointed time, he would acquire immortality. If, however, he were to reject his teacher and fail to renounce the world, he would die instantly.

Gopicandra was brought up in luxury free from worldly cares and became a successful ruler. In the twelfth year of his reign, Jalandhari arrived at the palace gardens demanding what was rightfully his. The queen mother broke the news to Gopicandra. After questioning her closely, he arrived at a decision. He went to Jalandhari and, to everyone's horror, threw him into a deep well. He blocked the well with a huge rock and then had seven hundred cartloads of horse manure dumped on top of the rock.

As prophesied, the minions of Yama, God of Death, arrived and dragged Gopicandra's psychical body into the sky. Suddenly Jalandhari materialized on the scene, quite unaffected by his disciple's cruel treatment. His superior power quickly convinced Yama's servants to release Gopicandra's soul. The young king instantly awoke in his body. Reluctantly he accepted the life of a renouncer. But Jalandhari had to intervene many more times in his disciple's life, because Gopicandra was strongly attached to his 1100 wives, 1600 slave girls, and their children, as well as the luxurious life, power, and glory of a regent. He is probably the most insubordinate disciple on record in the history of Yoga. But he also won the supreme prize of liberation in his life.

Matsyendra's name is specifically associated with the Kaula sect of the Siddha movement, of which he may have founded the Yogini-Kaula branch. This obscure Tantric sect derives its name from its primary doctrinal tenet, the kula. Kula is the ultimate Reality in its dynamic or feminine aspect as Shakti, specifically kundalini-shakti. The literal meaning of *kula* is, curiously, "flock" or "multitude" but also, more significantly, "family" and "home." Thus, it evokes both the sense of differentiation and protectedness, which of course apply to the serpent power; the kundalini is both the source of the multitudinous universe and the ultimate security for the yogin who knows the kula secret. In this school, Shiva is often referred to as akula—the principle that transcends differentiation.

The related concept of kaula stands for the condition of enlightenment or liberation, gained through the union of Shiva and Shakti. The word also refers to the practitioner of this esoteric path.

Matsyendra ("Lord of Fish") is also known as Minanatha, which has the same connotation. This may be a reference to his trade as a fisherman. According to the legendary account given in the Kaula-Jnana-Nirnaya ("Ascertainment of Kaula Knowledge"), which belongs to the eleventh century and is the oldest available source of information about Kaulism, Matsyendra recovered the canon of the Kaulas (called kula-agama) from a large fish that had swallowed it. Some scholars understand Matsyendra's name symbolically and argue that it suggests a spiritual grade; this need not conflict with the conclusion that he earned his living from the sea. Some traditions state that a person who carries the title *matsyendra* has mastered the practice of suspending breath and mind by means of the "space-walking seal," khecari-mudra, one of the most important bodily "seals" of the Nathas.

Legend has it that a peasant woman once implored Shiva to grant her a son. Touched by her fervent prayers, the great god gave her magical ash to eat, which would ensure her pregnancy. In her ignorance the woman discarded the priceless gift on a dung heap. Twelve years later, Matsyendra happened to overhear a conversation between Shiva and his divine spouse Parvati. Wishing to see the child granted to the peasant woman, Matsyendra went to visit her. She sheepishly confessed what had happened to Shiva's graceful gift. Unperturbed, the siddha asked her to search the dung heap again. There she found a twelve-year-old boy, whom she named Goraksha ("Cow Protector").

Matsyendra adopted Goraksha as his disciple, and soon the student's fame exceeded that of his teacher. In some stories, Goraksha is portrayed as using his considerable magical powers for the benefit of his guru. Thus, according to one legend, Matsyendra went to visit Ceylon, where he fell in love with the queen. She invited him to stay with her in the palace, and before long Matsyendra was thoroughly ensnarled in courtly life. When Goraksha heard about his teacher's fate, he at once went to rescue him. Goraksha assumed a female form so that he could enter the king's harem and confront him. Thanks to his disciple's timely intervention, Matsyendra came to his senses and returned to India, accompanied by his two sons Parasnath and Nimnath.

Later, another story relates, Goraksha killed Matsyendra's sons, only to restore them to life. All these legends, of course, have deep symbolic significance. For instance, the murder of the two boys can be interpreted as the yogic act of withdrawing the life-force (prana) from the ida- and the pingala-nadi, the currents to the left and right of the axial current (sushumna-nadi), and gathering it in the esoteric energy center at the base of the spine, from where the awakened kundalini ascends to the crown center.

Goraksha, who lived in the late tenth and early eleventh centuries A.D., is remembered as a miracle worker second to none. He was obviously a realized adept and a charismatic personality of considerable social influence. Yet, according to most traditional accounts, he hailed from the lower, if not the lowest, social strata. Accounts agree that he embraced the ascetic life at an early age and practiced lifelong celibacy. He was apparently a very handsome man who traveled widely in India.

The invention of Hatha-Yoga is attributed to Goraksha alone, though many of the tenets and practices of this school were in existence long before his time.[8] Goraksha is also said to have founded the Kanphata ("Split-ear") order of the Nathas, which gets its curious name from one of the distinguishing marks of its members, namely their split earlobes into which they inserted large rings (called mudra). Some members claim that this custom affects an important current (nadi) of life-force at the ear, which facilitates the acquisition of certain magical powers.

The Kanphata order is scattered throughout India and includes hermits and monastic groups as well as a small number of married men and women. The 1901 census of India reported 45,463 Nathas, almost half of whom were women. They generally have a low social status; as George Weston Briggs reported, they

> . . . make charms for themselves, and some sell them to others; they pronounce spells and practice palmistry and juggling, tell fortunes, and interpret dreams; they sell a woollen amulet to protect children from the evil eye; and they pretend [?] to cure disease, muttering texts over the sick and practising medicine and exorcism, and vending drugs.[9]

The picture painted by Briggs and others suggests that the order founded by Goraksha is in a state of decline, and many of its members are both despised and feared for their actual or putative magical powers and ever-ready curses. But there are those who continue to instruct the villagers in spiritual and worldly matters and who, like the lineage of Bhartrinatha, entertain and edify through their music and songs. While it is true that the danger of narcissism lurks in all body-centered paths, it is also true that self-transcending love is not absent from any genuine spiritual approach, including Hatha-Yoga.

WALKING THE RAZOR'S EDGE: THE HATHA-YOGIC PATH

> The body is the abode (alaya) of God, O Goddess. The psyche (jiva) is God Sada-Shiva. [The yogin] should abandon the offering-remains of ignorance. He should worship with the conviction "I am He."

This quote from the Kularnava-Tantra (IX.41) states the ultimate purpose of Hatha-Yoga, which is God-realization, or enlightenment, here and now, in a divinized or immortal body. This is often expressed as the state of balance or harmony (samarasa) in the body, when the ordinarily diffuse life-energy is stabilized in the central channel. This idea is present in the term *hatha-yoga*, which is esoterically explained as the union between "sun" and "moon," the conjunction of the two great dynamic principles or aspects of the body-mind.

The life-force (prana) is polarized along the spinal axis, where the dynamic pole (represented by Shakti) is said to be at the base of the spine and the static pole (represented by Shiva) at the crown of the head. The hatha-yogin's work consists in uniting Shakti with Shiva. For this marriage to come about, however, he must first stabilize the alternating life-current animating the body. This dynamic flow is polarized positively and negatively, rushing up and down on the left and right sides of the body. The positive current is experienced as heating, the negative as cooling. On the material level they correspond to the sympathetic and the parasympathetic nervous system respectively.

According to the Tantric model of the human body, the axial channel (called sushumna) is entwined by the helical ida- and pingala-nadis. The ida is the carrier or flow of the lunar force on the left of the bodily axis, and the pingala is the conduit or flow of the solar force on the right. The syllable *ha* in the word *hatha* represents the solar force of the body; the syllable *tha* represents the lunar force. The term *yoga* stands for their conjunction, which is the ecstatic state of identity between subject and object.

The hatha-yogin's primary objective is to intercept the left and right current and draw the bipolar energy into the central channel, which commences at the anal center, the muladhara-cakra, where the kundalini is thought to be asleep. This persistent effort to redirect the life-force acts upon the kundalini, mobilizing it. This action can be compared to a hammer striking an anvil, and hence the exoteric meaning of the word *hatha* is "force." Hatha-Yoga is a forceful enterprise in which the body's innate life-force is utilized for the transcendence of the self.

Purificatory Techniques

Breath control, which is the most immediate way of affecting the life-force, is at the heart of Hatha-Yoga practice. However, in their long experimentation with the breath, the yogins found that most aspirants should undergo more or less extensive purification prior to embarking on breath control. Thus, they invented a large array of cleansing techniques in order to prepare the body for the demands of the higher stages of practice. The Gheranda-Samhita has the following pertinent stanzas:

> Purification, strengthening, stabilizing, calmness, lightness, perception [of the Self], and the untainted [condition of liberation] are the seven means of [the Yoga of] the pot (gatha) [i.e., the body]. (I.9)

> Purification [is accomplished] by the six acts; [the yogin] becomes strong through postures (asana); stability [is acquired] through the seals (mudra), and calmness through sense-withdrawal (pratyahara). (I.10)

> Lightness [results] from breath control (pranayama), perception of the Self from meditation (dhyana), and the untainted [state] from ecstasy (samadhi); [this last state] is undoubtedly liberation (mukti). (I.11)

Sage Gheranda continues to describe the six acts (shat-karman), which comprise the following six purificatory practices:

1. Dhauti ("cleansing"), consisting of the following four techniques:
   i. Antar-dhauti ("inner cleansing") is of four types: The first technique is performed by means of swallowing the breath and expelling it through the anus; the second by means of completely filling the stomach with water; the third by stimulating the "fire" in the abdomen through repeatedly pushing the navel back toward the spine; the fourth is executed by washing the prolapsed intestines.
   ii. Danta-dhauti ("dental cleansing") includes cleaning teeth, tongue, ears, and frontal sinus.
   iii. Hrid-dhauti ("heart cleansing") consists in the cleansing of the throat by means of a plantain stalk, turmeric, cane, or a piece of cloth, or by self-induced vomiting, which is beneficial for those suffering from diseases of the chest ("heart").
   iv. Mula-shodhana ("root purification") is the cleansing of the anus manually, with water, or with a turmeric stalk, which heals gastrointestinal diseases and increases bodily vigor.
2. Vasti ("bladder") consists in the contraction and dilation of the sphincter muscle to cure constipation, flatulence, and urinary ailments. It can be performed while standing in water.
3. Neti (untranslatable) refers to a thin thread around nine inches in length that is inserted into the nostrils and passed through the mouth to remove phlegm and, because of its action upon the ajna-cakra, to induce clairvoyance (divya-dristhi).
4. Lauli ("to-and-fro movement"), also called nauli, consists in rolling the abdominal muscles sideways to massage the inner organs, which is thought to cure a variety of diseases.
5. Trataka (untranslatable) is the steady, relaxed gazing at a small object until tears begin to flow, which is said to cure diseases of the eye and also induce clairvoyance.
6. Kapala-bhati ("skull-lustre") comprises three practices, which are said to remove phlegm; the last is additionally said to make the yogin as attractive as the God of Love, Kamadeva:
   i. The "left process" (vama-krama), consisting in breathing through the left nostril and expelling the air through the right, and vice versa.
   ii. The "inverted process" (vyut-krama), consisting in drawing water up through the nostrils and expelling it through the mouth.
   iii. The "shit process" (shit-krama), consisting in sucking water up through the mouth and expelling it through the nose. The phrase shit is onomatopoeic for the sound produced by this practice.

Other texts occasionally give different definitions of the above practices, and some scriptures mention further techniques for purifying the body and preparing it for the advanced art of breath control. Noteworthy is the Sat-Karma-Samgraha (also titled Karma-Paddhati) of Cidghanananda, which is a manual perhaps dating back to the eighteenth century and comprising 149 stanzas. It deals extensively with purificatory techniques and ailments resulting from faulty Yoga practice. According to the Hatha-Yoga-Pradipika (II.21), only those who are flabby and phlegmatic need to resort to the "six practices" to purify the body.

Postures

Sage Gheranda treats Hatha-Yoga as having seven rather than eight limbs, whereby the postures (asana) and the seals (mudra) are respectively the second and third limbs, while the ethical rules (yama and niyama) are not regarded as independent aspects. The Gheranda-Samhita (II.1) makes the point that there are as many asanas as there are animal species. Gheranda claims that Shiva taught as many as 840,000 postures, of which eighty-four are considered important by yogins. According to the Hatha-Yoga-Pradipika (I.33), however, Shiva taught only eighty-four postures.

Of these postures, the following thirty-two are described in the Gheranda-Samhita: (1) Siddha-asana ("adept posture"); (2) padma-asana ("lotus posture"); (3) bhadra-asana ("auspicious posture"); (4) mukta-asana ("liberated posture"); (5) vajra-asana ("diamond posture"); (6) svastika-asana ("cross posture"); (7) simha-asana ("lion posture"); (8) gomukha-asana ("cow-face posture"); (9) vira-asana ("hero posture"); (10) dhanur-asana ("bow posture"); (11) mrita-asana ("corpse posture"); (12) gupta-asana ("hidden posture"); (13) matsya-asana ("fish posture"); (14) matsyendra-asana ("Matsyendra's posture"); (15) goraksha-asana ("Goraksha's posture"); (16) pashcimottana-asana ("back-stretch posture"); (17) utkata-asana ("extraordinary posture"); (18) samkata-asana ("dangerous posture"); (19) mayura-asana ("peacock posture"); (20) kukkuta-asana ("cock posture"); (21) kurma-asana ("tortoise posture"); (22) uttana-kurmaka-asana ("extended tortoise posture"); (23) uttana-manduka-asana ("extended frog posture"); (24) vriksha-asana ("tree posture"); (25) manduka-asana ("frog posture"); (26) garuda-asana ("eagle posture"); (27) vrisha-asana ("bull posture"); (28) shalabha-asana ("locust posture"); (29) makara-asana ("shark posture"); (30) ushtra-asana ("camel posture"); (31) bhujanga-asana ("cobra posture"); and (32) yoga-asana ("Yoga posture"). In place of lengthy descriptions, which can be found in numerous books, the illustration depicts some of these posture. Contemporary manuals describe as many as 200 postures.

Obviously, some of these postures, are intended for prolonged sitting in meditation. Most of them, however, are designed to regulate the life-force in the body in order to balance, strengthen, and heal it. But even the meditation

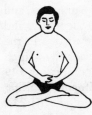 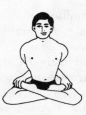 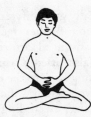 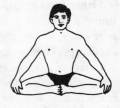

Siddha   Baddha-Padma   Padma   Bhadra

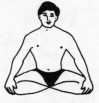 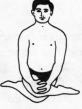 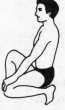 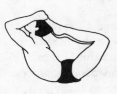

Simha   Gomukha   Vira   Dhanur

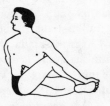 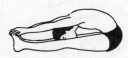

Matsyendra   Goraksha   Pashcimottana

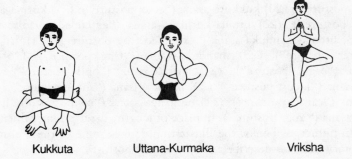

Kukkuta   Uttana-Kurmaka   Vriksha

Some of the thirty-two principal postures (asana) of Hatha-Yoga according to the Gheranda-Samhita.

postures are said to have therapeutic value, and in some instances rather exaggerated claims are made. In both Eastern and Western Yoga circles, this aspect of Hatha-Yoga is often overemphasized. The following observation found in the Kularnava-Tantra (IX.30) applies:

> Yoga is not [attained] through the lotus posture and not through glancing at the tip of the nose. It is the identity of the self (jiva) and the Self (atman) which the Yoga experts (visharada) call "Yoga."

Seals and Locks

Related to the postures are the seals (mudra) and locks (bandha), which form the third limb of Hatha-Yoga. The seals represent more advanced techniques; as is clear from the last five mudras, they even merge with meditative practices. "They are divine," declares Svatmarama, the author of the Hatha-Yoga-Pradipika (III.8), "and bestow the eight [great paranormal] powers. They are favored by all the adepts and are difficult to obtain even by the gods." Svatmarama further states that they should be kept secret, just as one would not divulge one's sexual intimacies with a well-bred woman.

The locks (bandha) are special bodily positions that are designed to restrain the life-force in the trunk and thereby stimulate it.

In the Gheranda-Samhita (III), twenty-five mudras are described in this sequence: (1) Maha-mudra ("great seal"), performed by pressing the left heel against the perineum and grasping the toes of the right outstretched leg, while contracting the throat; (2) nabho-mudra ("sky seal"), which can be done during any activity, is executed by turning the tongue upward against the palate; (3) uddiyana-bandha ("Uddiyana lock"), performed by drawing back the abdomen; (4) jalandhara-bandha ("Jalandhara's lock"), done by contracting the throat; (5) mula-bandha ("root lock"), executed by contracting the anal sphincter muscle; (6) maha-bandha ("great lock"), performed by pressing the left ankle against the perineum, while placing the right foot on top of the other and contracting the anal sphincter muscle; (7) maha-vedha ("great penetrator"), executed by engaging the uddiyana-bandha during the maha-mudra; (8) khecari-mudra ("space-walking seal"), a very important technique, performed by inserting the elongated tongue into the passage above the upper palate and by fixing the gaze on the spot between the eyebrows; this is said to release the "nectar of immortality" (amrita), sweet-tasting saliva, which leads to health, longevity, and a host of paranormal powers; (9) viparita-karani-mudra ("inverted action seal"), colloquially known as the headstand, which prevents the ambrosia (amrita, soma) from dripping into the "fire" at the navel; (10) yoni-mudra ("womb seal"), performed by sitting in the adept posture and closing the eyes, ears, nostrils, and mouth with the fingers, followed by breath retention and simultaneous contemplation of the six centers (cakra); (11) vajroli-mudra ("thunderbolt seal"), executed by raising oneself off the ground while winding the legs around the neck; however, other texts provide a completely different explanation of this practice, which involves drawing up liquids through the penis; (12) shakti-calani-mudra ("power-stirring seal"), performed by forcibly joining the life-force in the chest with that in the abdomen while contracting the anal sphincter muscle by means of ashvini-mudra and while sitting in the adept's posture; (13) tadagi-mudra ("pond seal"), performed by pulling back the abdomen while lying prone; (14) manduki-mudra ("frog seal"), done by moving the tongue until the "nectar" flows profusely, which is then swallowed; (15) shambhavi-mudra ("Shambhu's seal"), a most important technique that consists in gazing at the spot between the eyebrows while inwardly contemplating the transcendental Self; Shambhu is another name for God Shiva, and the yogin who has mastered this technique is said to resemble the great god himself; (16) ashvini-mudra ("dawn-horse seal"), performed by repeatedly contracting the anal sphincter muscle; (17) pashini-mudra ("bird-catcher seal"), executed by crossing the legs behind the neck, though not raising the body off the ground as in the vajroli-mudra; (18) kaki-mudra ("crow seal"), done by slowly inhaling through the mouth, which is held in a position resembling a crow's beak; (19) matangi-mudra ("elephant seal"), performed by standing neck-deep in water and sucking up water through the nose and expelling it through the mouth; (20) bhujangini- or bhujagi-mudra ("serpent seal"), executed by drawing in air through the mouth while making a slight rasping noise with the throat; and (21–25) the five concentrations (dharana) upon the material elements, which involve focusing the life-force and the mind on each respective element for two hours while imaging the various symbolic forms associated with it (such as the presiding deity of each element, its seed mantra, and so on); the five elements are earth, water, fire, air, and ether (akasha, kha).

Sense-Withdrawal

According to Gheranda's path, the fourth limb of Hatha-Yoga is sense-withdrawal (pratyahara), which he deals with only cursorily. It simply consists in withdrawing attention from external, sensory objects. The fact that this practice is placed before breath control, the fifth limb, indicates that yogic breathing presupposes a great measure of mental discipline.

Breath Control

Breath control (pranayama) is the careful regulation of the life-force (prana) in its different forms. From the point of view of the hatha-yogin, the work of Yoga is impossible to accomplish without mastery of the breath/life-force. As the Yoga-Bija (77) puts it:

He who desires union (yoga) without controlling the breath (pavana) is, to yogins, like someone who wants to cross the ocean in an unbaked [earthen] pot.

In the words of the Hatha-Yoga-Pradipika (II.2-3):

When the breath moves, consciousness (citta) [also] moves. When it is immobile, [consciousness is also] immobile, and the yogin obtains stability. Therefore, one should restrain the breath.

It is said that so long as there is breath in the body, so long there is life. Its departure is death. Therefore, one should restrain the breath.

Before describing the various techniques of breath control, Sage Gheranda stresses the importance of proper diet and environment. Among other things, he states that the yogin should commence pranayama during the spring or autumn season, when the weather is neither extremely hot nor excessively cold. He also emphasizes the importance of purifying the channels (nadi) along which the life-force flows. This purification process is said to be of two kinds, which are technically (and untranslatably) known as samanu and nirmanu respectively. The former is a meditative exercise by means of which the presiding deities of the various occult bodily centers (cakra) are invoked and installed in the body. This is combined with the recitation of their respective bija-, or seed, mantras. The nirmanu type of purification is the practice of cleansing (dhauti), as described under the "six practices."

Gheranda distinguishes the following eight types of breath control, which he calls retentions (kumbhaka; lit., "pot"):

1. Sahita-kumbhaka ("joined retention"), a complex breathing technique involving visualization of different deities in conjunction with inhalation, retention, and exhalation; the rhythm is 1:4:2. Thus, if inhalation lasts five seconds, the breath has to be held for twenty seconds, while exhalation extends over ten seconds. The rhythm is measured in matras, a matra being several seconds long. The maximum duration is given as 20:80:40 matras, which, depending on the system used, can total more than seven minutes. The breathing is done alternately through the left and the right nostril; after inhalation and prior to retention, the yogin performs the abdominal lock (uddiyana-bandha). Svatmarama, the author of the Hatha-Yoga-Pradipika, understands sahita-kumbhaka differently. He uses it as a generic term for all forms of pranayama that entail inhalation and exhalation, contrasting them with kevala-kumbhaka, or full-blown retention of the breath, which skilled yogins can perform for several hours at a time. According to the Gheranda-Samhita, however, sahita-kumbhaka is of two kinds: sagarbha ("with seed"), performed while mentally repeating a bija-, or seed,

mantra, such as *om, ram,* or *yam;* and nigarbha ("without seed"), performed without the aid of a bija-mantra.

2. Surya-bheda-kumbhaka ("sun-piercing retention"), which gets its name from the fact that in this technique the yogin inhales exclusively through the right (solar) nostril and exhales only through the left (lunar) nostril; in between he practices the neck lock (jalandhara-bandha) while forcibly retaining the air in his lungs, until he experiences heat in the roots of his hair and fingertips.

3. Ujjayi-kumbhaka ("victorious retention"), executed by inhaling through both nostrils, retaining the air (or life-force) in the nose, then drawing it further into the mouth and holding it there for as long as is comfortable by means of the throat lock (jalandhara-bandha). According to the Hatha-Yoga-Pradipika (II.51), this practice is performed in such a way that a sonorous sound is produced in the throat during inhalation.

4. Shitali-kumbhaka ("cooling retention"), executed by drawing in air through the mouth and exhaling it through both nostrils after a short period of breath retention. In the Hatha-Yoga-Pradipika (II.54), this technique is to be done by curling the tongue. A related technique, also described in the Pradipika (II.54), is sitkari ("*sit*-maker"), which is executed by making a hissing sound (i.e., *sit*) during inhalation through the mouth; exhalation should be through the nostrils.

5. Bhastrika-kumbhaka ("bellows retention"), performed by rapid inhalation and exhalation through both nostrils simultaneously; the cycle should be repeated three times in all. This practice is said to awaken the kundalini force very quickly.

6. Bhramari-kumbhaka ("beelike retention"), performed by inhalation and prolonged retention of the breath while blocking the ears and intently listening to the various inner sounds generated in the right ear. According to the Hatha-Yoga-Pradipika (II.68), a beelike sound is produced during inhalation and exhalation.

7. Murccha-kumbhaka ("swooning retention"), which consists in gentle retention effected by the throat lock (jalandhara-bandha) while fixing attention on the spot between the eyebrows and detaching oneself from all objects; this is followed by slow exhalation. This technique produces a euphoric state.

8. Kevali-kumbhaka ("absolute retention"), which is simply retention of the breath for as long as possible. It should be performed five to eight times a day, with one to sixty-four repetitions per session.

Breath control has a range of physiological and psychomental effects, and Gheranda differentiates between three levels of mastery: At the lowest level, pranayama generates heat in the body. At a higher level, it causes tremor in the limbs, especially in the spinal column. At the highest level, it leads to actual levitation. Pranayama is also held to cure a great variety of diseases, to awaken the serpent power, and to create blissful states of consciousness.

Meditation

The last-mentioned function of breath control leads into meditation (dhyana). In Hatha-Yoga and Tantrism in general, dhyana is characteristically understood as visualization. The Gheranda-Samhita (VI.1) speaks of three types of dhyana: (1) visualization having a "coarse" (sthula) object, such as a carefully visualized deity; (2) visualization having a "subtle" (sukshma) object, namely the Absolute in the form of the transcendental point-origin (bindu) of the universe, as explained in connection with Tantrism; and (3) contemplation of the Absolute as light (jyotis). The Gheranda-Samhita (VI.21) states:

> The contemplation of light (tejo-dhyana) is understood to be a hundred times better than coarse visualization (sthula-dhyana). Subtle visualization (sukshma-dhyana), the greatest of all, is a hundred thousand times better than the contemplation of light.

In subtle visualization or contemplation, attention is simply introverted upon the inner essence, the Self (atman), and a degree of unitive consciousness is achieved. Sage Gheranda explains this process in terms of the awakened kundalini uniting with the Self and rising to the center at the crown of the head, which brings us to the crowning accomplishment of the hatha-yogin, samadhi.

Ecstasy

The ascent of the kundalini to the top center signals the yogin's transcendence of the ego-consciousness in ecstatic unity, or samadhi, which is the seventh and final limb of Hatha-Yoga. The Gheranda-Samhita (VII.3–4) features these pertinent definitional stanzas:

> Separating the mind from the "pot" [i.e., the body], one should identify it with the transcendental Self (parama-atman): This is to be known as ecstasy (samadhi), which means liberation from the states [of consciousness], and so on.[10]

> "I am the Absolute. I am no other. Verily, I am the Absolute, not an experiencer of grief. I am of the form of Being-Consciousness-Bliss, ever free, self-existent (svabhavavan)."

The Hatha-Yoga-Pradipika (IV.5–7) offers the following helpful explanations:

Just as salt enjoys sameness with water through union [with it], so the identity (aikya) of mind and Self is named "ecstasy" (samadhi).

When the mind and the life-force merge and dissolve, the [resulting state of] balance (samarasatva) is named "ecstasy."

That [state of] balance (sama), which is the identity of the individuated self (jiva-atman) and the transcendental Self (parama-atman), in which all conceptualization (samkalpa) is vanished, that is named "ecstasy."

It is clear that ecstasy refers here not to one of the lower types of samadhi, which are associated with spontaneously arising thought forms and imagery, but to the ultimate realization of perfect identity with the transcendental Reality. That is to say, the samadhi intended is nirvikalpa-samadhi, "formless ecstasy," which is thought to be synonymous with liberation or enlightenment itself. Thus, at the end of the long and arduous journey the hatha-yogin enjoys the same condition of utter simplicity to which the raja-yogin also aspires. But the apparent detour of Kundalini-Yoga, which seeks to realize the psychospiritual potential of the body, was not futile. For the yogin does not view Self-realization as an event that is separate from life in the physical realm.

The realization of the hatha-yogin is portrayed as being more complete than that of the raja-yogin, simply because it includes the body. The high risks and difficulties of Kundalini-Yoga are compensated by the advantage of extending enlightenment to the body and to physical existence in general, which is expressed in the Tantric formula that liberation (mukti) and enjoyment (bhukti) are fully compatible. For the Tantric yogin, the body is indeed a manifestation of the ultimate Reality. As Sir John Woodroffe, the pioneer of Tantric studies, put it:

He [the yogin] realises in the pulsing beat of his heart the rhythm which throbs through, and is the sign of, the universal life. To neglect or to deny the needs of the body, to think of it as something not divine, is to neglect and deny that greater life of which it is a part, and to falsify the great doctrine of the unity of all and of the ultimate identity of Matter and Spirit. Governed by such a concept, even the lowliest physical needs take on a cosmic significance. The body is Shakti. Its needs are Shakti's needs; when man enjoys, it is Shakti who enjoys through him. In all he sees and does it is the Mother who looks and acts. His eyes and hands are Hers. The whole body and all its functions are Her manifestation. To fully realize Her as such is to perfect this particular manifestation of Hers which is himself.[11]

In Hatha-Yoga, humanity's hope for physical immortality merges with the spiritual impulse toward liberation from the shackles of the ego-ensconced mind. While the dream of an incorruptible earthly body is only a dream, the tradition of Hatha-Yoga has an immense wealth of hard-won information about the hidden potential of the human body-mind from which we can greatly benefit in our own quest for ultimate meaning and happiness. Modern medicine and psychology, aided by advanced scientific concepts, methods, and instrumentation, are gradually rediscovering some of the amazing facts that yogins have talked about and demonstrated for centuries. It is obvious that, once the materialistic bias of mainstream science is overcome, we will not only be able to confirm many yogic theories and validate their associated practices, but also improve on them and move beyond them.

I believe that a careful study of Hatha-Yoga, in particular the kundalini phenomenon, can greatly extend our understanding of the human body-mind and its surprising abilities. Of course, we must be willing to step into the yogin's laboratory and replicate his experiments on our own person. Subjective testing is, in this case, a reasonable approach; it also happens to be the only logical way of meeting the current scientific ideal of "objectivity."

THE LITERATURE OF HATHA-YOGA

Yogins have always been wary of the written word, and those who wrote down their insights and experiences were the exception rather than the rule. But, as I have tried to show in this volume, there is a considerable Yoga literature nonetheless. Mostly it exists in manuscript form only, and editions and translations represent a mere fraction of what is available in the libraries and learned homes of India. Not a few of these works deal with Hatha-Yoga. I have already introduced the Yoga-Upanishads, some of which treat of Kundalini-Yoga, which overlaps with Hatha-Yoga insofar as the serpent power (kundalini-shakti) is at the core of higher Hatha-Yoga practice. In the following I will briefly describe the most important Hatha-Yoga scriptures that exist in addition to those Upanishads.

Goraksha's Writings

Perhaps the earliest work of this branch of the Yoga tradition is the text entitled Hatha-Yoga, attributed to Goraksha himself. Unfortunately it is no longer available, though some of its stanzas may well have survived in other works. Goraksha is also credited with the authorship of a number of other texts, including the Goraksha-Paddhati ("Track of Goraksha"), which consists of 200 stanzas outlining the Hatha-Yoga path; the Goraksha-Shataka ("Goraksha's Century"), a fragment of the former work; the Goraksha-Samhita ("Goraksha's Collection"), which appears to be identical with the Paddhati; the Hatha-Dipika ("Lamp of Hatha"), about which nothing is known; the Jnana-Amrita ("Nectar of Wisdom"), a work dealing with the sacred duties of a hatha-yogin; the Amanaska-Yoga ("Transmental Yoga"), which has 211 stanzas; the Amaraugha-Prabodha ("Understanding the Immortal Flood"), a work of 74 stanzas that defines Mantra-, Laya-, Raja-, and Hatha-Yoga and speaks of the bindu and the nada as the two great remedies present in every human body, which alone can save the yogin from death; and the Yoga-Martanda ("Sun-Bird of Yoga"), which has 176 stanzas, many of which are similar to those found in the Hatha-Yoga-Pradipika.

Siddha-Siddhanta-Paddhati

Another important text ascribed to Goraksha is the Siddha-Siddhanta-Paddhati ("Track of the Doctrine of the Adepts"), a comprehensive work of six chapters with a total of 353 stanzas.[12] It develops the Natha philosophy of the body (pinda). In the first chapter, six types or levels of embodiment are distinguished, beginning with the transcendental (para) body and ending with the "embryonic" (garbha) or physical body. The esoteric anatomy of the last-mentioned body is explained in the second chapter. In one stanza (II.31), a genuine yogin is defined as someone who knows firsthand the nine "wheels" (cakra), the sixteen "props" (adharas) or loci of concentration, the three "signs" (lakshya), and the five ether-spaces (vyoman).

The nine cakras include the well-known series of seven, except that the sahasrara is called nirvana-cakra. The eighth center is the talu-cakra, which is situated at the palate and is the location of the mysterious "bell" (ghantika), or uvula, and the "royal tooth" (raja-danta), the point from which the divine nectar (amrita) oozes. The ninth cakra is the akasha-cakra, which is said to have sixteen spokes and is to be found at the "brahmic fissure" at the crown of the head.

The sixteen props are locations in the body on which attention can be fixed during concentration; the toes, the muladhara-cakra at the base of the spine, anus, penis, lower abdomen, navel, heart, throat, uvula, palate, tongue, the middle spot between the eyebrows (the location of the ajna-cakra), the "root" of the nose, the forehead, and the akasha-cakra.

The three signs are the experience of light outside the body, light inside the body, and purely mental light phenomena of different kinds. The signs are respectively called bahya-lakshya, antar-lakshya, and madhya-lakshya. These have been mentioned, together with the five types of ether or consciousness-space (akasha), in the section on photistic Yoga in Chapter 11.

The third chapter of the Siddha-Siddhanta-Paddhati continues this treatment and particularly speaks of the body as a microcosmic mirror image of the cosmos. The fourth chapter introduces the kundalini-shakti, which is said to exist in two conditions—unmanifest (cosmic) and manifest (individuated). In the former state it is known as akula, in the latter as kula. Furthermore, the kula-kundalini can either be awakened or dormant. While the kundalini-shakti is one force, it is present as minor forces in the different centers. Also, the text makes a distinction between the lower, the middle, and the upper force (shakti), which are respectively located at the basal center, the navel center, and the crown center.

The fifth chapter makes the point that success in Yoga depends on the teacher's grace. It enables the yogin to renounce all the paranormal powers (siddhi) that he has obtained in the course of his kundalini practice and proceed to the "nonemergent" (nirutthana) state where the body unites with the "supreme estate" (param-pada)—that is, Shiva.

The sixth chapter contains brief definitions of various types of ascetics and, among other things, lists the distinguishing characteristics of the avadhuta-yogin, the adept who has "shaken off" (*ava* + *dhuta*) all attachments and concerns.

Other Works Attributed to Goraksha

Another work attributed to Goraksha is the Gorakh-Bodh ("Instruction by Gorakh"), a treatise of 133 stanzas composed in archaic Hindi. It consists of a fictitious dialogue between Matsyendra and Goraksha, which perhaps dates back to the fourteenth century A.D.

The Goraksha-Upanishad, written in a mixture of Hindustani and Rajasthani, may date from the fifteenth century. Among other things, it lists the requisite qualities of a competent teacher and a fit disciple.

The Goraksha-Vacana-Samgraha ("Collection of Goraksha's Sayings"), consisting of 157 verses, claims to give out authentic teachings by Goraksha but was probably authored in the seventeenth century. The fact is that we do not have a single work we can definitely regard as Goraksha's creation. Often the followers of a great master credited their own writings to him, as was still the case with Swami Shivananda of Rishikesh, who "authored" several hundred works. The vernacular literature on Hatha-Yoga, which also includes the Hindi poems ascribed to Goraksha, is ill researched.

Ananda-Samuccaya

A little-known but significant Hatha-Yoga work that may date back to the thirteenth century A.D. is the Ananda-Samuccaya ("Mass of Bliss"), which has 277 stanzas distributed over eight chapters. It introduces many esoteric concepts that do not appear elsewhere in the extant Yoga literature. The style of this Sanskrit text has been described as "very lucid and marked with high literary merits,"[13] which is rare for this literary genre. Unfortunately, we do not know the author.

Carpata-Shataka

Another old work is the Carpata-Shataka. As the title indicates, it consists of a century of verses by the adept Carpata (or Carpati). This text emphasizes discrimination (viveka) and renunciation as well as the moral foundation of

Yoga. The author's conceptual world appears to be closer to Jainism than to Hatha-Yoga, which makes this Shataka of great historical interest.

Yoga-Yajnavalkya and Brihad-Yogi-Yajnavalkya

The Yoga-Yajnavalkya ("Yajnavalkya's Yoga"), which is also known as the Yoga-Yajnavalkya-Gita, is a work of 485 stanzas distributed over twelve chapters. It is attributed to Yajnavalkya, who is different from the famous Upanishadic sage by that name. The editor of this text regarded it as "the earliest available book on Hathayoga for the common man."[14] He mentioned the period between 200 and 400 A.D. as a possible date for the Yoga-Yajnavalkya. This is unlikely, however. It is true that this scripture does not refer to the seven occult centers (cakra) of the body and only speaks of drawing the serpent power into the lotus of the heart, but this need not necessarily imply that it antedates the typical cakra model of Hatha-Yoga and Tantrism. It is, nevertheless, quite likely that this is a fairly early work, perhaps belonging to the twelfth century A.D.

The Brihad-Yogi-Yajnavalkya-Smriti ("Great Treatise on Yogin Yajnavalkya's [Yoga]") was probably composed several centuries after the Yoga-Yajnavalkya and appears to be an expanded version of that text. It is a fairly substantial treatise of 886 stanzas that describes many ritual practices to be followed by the yogin. Much space is given to the philosophy and practice of Mantra-Yoga, consisting in the recitation of the sacred syllable *om* combined with breath control. The teacher is presumably the same Yajnavalkya who is the authority in the Yoga-Yajnavalkya.

The Yoga-Vishaya ("Object of Yoga"), misleadingly ascribed to Matsyendra, is a short work of 33 verses. It covers such basic topics as the nine centers (cakras), the three "knots" (granthi), and the nine "gates" (dvara). The nine centers have already been discussed. The three knots are constrictions of the life-force inherent in the unenlightened body-mind. Known as rudra-granthi, vishnu-granthi, and brahma-granthi, they are located respectively at the base of the spine, the heart, and the throat. The objective of breath control is to have the life-force (prana) pierce through these knots so that the kundalini can fully ascend along the spinal axis.

Hatha-Yoga-Pradipika

The Hatha-Yoga-Pradipika ("Torch of Hatha-Yoga") was composed by Svatmarama (or Atmarama) in the middle of the fourteenth century A.D. This is undoubtedly *the* classic manual on Hatha-Yoga. It comprises 389 stanzas organized into four chapters. Svatmarama Yogendra, a follower of the Shaiva Yoga tradition of Andhra, expounds Hatha-Yoga as a means to Raja-Yoga.

One is not successful in Raja-Yoga without Hatha-[Yoga], nor in Hatha-[Yoga] without Raja-Yoga. Hence one should practice both for [one's spiritual] maturation. (II.76)

The first chapter is dedicated primarily to a description of the principal postures (asana), while the second chapter speaks of the cleansing practices as well as the life-force (prana) and its regulation through breath control (pranayama). In the third chapter, Svatmarama introduces the subtle physiology and techniques such as the seals (mudra) and locks (bandha) by which the life-force can be properly contained in the body in order to awaken the kundalini. The concluding chapter deals with the higher stages of yogic practice, including the ecstatic condition (samadhi).

The Hatha-Yoga-Pradipika has an excellent commentary entitled Jyotsna ("Light"), by Brahmananda.

Hatha-Ratna-Avali

The Hatha-Ratna-Avali ("String of Pearls on Hatha") of Shrinivasa Bhatta, which may have been composed in the mid-seventeenth century A.D. and appears to have at least one commentary, is a work of 397 verses. Shrinivasa, who also wrote works on Vedanta, Nyaya, and Tantra, offers a masterly treatment of Hatha-Yoga, which expands on the information contained in the Hatha-Yoga-Pradipika.

Gheranda-Samhita

Gheranda-Samhita ("Gheranda's Collection"), which was probably composed toward the end of the seventeenth century A.D., is one of the best known works on Hatha-Yoga. The author of the Gheranda-Samhita followed the Vaishnava Yoga tradition of Bengal. This work has seven chapters with 317 verses in all, though some manuscripts have additional stanzas. It describes no fewer than 102 yogic practices, including twenty-one hygienic techniques, thirty-two postures, and twenty-five seals (mudra). It speaks of seven limbs of Yoga and curiously treats breath control (pranayama) *after* sense-withdrawal (pratyahara).[15]

Yoga-Karnika

Yoga-Karnika ("Ear-Ornament of Yoga") of Aghoranananda was composed sometime in the eighteenth century A.D. It has thirteen chapters with well over 1200 verses. The arrangement of the content is far from systematic, nor is the work particularly original. Its value lies in the many quotations it provides from other Hatha-Yoga scriptures, including some texts not readily available.

Shiva-Samhita

After the Hatha-Yoga-Pradipika and the Gheranda-Samhita, the Shiva-Samhita ("Shiva's Collection") is the most important manual of Hatha-Yoga. It comprises 645 stanzas distributed over five chapters. This scripture is particularly valuable because it includes a fair amount of philosophical matter. Its date is unknown, but it appears to be a work of the late seventeenth or early eighteenth century A.D.

The entire first chapter is devoted to expounding Vedantic nondualism:

Illusion (maya) is the mother of the world; not by any other principle is it established. When [this maya] is destroyed, then the world surely ceases to exist as well. (I.64)

He for whom this entire [universe] is the play of maya, which is to be overcome—he has no delight in things and no pleasure in the body. (I.65)

When a person is free from all superimpositions (upadhi), then he can claim to be of the form of untainted, indivisible wisdom (jnana). (I.67)

The second chapter contains descriptions of some of the esoteric structures of the human body. The third chapter opens with a discussion of the teacher and the qualified students, and then goes on to discuss breath control and the three levels of yogic accomplishment: (1) the "pot state" (ghata-avastha), where the life-forces in the body (called the "pot") collaborate with the universal Self; (2) the "accumulation state" (paricaya-avastha), where the life-force is immobilized along the bodily axis (sushumna); (3) and the "maturation state" (nishpatty-avastha), where the yogin has destroyed the seeds of his karma and "drinks from the water of immortality" (III.66).

In the fourth chapter the anonymous author describes the various locks (bandha) and seals (mudra) for awakening the kundalini. The fifth chapter is a treatment of the obstacles on the yogic path, followed by a discussion of the secret bodily centers (cakra), especially the crown center, and of the higher stages of Yoga. The text concludes by affirming that even householders can attain liberation, so long as they observe the duties of a yogin with diligence and give up all attachments.

The older literature on Hatha-Yoga has barely been researched. We know of many more titles than those introduced here, but they are manuscripts, seen by few, that are buried in dusty libraries where they are slowly deteriorating in the humid climate of India. But I believe that the salvaged literature contains the substance of the Hatha-Yogic tradition. If we wish to dig deeper, we must be willing to sit at the feet of the few masters who are still teaching the forceful Yoga.

Epilogue

Yoga is like an ancient river with countless rapids, eddies, loops, tributaries, and backwaters, extending over a vast, colorful terrain of many different habitats. In this volume I have provided a bird's-eye view, giving the reader the broader picture and, I hope, a deeper appreciation of the inviting waters of Yoga and also of the checkered cultural landscape through which the river of Yoga has flowed in the course of its millennia-long development. Occasionally, however, I have zeroed in on a particularly relevant feature, exploring it as space permitted.

Our last glance fell on the riverine current of Hatha-Yoga, the Tantric tradition seeking to accomplish both spiritual enlightenment and bodily immortality. It is this branch of the meandering river of Yoga that carries us to the ocean, the world beyond India. For Yoga has definitely come West. There are today hundreds of thousands of Hatha-Yoga practitioners around the world who benefit from this age-old technology of bodily wholeness and personal growth. There are even more practitioners of meditation, especially "transcendental meditation," which is a form of Mantra-Yoga. They enjoy glimpses of the secrets of consciousness and its astonishing capacity to lift itself up by its own bootstraps—that is, to go beyond its own conditioning.

Yet only a few people deeply and consistently commit themselves to exploring the intricate psychotechnology of the different branches of the Yoga tradition. It is they who are discovering that consciousness, the human body-mind, is a well-equipped laboratory in which can be found, through ecstatic self-transcendence, the philosopher's stone, the alchemical elixir of enlightenment. Admittedly, not everyone is able to follow their example, nor is this necessarily desirable.

Nonetheless, the tradition of Yoga, of which there are still representative masters to be found, offers a wonderful opportunity to delve into the psychic and spiritual dimensions that our postindustrial civilization has tended to neglect and shun. We can study the scriptures of Yoga, both ancient and modern, and allow their esoteric knowledge and wisdom to enrich our understanding of human nature. With guidance, we can even try to verify on our own person some of the claims made by Yoga authorities past and present. This should of course never be a matter of merely imitating the East; but we can learn from its triumphs and its failures.

Certainly, Yoga deserves far more careful attention from scientists than it has so far been granted. Our modern Western civilization, which now exerts a strong influence in all reaches of the globe, is in desperate need of a psychotechnology that can counterbalance the baneful effects of the excesses of scientific technology developed in the Euro-American countries during the past century. Scientists, who are after all committed to understanding "reality," have a special obligation to explore the great intuitions of the spiritual traditions of the East, which vigorously challenge the current scientific view of the world.

The limitations of the materialistic paradigm have become increasingly apparent over the last several decades. More and more scientists are less and less certain of what it is they are trying to observe, measure, describe, and comprehend. This newly won virtue of uncertainty is a possible open door to a more spacious world-view that also accommodates the psychospiritual aspects of existence. The insights and findings of India's spiritual traditions, painstakingly gathered over more than three millennia, can give us a glimpse of what we are likely to find on the other side of the door once present scientistic dogmas have been transcended.

Practitioners of such a reformed science will then be able to sift reality from fiction, and creative imagination (mythology) from mere wishful thinking. They will also be in a position to create the new language that is undoubtedly necessary to describe what they will encounter. Above all, they will learn to stand again in awe of the great Mystery of existence and be humbled and transformed by it. This challenge of the spirit confronts us all, and today it confronts us more pressingly than ever before in human history.

Collectively and individually we will definitely have to find our own answers—our own Yoga.

Chronology

B.C.

c. 2500–1800 Indus civilization

c. 1800–1300 Gradual invasion of India by the Vedic Aryans, hailing from central Russia

c. 1200 Probable date of the legendary Rishabha, the first "ford-maker" of Jainism

c. 1200–1000 Composition of the hymns of the Rig-Veda in archaic Sanskrit

c. 1000 The great war between the Pandavas (Arjuna's clan) and the Kauravas reported in the Mahabharata epic

c. 1000–900 Composition of the magical hymns of the Atharva-Veda

c. 1000–800 Composition of the Brahmanas, works explaining and serving the sacrificial ritualism of the priestly estate of the Vedic society

c. 850 Yajnavalkya, ancient India's most famous sage

c. 800 Vedic Aryan society spreads to northeast India; composition of the earliest Upanishads, such as the Brihad-Aranyaka and the Chandogya

c. 700 Beginnings of the medical teachings of the Sushruta-Samhita, a principal work on Ayur-Veda, north India's native medical system

c. 600 The rise of the culture of Magadha (in the

	northeastern corner of the Indian peninsula), which spawned the great heterodox traditions of Buddhism and Jainism; era of the sage Kapila, founder of the Samkhya tradition
c. 599–527	Vardhamana Mahavira, founder of historical Jainism
c. 563–483	Gautama Siddhartha, the Buddha, founder of Buddhism, whose dates are sometimes given as 558–478 B.C.
c. 500 or 600	Kanada, author of the Vaisheshika-Sutra, principal work of the Vaisheshika tradition within Hinduism; also probably time of Gautama, founder of the Nyaya tradition and composer of the Nyaya-Sutra
c. 500	Earliest portions of the Mahabharata epic
c. 400–450	Composition of the Katha-Upanishad, oldest Upanishadic work dealing explicitly with Yoga
c. 350	Composition of the original Bhagavad-Gita, which was later incorporated into the Mahabharata epic
c. 327–325	Invasion of India by Alexander the Great
c. 300	Jaina Council of Pataliputra, after which occurred the split into Digambaras (nude followers) and Shvetambaras (followers dressed in white)
c. 300 B.C.–A.D. 300	Composition of the didactic passages of the Mahabharata epic, notably the Moksha-Dharma
c. 269 (or 273)–232	Emperor Ashoka, who greatly furthered the dissemination of Buddhism; alternative dates are 268–231 B.C.
c. 200 B.C.	Composition of Jaimini's Mimamsa-Sutra
c. 200 B.C.–A.D. 200	Era of greatest influence of Buddhism
c. 200 B.C.–A.D. 200	Date of origin of the hymns of the Tirumurai, the Tamil equivalent of the Vedas, collected as an anthology by Nambiandar Nambi in the eleventh century A.D.
c. 150	Patanjali the grammarian, traditionally regarded as author of the Yoga-Sutra; probable date of Lakulin or Lakulisha, legendary founder of the Yoga-prac-

ticing Pashupatas and author of the Pashupata-Sutra

c. 100 B.C.–A.D. 200   Rise of Mahayana Buddhism; composition of the earliest Mahayana-Sutras, such as the Ashta-Sahasrika, the Lankavatara, and the Sad-Dharma-Pundarika

A.D.

c. 50   Arrival of Buddhism in China; period of the renowned Buddhist teacher Ashvaghosha

c. 100   Probable date of Caraka, great authority on Ayur-Veda

c. 150   Probable date of composition of the Yoga-Sutra; period of the great Buddhist adept Nagarjuna; final redaction of the Manava-Dharma-Shastra

c. 200   Composition of the Brahma-Sutra of Badarayana, one of the fundamental works of the Vedanta tradition

c. 350   Composition of the Markandeya-Purana, one of the earliest works of this literary genre; probable date of the Jaina philosopher Kunda-Kunda; founding of the Buddhist Yogacara school by Asanga and of the Vijnanavada school by Asanga's brother Vasubandhu; Ishvara Krishna, author of the Samkhya-Karika

c. 400–500   Foundation of Nalanda, most renowned of all Buddhist monasteries; composition of the Ahirbudhnya-Samhita, an early Pancaratra (Vaishnava) work

c. 450   Composition of the Yoga-Bhashya, the oldest extant commentary on the Yoga-Sutra; probable date of origin of the Kapalika order of Shaivism

c. 470–543   Bodhidharma, founder of the Buddhist meditation (chán) tradition in China

c. 550–800   Gradual expansion of the Pancaratra (Vaishnava) tradition into south India

c. 600   Composition of the earliest Tantras, such as the Buddhist Guhya-Samaja and the Hevajra

c. 606–647	King Harsha, a patron of the arts, immortalized by the court poet Bana
c. 638–713	Hui-Neng, sixth and last patriarch of Chinese Buddhism
c. 650	Tirumular, renowned adept-bard of south India, author of the Tirumantira
c. 750	Padma Sambhava, the "precious guru," who introduced Tantrism into Tibet; probable date of the Jaina philosopher Haribhadra, who authored several works on Yoga
c. 700	Gaudapada, author of the Mandukya-Karika and teacher of Shankara's teacher Govinda
c. 750	Composition of the original version of the Yoga-Vasishtha
c. 750–850	Composition of the devotional Tamil poems of the twelve south Indian Alvars
c. 788–820	Shankara, the most renowned propounder of radical nondualism (Advaita Vedanta)
c. 800	Emergence of the Buddhist Sahajayana; final composition of the Caraka-Samhita, one of the principal works on Ayur-Veda; probable date of the Tamil adept-bard Namm Alvar (Shatakopa); composition of the bulky Shakti-Sangama-Tantra
c. 825	"Discovery" of the Shiva-Sutra by the Kashmiri adept Vasugupta, who also authored the Spanda-Sutra
c. 850	Composition of Vacaspati Mishra's Tattva-Vaisharadi, an important subcommentary on the Yoga-Sutra
c. 900	Composition of the Bhagavata-Purana; date of Nathamuni, great Vaishnava practitioner of Yoga
c. 950	Matsyendra, great adept (siddha) and reputed teacher of Goraksha; thought to have founded the Yogini branch of the tradition of Kaula Tantrism; composition of Shandilya's Bhakti-Sutra; composition of the expanded version of the Yoga-Vasishtha
c. 950–970	Birthdate of the great Buddhist scholar and adept Abhinavagupta

c. 988–1069	Tilopa, great Buddhist adept and teacher of Naropa
c. 1000	Composition of King Bhoja's Raja-Martanda, well-known commentary on the Yoga-Sutra; composition of Narada's Bhakti-Sutra; emergence of the Buddhist Kalacakrayana, an offshoot of Mahayana Buddhism; beginnings of the Kalamukha order of Shaivism
c. 1000–1200	Gradual disappearance of Buddhism from India
c. 1000–1400	Composition of Upanishads with a strong Shakta orientation
c. 1012–1097	Marpa, founder of the Kagyupa school of Tibetan Buddhism and teacher of Milarepa
c. 1016–1100	Naropa, great Buddhist adept and teacher of Marpa
c. 1017–1137	Ramanuja, one of the great preceptors of medieval Vaishnavism, teacher of Qualified Nondualism (Vishishta-Advaita) and proponent of Bhakti-Yoga
c. 1025	Composition of al-Biruni's partial translation into Arabic of Patanjali's Yoga-Sutra
c. 1040–1123	Milarepa, Tibet's most famous yogin-saint
c. 1050	Composition of Sekkirar's Peria-Purana in Tamil
c. 1050	Goraksha, founder of the Kanphata sect and author of lost treatise entitled Hatha-Yoga
c. 1089–1172	Hemacandra, famous Jaina philosopher and author of Yoga-Shastra
c. 1100	Composition of the Mahanirvana-Tantra
c. 1106–1167	Basava or Basavanna, reputed founder of the Lingayat tradition of south India, which is also known as Vira-Shaivism
c. 1190–1276	Madhva, founder of the dualist branch of Vedanta; his dates are sometimes given as A.D. 1199–1278
c. 1200–1900	Composition of a range of Hatha-Yoga scriptures, including the Yoga-Yajnavalkya (c. 1200), the Ananda-Samuccaya (c. 1300), the Carpata-Shataka (c. 1300), and the Goraksha-Upanishad (c. 1400)

c. 1250	Meykandar, author of the Shiva-Jnana-Bodha, important Shaiva work in Tamil
c. 1275–1296	Jnanadeva, Maharashtra's most renowned Yoga adept and author of the beautiful Jnaneshvari, a poetic Marathi commentary on the Bhagavad-Gita
c. 1300	Possible date of origin of the Aghori order of Shaivism
c. 1350	Composition of the Hatha-Yoga-Pradipika, one of the standard works on Hatha-Yoga; composition of the Samkhya-Sutra ascribed to the ancient sage Kapila
c. 1440–1518	Kabir, a popular poet-saint of north India, who was instrumental in integrating Hinduism with Moslem teachings
c. 1450	Vidyaranya, author of the Jivanmukti-Viveka, a Vedanta work on the ideal of liberation during the embodied condition
c. 1455–1570	Drukpa Kunley, famous crazy-wisdom adept of Tibet
c. 1469–1539	Nanak, founder of the Sikh tradition and author of the Adi-Granth
c. 1479–1531	Vallabha, a renowned teacher of Bhakti-Yoga centering on worship of God Krishna
c. 1485–1533	Caitanya, one of the foremost Vaishnava teachers of Bengal and a great bhakti-yogin
c. 1500	Composition of the Avadhuta-Gita
c. 1532–1623	Tulsi Das, a widely influential north Indian poet-saint, composer of the Hindi Ramayana
c. 1550	Vijnana Bhikshu, author of numerous philosophical works, including commentaries on the Yoga-Sutra, notably his Yoga-Varttika
c. 1556–1605	Emperor Akbar, greatest of India's Moslem rulers
c. 1650	Composition of the Gheranda-Samhita, a popular manual on Hatha-Yoga
c. 1718–1775	Ram Prasad Sen, celebrated Bengali poet and Kali worshipper
c. 1750	Composition of the Shiva-Samhita, a widely studied work on Hatha-Yoga

c. 1760	Beginning of the British raj in India
c. 1772–1833	Rammohun Roy, founder of the influential Brahma Samaj organization, who has been called the "father of modern India"
1834–1886	Sri Ramakrishna, one of the great mystics of modern India
c. 1861–1941	Rabindranath Tagore, poet laureate of Bengal, a representative of the new Indian humanism
c. 1862–1902	Vivekananda, chief disciple of Sri Ramakrishna and founder of the Ramakrishna Mission, a key figure in the dissemination of Hinduism in Europe and America
c. 1869–1948	Mohandas Karamchand Gandhi, advocate of the principle of nonharming (ahimsa) in all areas of life, especially politics
c. 1872–1950	Sri Aurobindo, founder of Integral Yoga
c. 1875	Founding of the Theosophical Society, which established its headquarters in Adyar, India, in 1882; thanks to the efforts of this organization, many Sanskrit texts were translated into English for the first time
c. 1879–1950	Ramana Maharshi of Tiruvannamalai in south India, one of modern India's most renowned sages and a staunch proponent of Advaita Vedanta
c. 1947	Political independence of India

Glossary of Key Words in Sanskrit

Agama ("Tradition"). A type of sectarian work of encyclopedic scope, dedicated to God Shiva.

Ahimsa ("Nonharming"). Abstention from harmful actions, thoughts, and words. An important moral discipline (yama) in Yoga, Buddhism, and Jainism.

Ajna-cakra ("Command wheel"). The psychic center located in the head, also known as the third eye. It is through this center that the guru communicates telepathically with the disciple.

Anahata-cakra ("Wheel of the unstruck [sound]"). The psychic center located at the heart, where the universal sound *om* can be heard in meditation.

Ananda ("Bliss"). (i) In Vedanta, the mind-transcending blissfulness of the ultimate Reality, or Self. This is not considered to be a quality but the very essence of Reality. (ii) In Patanjali's Yoga, an experimental state associated with a lower type of ecstasy; i.e., samprajnata-samadhi.

Arjuna. The hero of the Bhagavad-Gita; disciple of Lord Krishna.

Asamprajnata-samadhi ("Supraconscious ecstasy"). The technique leading to, and the experience of, unified consciousness, in which the subject becomes one with the experienced object, without any thoughts or ideas being present. In Vedanta, this is known as nirvikalpa-samadhi. Cf. also **samprajnata-samadhi.**

Asana ("Seat"). Posture, which is the third limb (anga) of the eightfold path of Patanjali's Yoga.

Ashrama. (i) Hermitage. (ii) Stage of life according to the Hindu model of society. Four stages are distinguished: pupilage (brahmacarya), householdership (garhasthya), forest-dwelling life (vana-prasthya), and renunciation (samnyasa).

Atharva-Veda ("Atharvan's Knowledge"). One of the four Vedic hymnodies, dealing primarily with magical spells but also containing several important documents of early Yoga.

Atman ("Self"). The transcendental Self according to the nondualist (Vedanta) schools of thought, which is identical with brahman. Cf. **purusha.**

Avadhuta ("Cast off"). A radical type of renouncer who abandons all conventions; a crazy adept.

Avatara ("Descent"). An incarnation of the Divine, such as Krishna and Rama.

Avidya ("Ignorance"). Spiritual nescience, which is the root of all human suffering and the cause of one's bondage to egoic states of consciousness.

Ayur-Veda ("Science of Life"). The native Hindu system of medicine.

Bandha ("Lock"). Special techniques used in Hatha-Yoga for confining the life-force (prana) in certain parts of the body.

Bhagavad-Gita ("Lord's Song"). The earliest and most popular scripture of Yoga, containing the teachings of Lord Krishna to Arjuna.

Bhagavata. (i) Adherent of Vishnu in the form of Krishna. (ii) Name of the sect of Krishna worshippers.

Bhagavata-Purana. A comprehensive tenth-century work containing, among other things, the mythical life story of Lord Krishna.

Bhakta ("Devotee"). A follower of Bhakti-Yoga.

Bhakti (Love, devotion). The spiritual sentiment of loving participation in the Divine.

Bhakti-Yoga ("Yoga of Love"). One of the principal schools of Hindu Yoga.

Bhuta ("Element"). Hindu cosmology distinguishes five elements: earth, water, fire, air, and ether (akasha).

Bindu ("Dot, drop"). (i) The dot placed above the letter *m* in the syllable *om,* indicating that the sound *m* is to be hummed. (ii) The hummed sound *m* in *om.* (iii) A special psychic center in the head, close to the ajna-cakra. (iv) The central point of a yantra or mandala. (v) In yogic experience, the objectless state of consciousness prior to the appearance of images and thoughts but not identical to the transcendental Being-Consciousness. (vi) In Hindu cosmology, the threshold between the unmanifest dimension of Nature and manifestation. (vii) Semen, which, according to Tantrism, should be mingled with the woman's ejaculate, called rajas.

Bodhisattva ("Enlightenment being"). In Mahayana Buddhism, the spiritual practitioner who has vowed to commit himself or herself to the liberation of all beings, postponing his or her own ultimate realization.

Brahma. The Creator-God of the famous medieval Hindu triad of gods. The other two are Vishnu (as Preserver) and Shiva (as Destroyer). Brahma must be carefully distinguished from the brahman, which is the eternal foundation of existence.

Brahmacarya ("Brahmic conduct"). The practice of chastity in thought, word, and deed, which is regarded as one of the fundamental disciplines (yama) of Yoga.

Brahman. The Absolute according to Vedanta; the transcendental Ground of the world. See also **sac-cid-ananda, atman.**

Brahmana. (i) A member of the priestly class of Hindu society, a brahmin. (ii) A type of ritual text explaining the hymns of the Veda as they are relevant to the sacrificial ritual.

Buddha ("Awakened"). Title of Gautama, founder of Buddhism.

Buddhi ("Wisdom"). The higher, intuitive mind, or wisdom-faculty. The term is also used occasionally in the sense of thought or cognition.

Cakra ("Wheel"). A psychic center of the body. Tantrism and Hatha-Yoga generally distinguish seven principal centers: muladhara, svadhishthana, manipura, anahata, vishuddha, ajna, and sahasrara. These are aligned along the spinal axis and form part of the body of the serpent power (kundalini-shakti).

Cit ("Consciousness"). Pure Awareness, or the transcendental Consciousness beyond all thought; the eternal Witness. See also **atman, purusha.**

Citta ("Consciousness"). The finite mind or consciousness, which is dependent on the play of attention. Cf. **buddhi, manas.**

Dattatreya. A early post-Christian sage connected with the Avadhuta tradition, who became deified as an incarnation of God Shiva.

Deva/devata ("Deity"). Usually this word refers to one of the many deities of the Hindu pantheon. They are envisioned as powerful beings in subtle dimensions of existence. Occasionally the term stands for the Divine itself.

Dharana ("Holding"). Concentration, the sixth limb of Patanjali's eightfold yogic path. It consists in the prolonged focusing of attention on a single mental object and leads to meditation (dhyana).

Dharma. (i) The cosmic law or order. (ii) Morality or virtue, as one of the legitimate concerns (purusha-artha) sanctioned by Hinduism. It is understood as a manifestation or reflection of the divine law. (iii) Teaching, doctrine.

Dharma-megha-samadhi ("Ecstasy of dharma cloud"). According to Patanjali, the highest form of supraconscious ecstasy (asamprajnata-samadhi), which is the doorway to liberation.

Dhyana ("Meditation"). Meditative absorption, or contemplation, the seventh limb of Patanjali's yogic path, which is understood as a deepening of concentration (dharana). See also **samadhi.**

Diksha ("Initiation"). An important feature of all yogic schools.

Duhkha ("Pain"). According to all liberation schools of India, conditioned or finite existence is inherently sorrowful or painful. It is this insight that provides the impetus for the spiritual struggle to realize the immortal, blissful Self.

Gautama the Buddha. The founder of Buddhism, who lived in the sixth century B.C.

Gautama. The mythical founder of the Nyaya school of thought.

Gita. See **Bhagavad-Gita.**

Gopa/gopi. Male/female shepherd. In Vaishnavism, these terms refer to the devotees of Lord Krishna.

Goraksha(natha). The founder of the Kanpatha order of Hatha-Yogins, who lived in the tenth century A.D.

Guna ("Quality"). (i) In Yoga, Samkhya, and many schools of Vedanta, one of three primary constituents of Nature (prakriti): sattva (principle of lucidity), rajas (principle of activity), and tamas (principle of inertia). The interaction between these three types creates the entire manifest and unmanifest cosmos, including all psychomental phenomena. (ii) Virtue, high moral quality.

Guru ("Heavy"). Spiritual teacher.

Hamsa ("Swan"). (i) The breath/life-force (prana). (ii) The transcendental Self (atman). (iii) A type of wandering ascetic (parivrajaka).

Hatha-Yoga ("Forceful Yoga"). The Yoga of physical discipline, aiming at the awakening of the serpent power (kundalini-shakti) and the creation of an indestructible "divine" body (divya-deha).

Hinayana ("Small vehicle"). The minority school of Buddhism, which has arhatship (or arhantship) as its leading ideal. Cf. **Mahayana.**

Hiranyagarbha ("Golden Germ"). The mythical founder of Yoga.

Ish/Isha/Ishvara ("Ruler"). God. In Patanjali's Yoga, the ishvara is defined as a special transcendental Self (purusha). His uniqueness is due to the fact that He never was, and never will be, under the spell of spiritual ignorance (avidya).

Ishvara Krishna. Author of the Samkhya-Karika, the principal text of Classical Samkhya. He lived probably in the third century A.D. See also **Kapila.**

Jaina. A member of Jainism, the religion founded by Mahavira, a contemporary of Gautama the Buddha.

Japa ("Recitation"). Meditative recitation of mantras.

Jiva ("Living being"). The psyche, or finite conscious human personality, which experiences itself as different from others and does not know the transcendental Self. Cf. **atman, purusha.**

Jivan-mukti ("Living liberation"). According to most Vedanta schools, it is possible to gain liberation, or full enlightenment, even while still embodied. The Self-realized adept who is thus liberated is known as a jivan-mukta.

Jnana-Yoga. The nondualist Yoga of self-transcending wisdom, which proceeds by careful discrimination (viveka) between the Real (i.e., the Self) and the unreal (i.e., the ego).

Kaivalya ("Aloneness"). The state of liberation, especially in Yoga and Jainism. See also **moksha.**

Kali ("Black"). The Hindu goddess of destruction.

Kali-yuga ("Dark Age"). According to Tantrism, the modern age of spiritual decline, which requires a new approach to Self-realization. It is thought to have started in 3012 B.C.

Kapila. The founder of the Samkhya tradition, who may have lived in the sixth century B.C. He is said to be the composer of the Samkhya-Sutra, which, however, belongs to a much later era.

Karma/karman ("Action"). (i) Activity in general; work. (ii) The subtle effect caused by the actions and volitions of an unenlightened individual, which is responsible for his or her rebirth and also for some of the experiences during that future life. The idea behind all Indian liberation teachings is to escape the effects of past karma and prevent the production of new karma, whether good or bad.

Karma-Yoga ("Yoga of Action"). A cardinal type of Yoga, which consists in the self-transcending performance of actions that are in consonance with one's innermost being (svabhava) and in keeping with one's appropriate lifestyle (svadharma).

Kosha ("Sheath"). This Vedantic term denotes a bodily envelope, of which there are five: the body composed of food (anna-maya-kosha), the body composed of life-force (prana-maya-kosha), the body composed of thought (mano-maya-kosha), the body composed of understanding (vijnana-maya-kosha), and the body composed of bliss (ananda-maya-kosha). The last-mentioned envelope is identical with the Absolute (brahman).

Krishna ("Puller"). An ancient adept who was later deified. As an incarnation of God Vishnu, he instructed Prince Arjuna in the Bhagavad-Gita.

Kshatriya. Member of the warrior class of Hindu society.

Kundali/kundalini-shakti ("Coiled power" or "serpent power.") The awakening of this power, which lies dormant in the lowest psychic center of the human body, is the goal of Tantrism and Hatha-Yoga. The ascent of the kundalini to the highest psychic center, at the crown of the head, brings about a temporary state of ecstatic identification with the Self (in nirvikalpa-samadhi).

Kundalini-Yoga. The Yoga specifically dedicated to the arousing of the kundalini-shakti.

Laya-Yoga ("Yoga of Dissolution"). The Yoga of meditative absorption, involving the gradual dismantling of the ordinary consciousness until there ensues the ecstatic identification with the Self beyond the mind.

Linga ("Mark"). (i) The phallus as the symbol of creativity, which is specifically associated with God Shiva.

Mahabharata. One of the two great Hindu national epics, recounting the war between the Pandavas (Arjuna's side) and the Kauravas. The epic contains many instructional passages, including the Bhagavad-Gita. Cf. **Ramayana.**

Mahavira ("Great hero"). The title of Vardhamana, the historical founder of Jainism. See also **Jaina.**

Mahayana ("Great vehicle"). The majority branch of Buddhism, which has the bodhisattva as its great ideal. Cf. **Hinayana, Vajrayana.**

Maithuna ("Intercourse"). The ritual practice of sexual congress in the left-hand branch of Tantrism.

Manas ("Mind"). The lower mind, which is understood as a relay station for the senses (indriya) and is itself regarded as a sense. Cf. **Buddhi.**

Manipura-cakra ("Wheel of the jeweled city"). The psychic center at the navel.

Mantra. Sound that empowers the mind for concentration and the transcendence of the ordinary states of consciousness. A mantra can consist of a single syllable, like *om,* or a string of meaningful or even conventionally meaningless sounds.

Mantra-Yoga. The yogic path that has the recitation (japa) of mantras as its primary means.

Matsyendra(natha). A great adept of the Kaula school of Tantrism and the teacher of Goraksha, who lived in the tenth century A.D.

Mimamsa ("Discussion"). One of the six classical schools of Hindu philosophy, which is concerned with the explanation of Vedic ritualism and its moral applications.

Moksha ("Release"). According to Hindu ethics, the highest of possible human pursuits (purusha-artha) is liberation, which is synonymous with Self- or God-realization. See also **kaivalya.**

Mudra ("Seal"). (i) A hand gesture or bodily posture, which has symbolic significance but is also thought to conduct the life-energy in the body in certain ways. Both Hinduism and Buddhism know many such gestures, as can be seen in their iconographies. (ii) A female initiate in the Tantric ritual, with whom sacred intercourse (maithuna) is practiced. (iii) Parched grain, which is used in the Tantric ritual and is thought to act as an aphrodisiac.

Muladhara-cakra ("Root-support wheel"). The lowest of the psychic centers in the human body, situated at the base of the spine. It is here that the serpent power (kundalini-shakti) lies dormant.

Nada ("Sound"). The primal sound of the universe, sometimes said to be the sacred mantra *om.* It has various forms of manifestation, which can be heard as an inner sound when meditation reaches a certain depth.

Nadi ("Conduit"). According to Hindu esotericism, the human body (or, rather, its subtle counterpart) consists of a network of channels along which flows the life-force (prana). Often the figure 72,000 is mentioned. Of these channels, three are most important, viz. the ida-, the pingala-, and the sushumna-nadi. The last-mentioned extends from the lowest psychic center to the crown of the head, and it is along this pathway that the aroused kundalini-shakti must travel.

Narada. A famous ancient sage teaching Bhakti-Yoga, to whom the authorship of the Bhakti-Sutra is ascribed.

Nirvana ("Extinction"). In Buddhism, the transcendence of the ego-self, which is occasionally also described in positive terms, as a condition that is untouched by space and time. In Hindu contexts, the term is mostly used interchangeably with the Absolute (brahman).

Nirvikalpa-samadhi ("Transconceptual ecstasy"). The Vedantic term for what in Patanjali's school is called asamprajnata-samadhi. See also **savikalpa-samadhi.**

Niyama ("Discipline"). The second limb of Patanjali's eightfold Yoga, which consists in the practice of purity, contentment, austerity (tapas), study (svadhyaya), and devotion to the Lord (ishvara-pranidhana). See also **yama.**

Nyaya ("Rule"). One of the six classical Hindu schools, which is concerned with logic and critical argument.

Ojas. The energy produced through asceticism, especially the practice of chastity (brahmacarya).

Om. The key mantra of Hinduism, symbolizing the Absolute.

Panca-makara ("Five m's"). The collective name for the five practices of the core ritual of Tantrism: the consumption of fish (matsya), meat (mamsa), parched grain (mudra), and wine (madya), all of which are regarded as aphrodisiacs. The fifth element is intercourse (maithuna). In the left-hand branch of Tantrism, these are understood literally, while the right-hand schools interpret them symbolically. See also **Tantra.**

Parama-atman ("Supreme self"). The transcendental Self, as opposed to the empirical, living self (jiva-atman), which is individuated. See also **atman.**

Patanjali. Author of the Yoga-Sutra, which is the source text of Classical Yoga (or yoga-darshana). He probably lived in the second century A.D.

Prakriti ("Creatrix"). Nature, which is multidimensional, consisting of an eternal, transcendental Ground (called pradhana or alinga), and levels of subtle (sukshma) and gross (sthula) manifestation. The lowest level is the visible material realm with its myriad objects. Nature is made up of three types of forces, called guna.

Prana ("Life"). (i) Life in general. (ii) The life-force sustaining the body which has five principal forms. (iii) The breath as the external manifestation of the life-force.

Pranayama ("Breath control"). The careful regulation of the breath, which is the fourth limb of Patanjali's eightfold path. This is the most important practice of Hatha-Yoga.

Pratyahara ("Withdrawal"). Sensory inhibition, which is the fifth limb of Patanjali's eightfold path and precedes concentration (dharana).

Puja(na) ("Worship"). An important aspect of Bhakti-Yoga, Tantrism, as well as all schools of Yoga and Vedanta that focus on a personal deity, or the ritual veneration of one's teacher as an embodiment of the Divine.

Purana ("Ancient"). A type of popular quasi-religious encyclopedia, of which there are many. Most are of post-Christian origin and dedicated to a deity of the Hindu pantheon, notably Vishnu and Shiva. They often contain passages dealing with Yoga.

Purusha ("Male"). In the Yoga and Samkhya traditions, the transcendental Self, Spirit, or pure Awareness (cit), as opposed to the finite personality (jiva).

Rajas. (i) The quality of activity, which is one of the three primary constituents (guna) of Nature. (ii) Menstrual blood, which holds special significance in Tantrism. The mingling of rajas with the male semen (bindu) is said to bring about the ecstatic condition. See also **sattva, tamas.**

Raja-Yoga ("Royal Yoga"). A late name for Patanjali's school of thought, invented to contrast it with Hatha-Yoga.

Rama. The main hero of the Ramayana, deified as an incarnation of God Vishnu.

Ramanuja. The eleventh-century founder of the school of Qualified Nondualism (Vishishta Advaita) and principal rival of Shankara.

Ramayana. One of India's two great national epics, telling the heroic story of Rama. Cf. **Mahabharata.**

Rig-Veda ("Praise Knowledge"). The oldest hymnody of the Veda, the most sacred scripture of the Hindus, comparable to the Old Testament. See also **Atharva-Veda**.

Rishi. A type of Vedic seer, who sees the hymns (mantra) of Veda.

Sac-cid-ananda ("Being-Consciousness-Bliss"). The ultimate Reality according to Vedanta. See also **brahman, sat, cit, ananda**.

Sadhana ("Realizing"). The Tantric path toward Self-realization.

Sahaja ("Twinned"). A medieval term denoting the fact that the transcendental Reality and the empirical reality are essentially "twinned"—i.e., one and the same. It is often rendered as "spontaneous" or "natural."

Sahaja-samadhi ("Natural ecstasy"). The effortless ecstasy, identical with liberation. See also **samadhi**.

Sahasrara-cakra ("Thousand-spoked wheel"). The psychic center at the crown of the head, which in Tantrism is the destination point of the aroused serpent power (kundalini-shakti).

Samadhi ("Ecstasy"). This is the eighth limb of Patanjali's eightfold Yoga. It consists in the temporary identification between subject and contemplated object and has two main forms: conscious ecstasy (samprajnata-samadhi), which includes a variety of spontaneous thoughts, and supraconsciousness ecstasy (asamprajnata-samadhi), in which all ideation is transcended. See also **dharma-megha-samadhi, sahaja-samadhi**.

Samkhya ("Number"). One of the six main Hindu schools of thought, which is concerned with the classification of the levels of reality.

Samnyasa ("Renunciation"). The practice of turning one's attention away from worldly things and toward the Divine, which is generally accompanied by an outward act of abandoning conventional life.

Samprajnata-samadhi ("Conscious ecstasy"). The lower type of ecstatic identification between subject and contemplated object, accompanied by spontaneous thoughts (called pratyaya).

Samsara ("Confluence"). The finite world of change. Cf. **nirvana**.

Samskara ("Activator"). Every action or violition produces a subliminal deposit in the depth of consciousness, which, in turn, leads to new psychomental activity. See also **karma, vasana**.

Sat ("Being"). The Real. The Being aspect of the transcendental Reality. See also **cit, ananda**.

Sat-sanga ("Relationship to the True"). The spiritual practice of frequenting the good company of saints, sages, Self-realized adepts, and their disciples.

Sattva ("Being-ness"). The principle of lucidity, which is the highest type of primary constituent (guna) of Nature (prakriti).

Savikalpa-samadhi ("Ecstasy with form/ideation"). In Vedanta, the state of conscious identification with the transcendental Reality, accompanied by thoughts and imagery. Cf. **nirvikalpa-samadhi;** see also **samprajnata-samadhi**.

Shabda ("Sound"). According to Hindu thought, sound is inextricably connected with cosmic existence. Thus, sound exists on various levels of manifestation. The ultimate sound is the sacred mantra *om*.

Shaiva. Designation for any process or literary work, etc., pertaining to Shiva, or a worshipper of this God. See also **Vaishnava**.

Shakta. A process, literary work, etc., pertaining to Shakti, or a worshipper of the Divine Power.

Shakti ("Power"). The feminine power aspect of the Divine, which is fundamental to the metaphysics and spiritual technology of Tantrism.

Shakti-pata ("Descent of the power"). The process of initiation, or spirit baptism, usually in Tantric schools, by which the guru empowers the disciple's spiritual practice.

Shankara. The greatest propounder of Hindu nondualism (Advaita Vedanta), who lived in the late eighth century A.D. He probably converted from Yoga to Vedanta.

Shanti ("Peace"). A desirable quality in yogins. Ultimate peace coincides with Self-realization, or enlightenment (bodha).

Shiva ("Benign"). The God who, more than any other deity of the Hindu pantheon, has served yogins as a model throughout the ages.

Shudra. A member of the servile class of Hindu society.

Siddha ("Accomplished, perfected"). A Self-realized adept, one who has reached perfection (siddhi).

Siddhi ("Accomplishment"). (i) Spiritual perfection; i.e., the attainment of flawless identification with the ultimate Reality. A synonym for liberation (moksha). (ii) Paranormal power, especially the eight great powers that come as a result of perfect adeptship.

Svadhishthana-cakra ("Self-based wheel"). The psychic center in the genital region.

Tamas. The principle of inertia, or darkness, which is one of the three primary constituents (guna) of Nature.

Tantra ("Loom"). (i) A type of sacred scripture pertaining to Tantrism and primarily dealing with ritual worship focusing on the feminine principle, Shakti. (ii) Tantrism, the many-branched religiocultural movement originating in the early post-Christian era and flourishing about 1000 A.D. Tantrism has a right-hand (conservative) and a left-hand (antinomian) branch.

Tapas ("Glow, heat"). Asceticism, thought to lead to great vitality.

Tirthankara ("Ford-maker"). A Self-realized teacher of Jainism.

Upanishad ("Sitting-near"). A type of sacred Hindu scripture that expounds the metaphysics of nondualism (Advaita Vedanta).

Vaisheshika ("Distinctionism"). One of the six major Hindu schools of thought, which is concerned with the categories of existence.

Vaishnava. Designation for any process or literary work, etc., pertaining to Vishnu, or a worshipper of this god. See also **Shaiva.**

Vaishya. Member of the merchant class of Hindu society.

Vajrayana ("Adamantine vehicle"). The Tantric branch of Buddhism, especially of Tibet, which evolved out of the Mahayana.

Vasana ("Trait"). In Patanjali's Yoga, the concatenation of subliminal activators (samskara) deposited in the depth of consciousness.

Vashishtha. The name of several ancient sages, notably the great authority of the Yoga-Vasishtha.

Vedanta ("Veda's end"). The dominant Hindu tradition, which teaches that Reality is singular. See **brahman, atman.**

Videha-mukti ("Disembodied liberation"). The ideal of some schools of Vedanta, which deny that full liberation can be gained while the body is still alive. Cf. **jivan-mukti.**

Vishnu ("Worker"). The God worshipped by the Bhagavatas. His most famous incarnation is Lord Krishna.

Vishuddha-cakra ("Wheel of purity"). The psychic center at the throat.

Vratya. Member of a sacred brotherhood in the Vedic era, in whose circles early yogic practices were developed.

Vyasa. The legendary composer of the Mahabharata, the many Puranas, and the Yoga-Bhashya commentary to the Yoga-Sutra.

Yajna ("Sacrifice"). The practice of ritual sacrifice is fundamental to Hinduism. In Upanishadic times, the external sacrificial ritual was internalized in the form of intense meditation, leading to the tradition of Yoga.

Yajnavalkya. The most renowned sage of the early Upanishadic era.

Yama ("Restraint"). The first "limb" of Patanjali's eightfold Yoga, comprising five moral precepts of universal validity.

Yantra ("Device"). A geometric design in Hinduism representing the body of one's chosen deity for external worship and inner concentration.

Yoga ("Union"). (i) Spiritual practice in general. (ii) One of the six principal Hindu schools of thought, codified by Patanjali.

Yoga-Sutra ("Yoga aphorisms"). The source text of Classical Yoga, authored by Patanjali.

Yoga-Vasishtha. A massive poetic treatment of nondualist Yoga, composed sometime in the tenth century A.D.

Yogin. A male practitioner of Yoga.

Yogini. A female practitioner of Yoga.

Yuga ("Age"). According to Hindu mythochronology, there are four yugas, each of several thousand years' duration. The present age is the kali-yuga.

Notes

INTRODUCTION

1. The term *Vedantic* stems from the Sanskrit word *vedanta*, which means literally "Veda's end." It refers to the great Hindu tradition of nondualism, which postulates that there is only the one Reality that constitutes all beings and things.
2. Sri Aurobindo, *The Life Divine* (Pondicherry, India: Sri Aurobindo Ashram, 1977), vol. 1, pp. 3–4.
3. Ken Wilber, *The Atman Project: A Transpersonal View of Human Development* (Wheaton, Ill.: Theosophical Publishing House, 1980), p. ix.
4. Gary Zukav, *The Dancing Wu Li Masters: An Overview of the New Physics* (New York: Morrow Quill Paperbacks, 1979), pp. 42–43.
5. Rabindranath Tagore, *Gitanjali* (New York: Macmillan, 1971), p. 44.
6. See Colin Norman, *The God That Limps: Science and Technology in the Eighties* (New York: W. W. Norton, 1981).
7. Freeman J. Dyson, *Infinite in All Directions* (New York: Harper & Row, 1988), p. 270.
8. Da Free John, *The Enlightenment of the Whole Body* (Middletown, Calif.: Dawn Horse Press, 1978), p. 377.
9. See below, pp. 250–276.
10. See C. G. Jung, *Psychology and the East* (Princeton, N.J.: Princeton University Press, 1978).
11. See Karl Jaspers, *Vom Ursprung und Ziel der Geschichte* (Frankfurt, West Germany: Fischer Bucherei, 1956).
12. I have explained this in some detail in my book *Structures of Consciousness: The Genius of Jean Gebser—An Introduction and Critique* (Lower Lake, Calif.: Integral Publishing, 1987).

PART ONE: FOUNDATIONS

1 BUILDING BLOCKS

1. This definition is found in the fifth-century Yoga-Bhashya (I.1) of Vyasa, which is the oldest available commentary on the Yoga-Sutra of Patanjali, the standard work on Classical Yoga. The Sanskrit equation runs *yogah samadhih*, "Yoga is ecstasy."

2. See M. Eliade, *Yoga: Immortality and Freedom* (Princeton, N.J.: Princeton University Press, 1973), p. 77.
3. Precisely what the Upanishads are is explained in Part Two, Chapter 5.
4. For a detailed historical survey of the Hindu pantheon, see S. Bhattacharji, *The Indian Theogony: A Comparative Study of Indian Mythology from the Vedas to the Puranas* (Cambridge, England: Cambridge University Press, 1970). See also A. Danielou, *Hindu Polytheism* (New York: Pantheon Books, 1964), and D. and J. Johnson, *God and Gods in Hinduism* (New Delhi: Arnold-Heinemann, 1972).
5. The "Fourth" (turya, turiya, or caturtha) is the transcendental Condition beyond the three modes of attention, namely deep sleep (sushupti), dream sleep (svapna), and waking consciousness (jagrat). It is the superconscious Ground of all that exists.
6. According to some maverick researchers, Jesus was educated in Kashmir, but this is mere conjecture. Others maintain, on literary and archaeological grounds, that he retired to Kashmir after surviving his crucifixion. See, e.g., A. Faber-Kaiser, *Jesus Died in Kashmir* (London: Gordon & Cremonesi, 1977) and H. Kersten, *Jesus Lebte in Indien* (Munich: Droemersche Verlagsanstalt, 1983) [German].
7. See, e.g., the Mahabharata (XII.293.30).
8. The term *yogini* also applies to a member of a group of female deities who are regarded as manifestations of the universal creative energy (shakti); they play an important role in certain schools of Tantrism. The cult of the sixty-four yoginis dates back to the sixth or seventh century A.D. See H. C. Das, *Tantricism: A Study of the Yogini Cult* (New Delhi: Sterling Publishers, 1981).
9. Tantrism, or Tantra, is explained in Chapter 12.
10. M. Eliade, *Yoga: Freedom and Immortality* (Princeton, N.J.: Princeton University Press, 1973), p. 5.
11. Ibid., p. 5.
12. See, e.g., the grammarian Patanjali's Maha-Bhashya, commenting on Panini's Sutra II.1.41.
13. See M. P. Pandit, *The Kularnava Tantra* (Madras, India: Ganesh, 1965), pp. 98–99.
14. See Swami Narayananda, trans., *The Guru Gita* (Bombay: India Book House, 1976).
15. See Ngawang Dhargyey, et al., *Fifty Verses of Guru-Devotion by Asvaghosa* (Dharamsala, India: Library of Tibetan Works and Archives, 1975).
16. C. Trungpa, *Cutting Through Spiritual Materialism* (Boulder, Colo.: Shambhala, 1973), p. 58.
17. The most detailed explanation of the enlightened adept's spontaneous spiritual transmission is found in the works of the contemporary teacher Da Free John, notably in *The Method of the Siddhas* (Clearlake, Calif.: Dawn Horse Press, 1978).
18. This is verse 69 (or 68, depending on the edition) of Umapati's Shata-Ratna-Samgraha ("Compendium of One Hundred Jewels"). The next verse explains the word *diksha* as connoting both "destruction" (kshapana) and "giving" (dana). What is destroyed is the state of "animality" (pashutva) of the unenlightened being, and what is given, by grace, is the supreme condition of "Shivahood" (shivatva).
19. The expression *parivraj* is curious here, because this type of avadhuta, also known as yati ("ascetic"), is charged with living the life of a householder. Only the parama-hamsa, or hamsa, wanders about unfettered by any restrictions.
20. This esoteric etymology, which divides the word *avadhuta* into its constituent syllables, is developed on the basis of a word play; i.e., many of the key descriptive terms in each verse begin with the syllable that is being explained. Thus in stanza

8, which expounds the significance of the syllable *dhu* , the melodious phrases *dhuli-dhusara-gatrani* ("limbs grey from dust") and *dharana-dhyana-nirmuktah* ("relieved of concentration and meditation") are found, and so on.

21. See R. Hauschild, *Die Aṣṭāvakra-Gītā* (Berlin: Akademie-Verlag, 1967), p. 55. Hauschild's is the only critical edition of this text. For an English translation see Swami Nityaswarupananda, *Ashtavakra Samhita* (Mayavati, India: Advaita Ashrama, 1953).

22. See H. S. Joshi, *Origin and Development of Dattātreya Worship in India* (Baroda, India: Maharaja Sayajirao University of Baroda, 1965).

23. Curiously, the Avadhuta-Gita attributed to Dattatreya contains a whole chapter (VIII) that has a decidely misogynous tone, for which reason it has often been regarded as a later interpolation.

24. This problem is discussed in depth in my book *Crazy Wisdom,* published by Paragon House Publishers (New York).

2 THE WHEEL OF YOGA

1. Swami Vivekananda, *Raja-Yoga or Conquering the Internal Nature* (Calcutta: Advaita Ashrama, 1962), p. 66.
2. Ibid., p. 11.
3. Bubba [Da] Free John, *The Enlightenment of the Whole Body* (Middletown, Calif.: Dawn Horse Press, 1978), p. 500.
4. J. W. Hauer, *Der Yoga* (Stuttgart, West Germany: Kohlhammer Verlag, 1958), p. 271.
5. N. K. Brahma, *Philosophy of Hindu Sadhana* (London: Kegan Paul, Trench, Trubner, 1932), p. 137.
6. Swami Satprakashananda, *Methods of Knowledge* (London: Allen & Unwin, 1965), p. 204.
7. In the Vedanta-Siddhanta-Darshana, which is a late medieval work, seven stages (bhumi) of gnosis are mentioned:

> The great seers have spoken of seven stages of wisdom. Of these the first stage of wisdom is designated as "good will" (shubha-iccha); the second is reflection (vicarana); the third is subtlety of mind (tanu-manasa); the fourth is the attainment of lucidity (sattva-apatti); the fifth is nonattachment (asamsakti); the sixth is the vanishing of all objects (pada-artha-abhavani) [in the state of ecstasy]; and the seventh is the entering into the "Fourth" [i.e., the ultimate Reality beyond waking, dreaming, and sleeping]. (190–192)

We will encounter these stages again in Chapter 10 ("The Nondual Approach to God"), which includes a discussion of the Yoga-Vasishtha, a mammoth work that is exclusively dedicated to Jnana-Yoga.

8. *Confessions* I.1.
9. See, e.g., Jiva Gosvami's Shat-Sandarbha, Sanskrit edition, p. 541.
10. According to a cosmological theory that is upheld by all spiritual schools of Hinduism, Nature is a web woven by three fundamental forces, which are called sattva, rajas, and tamas. These stand respectively for the principles of lucidity, dynamism, and inertia. Their interaction is responsible for the immense variety of forms in the known universe, and they also underlie our different emotional dispositions. Thus, even our attitude toward the Divine is determined by the predominance of one or another of these three qualities.

11. S. N. Dasgupta, *Hindu Mysticism* (Chicago: Open Court Publishing, 1927), p. 126.
12. The importance of the Vratyas in the development of Yoga is discussed in Part Two, Chapter 4.
13. Some scholars regard the Bhagavad-Gita as older than the Shvetashvatara-Upanishad.
14. There is a late Shaiva counterpart to the Vaishnava Bhagavad-Gita, and that is the Ishvara-Gita, which is embedded in the second part of the Kurma-Purana (chapter 11). This composition, which is later than the Bhagavata-Purana (c. A.D. 900), belongs to an era in which the path of bhakti was broadened to a cultural movement that swept across the entire Indian peninsula. A comparable event occurred in medieval Europe in the thirteenth and fourteenth centuries when thousands of Christian women discovered the power of the heart through Jesus-oriented mysticism.
15. See G. Feuerstein, *The Essence of Yoga* (New York: Grove Press, 1976). See also G. Feuerstein, *The Bhagavad-Gita: Its Philosophy and Cultural Setting* (Wheaton, Ill.: Quest Books, 1983).
16. For a fascinating speculative account of the soma plant used in the Vedic ritual, see R. Gordon Wasson, *Soma, Divine Mushroom of Immortality* (New York: Harcourt, Brace and World, 1968).
17. Sir John Woodroffe, *The Garland of Letters: Studies in the Mantra-Śāstra* (Madras, India: Ganesh, 6th ed., 1974), p. 228.
18. The Sanskrit edition by Ramkumar Rai wrongly reads *jaya* for *japa*. Texts of this kind are often gramatically defective. See R. Rai, ed. and trans., *Mantra-Yoga-Samhitā* (Varanasi, India: Chaukhambha Orientalia, 1982).
19. Other popular but relatively recent works are the Mantra-Maharnava, Mantra-Muktavali, Mantra-Kaumudi, and Tattva-Ananda-Tarangini of Purnananda, which are as yet untranslated.
20. The Sanskrit edition by Ramkumar Rai (1982) wrongly reads *yoga* for *yaga*.

3   YOGA AND OTHER HINDU TRADITIONS

1. For a translation of, and a fine commentary on, the "hymn of creation" (nasadiya-sukta) of the Rig-Veda (X.129), see J. Miller, "The Hymn of Creation: A Philosophical Interpretation," in G. Feuerstein and J. Miller, *A Reappraisal of Yoga: Essays in Indian Philosophy* (London: Rider, 1972), pp. 64–85. Miller translates the word *tapas* here with "flame-power": "Darkness there was; at first hidden in darkness this all was undifferentiated depths. Enwrapped in voidness, that which flame-power kindled to existence, emerged" (verse 3).
2. See T. S. Anantha Murthy, *Maharaj: A Biography of Shriman Tapasviji Maharaj, A Mahatma Who Lived for 185 Years* (San Rafael, Calif.: Dawn Horse Press, 1972). Foreword, entitled "Penance and Enlightenment," by G. Feuerstein.
3. J. F. Sprockhoff, *Samnyāsa: Quellenstudien zur Askese im Hinduismus*. Vol. 1: *Untersuchungen über die Samnyāsa-Upaniṣads* (Wiesbaden, West Germany: Kommissionsverlag Franz Steiner, 1976), p. 2.
4. The somewhat obscure phrase "the senses move among their [appropriate] sense objects" of stanza V.9 means that the yogin is aware that the senses are doing their proper business, which is to roam among the sense objects, and that this is a spontaneous activity that does not depend on the illusion of there being an ego in charge.
5. The closest synonym for "philosophy" in Sanskrit is *anvikshiki-vidya* ("sci-

ence of examination"). The related term *tarka-shastra* ("discipline of reasoning") is generally applied only to the Nyaya school of thought, which deals with logic and dialectics. Modern pandits use the term *tattva-vidya-shastra* ("discipline of knowing reality") to express what we mean by "philosophical thinking." The concept of "religion," again, is captured in the Sanskrit term *sanatana-dharma,* which means the "eternal law," but it refers specifically to Hinduism rather than religion in general.

6. S. Radhakrishnan, *Indian Philosophy* (New York: Macmillan; London: Allen & Unwin, 1951), vol. 2, p. 429.

7. Max Müller, *The Six Systems of Indian Philosophy* (New York: Longmans, Green and Co., 1916), p. 263.

8. Self-actualization refers to the realization of our potential for such higher values as self-transcendence, love, compassion, integrity, creativity, and wholeness.

9. Some modern Ayur-Vedic specialists object to translating the three humors as "wind," "bile," and "phlegm" respectively. They argue that these terms are misleading, because vata, pitta, and kapha refer to whole functional systems of the body-mind. Thus, vata is responsible for all sensory and motor activities; pitta is responsible for all biochemical activities; kapha underlies skeletal and anabolic processes. It is obvious that the three doshas are related to the three gunas—sattva, rajas, and tamas.

PART TWO: FIVE THOUSAND YEARS OF GLORIOUS HISTORY

1. K. Jaspers, *Way to Wisdom: An Introduction to Philosophy* (New Haven, Conn.; London: Yale University Press, 1954), p. 96.

4 YOGA IN ANCIENT TIMES

1. See M. Harner, *The Way of the Shaman* (New York: Harper & Row, 1980). See also Joan Halifax, *Shamanic Voices: A Survey of Visionary Narratives* (New York: Dutton, 1979).

2. This psychohistorical movement toward individuation is explained in my book *Structures of Consciousness* (Lower Lake, Calif.: Integral Publishing, 1987).

3. Even the Buddhist ideal of the bodhisattva ("enlightenment being"), who vows to postpone his own ultimate enlightenment until all other beings are liberated, is not a social ideal. The bodhisattva is not a social-welfare worker but a spiritual aspirant or an adept whose only purpose is the *spiritual* welfare of others.

4. M. Eliade, *Yoga: Immortality and Freedom* (Princeton, N.J.: Princeton University Press, 1973), p. 320. See also his *Shamanism: Archaic Techniques of Ecstasy* (Princeton, N.J.: Princeton University Press, 1972).

5. See J. W. Hauer, *Der Yoga* (Stuttgart, West Germany: Kohlhammer Verlag, 1958), and M. Falk, *The Unknown Early Yoga and the Birth of Indian Philosophy* (Madras, India, 1941).

6. S. Piggott, *Prehistoric India* (Harmondsworth, England: Penguin Books, 1950), p. 138. See also B. Allchin and R. Allchin, *The Birth of Indian Civilization: India and Pakistan before 500 B.C.* (Harmondsworth, England: Penguin Books, 1968); J. Marshall, *Mohenjo Daro and the Indus Civilization* (London, 1931), 3 vols.; and R. E. Mortimer Wheeler, *Civilizations of the Indus Valley and Beyond* (London: Thames & Hudson, 1966).

7. S. Piggott, op. cit., p. 203.

8. The Vedic era can be assigned roughly to the time from 1500 to 1000 B.C. Thereafter follows the post-Vedic age.

9. The Vedic pantheon is said to comprise "thrice eleven" deities. The principal gods are Indra (God of War), Agni (God of Fire), Soma (God of the Soma plant), Varuna (God of Sky and Heaven, who upholds the universal order), and Surya (God of the Sun). The well-known Hindu triad consisting of gods Brahma, Vishnu, and Shiva belongs to the post-Christian era. Vishnu and Shiva are mentioned in the Vedas but do not figure prominently; Brahma, the Creator-God, is a post-Vedic creation.

10. J. Miller, *The Vedas: Harmony, Meditation and Fulfilment* (London: Rider, 1974), p. 45.

11. S. Aurobindo, *On the Veda* (Pondicherry, India: Shri Aurobindo Ashram, 1956), p. 384.

12. J. Miller, op. cit., p. 49.

13. Ibid., p. 97. Miller concedes that the full meaning of this fourth stage is not given in the Rig-Veda itself, but that it is one of the key teachings of the Upanishads, especially the Mandukya-Upanishad, which speaks of the Absolute as the "Fourth" (turiya).

14. For a translation of this remarkable hymn, see G. Feuerstein and J. Miller, *A Reappraisal of Yoga: Essays in Indian Philosophy* (London: Rider, 1972).

15. Further references are given in T. G. Mainkar, *Mysticism in the Rgveda* (Bombay: Popular Book Depot, 1961).

16. V. S. Agrawala, *The Thousand-Syllabled Speech. I. Vision in Long Darkness* (Varanasi, India: Vedaranyaka Ashram, 1963), p. i.

17. These renderings from the Atharva-Veda are based on the academic translation by W. D. Whitney, *The Atharva-Veda Saṃhitā* (Delhi: Motilal Banarsidass, reprinted 1962), 2 vols. This translation was first published in 1905.

18. For a treatment of Atharva-Vedic magic, see M. Stutley, *Ancient Indian Magic and Folklore: An Introduction* (Boulder, Colo.: Great Eastern Book Co., 1980).

19. The materials on the Vratyas consist of fragments written in archaic Sanskrit and of scattered references in the works of ancient writers who had a vested interest in being critical of the Vratyas. Little wonder that most scholars have shied away from studying them. The only really comprehensive study is that by the German Yoga researcher Jakob Wilhelm Hauer; however, he never completed the announced second volume. See J. W. Hauer, *Der Vrātya.* Vol. 1: *Die Vrātya als nichtbrahmanische Kultgenossenschaften arischer Herkunft* (Stuttgart, Germany: Kohlhammer Verlag, 1927).

20. This view, which was extensively documented by J. W. Hauer (1927), is challenged by J. C. Heesterman, "Vrātya and Sacrifice," *Indo-Iranian Journal,* 6 (1962–63). Heesterman sees in the Vratyas "authentic Vedic Aryas."

21. The Vratyas' connection with the Sama-Veda, containing the hymns that were sung during the Vedic rituals, was shown by J. W. Hauer. They were also connected with the recitation of epic sagas (the "Fifth Veda"), some of whose materials are to be found in the later Purana literature.

22. The seven pranas are (1) agni, fire; (2) aditya, sun; (3) candrama, moon; (4) pavamana, wind; (5) apa, the waters; (6) pashava, cattle; and (7) praja, creatures. The seven apanas are (1) paurnamasi, full moon; (2) ashtaka, the day of the moon's quarter; (3) amavasya, the day of the new moon; (4) shraddha, faith; (5) diksha, consecration; (6) yajna, sacrifice; and (7) dakshina, sacrificial gift. The seven vyanas are (1) bhumi, earth; (2) antariksha, mid-region; (3) dyau, sky; (4) nakshatra, stellar constellations; (5) ritu, the seasons; (6) artava, that which pertains to the seasons; and (7) samvatsara, the year.

5 THE WHISPERED WISDOM OF THE EARLY UPANISHADS

1. The notion of many scholars that this sacrifice was performed primarily by renouncers is not borne out by the available evidence, as was made clear by the Dutch indologist H. W. Bodewitz in *Jaiminīya Brāhmaṇa I, 1–65: Translation and Commentary, With a Study of Agnihotra and Prāṇāgnihotra* (Leiden, Holland: E. J. Brill, 1973).

2. The following books can be recommended for general study: K. N. Aiyar, *Thirty Minor Upanishads, Including the Yoga Upanishads* (El Reno, Okla.: Santarasa Publications, 1980); this is a facsimile reprint of the 1914 edition. P. Deussen, *Sixty Upanisads of the Veda,* translated from German by V. M. Bedekar and G. B. Palsule (Delhi: Motilal Banarsidass, 1980), 2 vols.; the German original was first published in 1897. R. E. Hume, *The Thirteen Principal Upanishads* (London: Oxford University Press, 1958). A. A. Ramanathan, *The Samnyāsa Upanisads (On Renunciation)* (Adyar, India: Adyar Library and Research Centre, 1978). T. R. Srinivasa Ayyangar, *The Yoga Upaniṣads* (Adyar, India: Adyar Library, 1952).

3. The phrase *shloka-krit* is ambiguous. *Shloka* can refer to a stanza, sound in general, or fame. It is derived from the verbal root *shru,* "to hear." I chose to render it here by "poetry." The underlying idea is that the sage, in the condition of ecstatic identification with the transcendental Reality, acknowledges that Reality as the source of his poetic exuberance.

4. In another section (III.10.3), the compound *yoga-kshema* is used, meaning "acquisition" and "preservation" respectively, which suggests that the technical denotation of the term *yoga* had not yet achieved preeminence.

6 JAINA YOGA: THE TEACHING OF THE VICTORIOUS FORD–MAKERS

1. According to the Jaina sources, Rishabha is said to have lived for no fewer than 8.4 million years. It is possible that he was a historical personage (who, to be sure, enjoyed an ordinary span of life), though nothing is known about him apart from the later legends. There are references to a certain seer Rishabha in the Rig-Veda and the Taittiriya-Aranyaka, but there is no reason to assume that the two were identical, though it is tempting to make that identification. It is especially noteworthy that Rishabha is mentioned in the Vratya Book of the Atharva-Veda, and that in the Jaina literature Rishabha is also called Keshi, "Long-hair." This possibly establishes a connection between him and early non-Vedic religious circles. Moreover, Rishabha's name, which means "bull," reminds one of the prominence given to that animal in the religion of the Indus civilization. Also of interest is the fact that the stories about Rishabha in the Bhagavata-Purana match those in the Jaina literature, and that while the author(s) of this Purana were respectful of Rishabha, they had few good words for his followers.

2. This aphorism is obscure. It appears that the third degree of pure meditation (shukla-dhyana) consists in bodily activity only. There is no consideration (vitarka) or reflection (vicara) at this level. Then, in the fourth and final stage, the already calmed bodily activity is utterly transcended.

7 YOGA IN BUDDHISM

1. C. Humphreys, *Buddhism* (Harmondsworth, England: Penguin Books, 1951), p. 27.
2. H. Beckh, *Buddha und seine Lehre* (Stuttgart, West Germany: Verlag Freies Geistesleben, 1958), p. 120. (Translated from the German)
3. Like Sanskrit, Pali is an invented language. It is the sacred language in which the earliest available pronouncements of the Buddha and his disciples are recorded.
4. This idea finds expression in the well-known Buddhist symbol of the wheel of life (bhava-cakra), which is said to have been the Buddha's unique discovery. The wheel of life has twelve links: (1) Ignorance (avidya) leads to (2) action-intentions (samskara); these give rise to (3) consciousness (vijnana), from which arise (4) name and form (nama-rupa); from this originates (5) the sixfold base (shad-ayatana)—that is, the objective world—which, in turn, yields (6) sense-contact (sparsha); this leads to (7) sensation (vedana), which effects (8) craving (trishna); this gives rise to (9) grasping (upadana), which leads to (10) becoming (bhava), from which results (11) birth (jati) and then (12) old age and death (jara-marana).

   This ancient formula bears the name pratitya-samutpada, "conditioned origination." It is important to remember that this whole process is thought to take place without a continuous entity, or soul, experiencing it. As the buddhologist Hans Wolfgang Schumann put it:

   Since there is no immortal Self which runs through the various lives like a silk thread through a string of pearls, it cannot be the same person who reaps the fruit of kammic [karmic] seeds of past existences in rebirth. On the other hand the reborn person is not completely different, for each form of existence is caused by, and proceeds from, its previous existence like a flame which is lit by another one. The truth lies between identity and isolation: in conditional dependence.

   The above quote stems from H. W. Schumann, *Buddhism: An Outline of Its Teachings and Schools,* trans. by Georg Feuerstein (London: Rider, 1973), p. 65.

8 THE FLOWERING OF YOGA

1. It is likely that this passage was added at a later stage, for it includes a description of a technique that gained particular importance in Hatha-Yoga. This is the khecari-mudra, which is executed by curling the tongue back against the palate and, according to later texts, even further back against the uvula. The purpose of this strange practice is to block off the life-force (prana) and breath, thereby stabilizing the mind.
2. M. K. Gandhi, *Young India* (Delhi, 1925), pp. 1078–1079. The immense popularity of the Gita is reflected in the numerous commentaries on it that have been composed in Sanskrit and the vernacular languages. The oldest available and most authoritative commentary is by Shankara (A.D. 788–820), the leading proponent of Hindu nondualism. Other well-known expositions of the Gita's teachings are by Ramanuja (eleventh century), the famous teacher of qualified nondualism; by the dualist Madhva (A.D. 1199–1276), who composed the Gita-Bhashya and the Gita-Tatparya; and by Jnanadeva (A.D. 1275–1296), whose Jnaneshvari, written in the Mara-

thi language, must be counted among the most beautiful poetic creations of India. In modern times, illuminating commentaries were composed by (among others) Mahatma Gandhi, the Bengali philosopher-yogin Sri Aurobindo Ghose, and philosopher and sometime-president of India Sarvepalli Radhakrishnan.

3. Swami Prabhavananda and Christopher Isherwood, *The Song of God: Bhagavad-Gita* (London: Phoenix House, 1947), p. 18.

4. G. Feuerstein, *The Bhagavad-Gita: Its Philosophy and Cultural Setting* (Wheaton, Ill.: Theosophical Publishing House, 1983), p. 162.

5. Thus, Bhishma, who is not only a heroic warrior but also a wisdom teacher, speaks of the meditation stages of vitarka (thinking), vicara (subtle reflection), and viveka (differentiation), without explaining them further. These stages are called codana (impeller), since they impel the mind to become absorbed in the objectless condition.

9 YOGA AS PHILOSOPHY AND RELIGION: CLASSICAL DUALIST YOGA

1. S. Dasgupta, *A History of Indian Philosophy* (Delhi: Banarsidass, 1975), vol. 1, p. 62.

2. As I have shown in my own detailed examination of the Yoga-Sutra, this great scripture could well be a composite of only two distinct Yoga traditions. On the one hand, there is the Yoga of eight limbs, or astha-anga-yoga, and on the other, there is the Yoga of action, or kriya-yoga. I have even suggested that the section dealing with the eight constituent practices is a quotation rather than a later interpolation. If this were indeed correct, the widespread equation of Classical Yoga with the eightfold path would be a historical curiosity, since the bulk of the Yoga-Sutra deals with kriya-yoga. But textual reconstructions of this kind are always tentative, and we must keep an open mind about this as about so many other aspects of Yoga and Yoga history.

   The advantage of this kind of methodological approach to the study of the Yoga-Sutra, which presumes the text's homogeneity or "textual innocence," is that it does not violate the work substantially, as is the case with those textual analyses that set out to prove that it is in fact corrupt or composed of fragments and interpolations. See G. Feuerstein, *Yoga-Sūtra: An Exercise in the Methodology of Textual Analysis* (New Delhi: Arnold-Heinemann, 1979).

3. A. Govinda, *The Psychological Attitude in Early Buddhist Philosophy* (London: Rider, 1969), p. 35.

4. See G. Feuerstein, *The Yoga-Sūtra: An Exercise in the Methodology of Textual Analysis* (New Delhi: Arnold-Heinemann, 1979).

5. These five "whirls" (vritti) of consciousness are: valid cognition (pramana), error (viparyaya), imagination (vikalpa), sleep (nidra), and memory (smriti). From their suspension ensues yogic ecstasy.

6. The Sanskrit commentators on the Yoga-Sutra take svadhyaya to also mean the meditative recitation (japa) of the sacred texts.

7. Swami Ajaya, *Yoga Psychology: A Practical Guide to Meditation* (Honesdale, Pa.: Himalayan International Institute, 1978), p. 73.

8. Gopi Krishna, *The Dawn of a Science* (New Delhi: Kundalini Research and Publication Trust, 1978), p. 223.

9. J. H. Clark, *A Map of Mental States* (London: Routledge & Kegan Paul, 1983), p. 29.

10. M. Eliade, *Yoga: Immortality and Freedom* (Princeton, N.J.: Princeton University Press, 1970), p. 39.

10 THE NONDUAL APPROACH TO GOD: POST–CLASSICAL YOGA

1. This excerpt is from chapter 6 of the Tejo-Bindu ("Fire-Point")-Upanishad.

2. This type of Yoga is to be distinguished from the Pashupata Yoga schools mentioned in the Puranas, which follow Patanjali's definition: "Yoga is the restriction of the fluctuations of consciousness." Kaundinya, for instance, explicitly rejects the dualistic metaphysics and methodology of both Samkhya and Patanjali's Yoga. He emphasizes that liberation is not so much dissociation from everything but association with the Divine.

3. Robert E. Svoboda, *Aghora: At the Left Hand of God* (Albuquerque, N.M.: Brotherhood of Life, 1986), p. 36.

4. Ibid., p. 22.

5. The translation is by A. K. Ramanujan, *Speaking of Siva* (Harmondsworth, England: Penguin Books, 1973), p. 28.

6. Paraphrase of a rendering by K. C. Pandey, *Abhinavagupta: An Historical and Philosophical Study* (Varanasi, India: Chaukhamba Amarabharati Prakashan, 1963), p. 21.

7. In this word the final *a* sound is long.

8. Here the long *a* is in the first syllable.

9. For a treatment of the twenty-four principles of the Samkhya tradition, see the "Yoga and Hindu Philosophy" section of Chapter 3 ("Yoga and Other Hindu Traditions").

10. See J. C. Pearce, *The Bond of Power* (New York: Dutton, 1981), pp. 30–31.

11. Noteworthy among these sacred Vaishnava scriptures are the Ahirbudhnya-, the Jayakhya-, the Vishnu-, the Parama-, and the Paushkara-Samhita, which are all untranslated. However, useful discussions of their contents are found in S. Dasgupta, *A History of Indian Philosophy,* (Delhi: Motilal Banarsidass, reprinted 1975), vol. 3.

12. S. Dasgupta, op. cit., vol. 3, pp. 83–84. I have modified the spelling of Sanskrit and Tamil words to make them consistent with the simplified transliteration adopted for this volume.

13. J. M. Sanyal, *The Srimad-Bhagvatam of Krishna-Dwaipayana Vyasa* (New Delhi: Munshiram Manoharlal, 1973), p. vi (publisher's note).

14. Sri Anirvan and Lizelle Reymond, *To Live Within: Teachings of a Baul* (High Burton, England: Coombe Springs Press, 1984), p. 252.

15. These are the different forms of the life-force in the body, which are briefly explained in Chapter 12 ("The Esotericism of Medieval Tantra Yoga"), in the section entitled "The Hidden Reality."

16. The name of the sage has two *sh* sounds, whereas Valmiki's work is correctly spelled *Vasishtha.*

17. Ram Tirtha, *In Woods of God Realization* (Delhi: Rama Tirtha Publication Trust Consortium, 1950), vol. 3, p. 295.

18. The phrase "triple universe" refers to the material dimension, the intermediate psychic dimension, and the higher psychic realms of Nature (prakriti).

19. This is one of three different versions.

11 GOD, VISIONS, AND POWER: THE YOGA–UPANISHADS

1. The Yoga-Upanishads are all available in reasonably reliable translations, published by the Theosophical Society of Adyar, India. Students of Yoga are greatly indebted to the Theosophical Society for making many Yoga scriptures available through their excellent publications program over the years.
2. J.-E. Berendt, *Nada Brahman: The World Is Sound—Music and the Landscape of Consciousness* (Rochester, Vt.: Destiny Books, 1987), p. 76.
3. Shyam Sundar Goswami, *Layayoga: An Advanced Method of Concentration* (London: Routledge & Kegan Paul, 1980), p. 13.
4. The practice of tarka probably refers to the careful evaluation of meditative states lest the yogin succumb to mere hallucinations.
5. J. M. Cohen and J.-F. Phibbs, *The Common Experience* (New York: St. Martin's Press, 1979), p. 141.
6. For a translation of other verses of this passage, see the section on Bhakti-Yoga in Chapter 2 ("The Wheel of Yoga").
7. The Yoga of "twelve measures" spoken of in verse 3 presumably refers to the retention of the breath for the duration of twelve repetitions of the syllable *om*.
8. Breath (shvasa) and life-force (prana) are, to the yogin, one and the same. Whereas one term emphasizes more the physical aspect, the other reminds us of the metaphysical dimension in which the breath participates.
9. The meaning of the phrase "three-by-three" (trayas-trayah) is not clear. It could refer to the three parts of the process of breath control, namely inhalation, retention, and exhalation, or to the repeated linking of vision, mind, and breath, as one Sanskrit commentator has it.
10. These three main channels of the life-force will be explained in connection with Hatha-Yoga (see Chapter 13).
11. For euphonic reasons, the word *kundali*, or *kundalini*, must be changed to *kundaly*, or *kundaliny*, when it is followed by a word beginning with a vowel, such as *upanishad*.
12. The word *cudamani* is changed to *cudamany* for the reasons stated in note 11 above.

12 THE ESOTERICISM OF MEDIEVAL TANTRA YOGA

1. Sometimes the terms *agama* and *tantra* are used interchangeably. The former term is explained as meaning "having come from (the mouth of God Shiva)."
2. Ananda Coomaraswamy, *The Dance of Shiva: Fourteen Indian Essays* (Bombay: Asia Publishing House, 1948), p. 140.
3. According to C. G. Jung, there are two key archetypal forces in the human psyche, which he called the anima and the animus. The former is feminine, the latter masculine. Their balanced copresence in each of us, whether male or female, is responsible for psychic harmony.
4. Adapted from the rendering given in Shashibhusan Dasgupta, *Obscure Religious Cults* (Calcutta: Firma KLM, reprinted 1976), p. 57.
5. Translated by Herbert V. Guenther, *The Royal Song of Saraha: A Study in the History of Buddhist Thought* (Berkeley, Calif.: Shambhala, 1973), p. 70.
6. Harold K. Schilling, *The New Consciousness in Science and Religion* (London: SCM Press, 1973), p. 113.

7. Bubba [Da] Free John, *The Paradox of Instruction* (San Francisco: Dawn Horse Press, 1977), p. 236.
8. See Arthur Avalon (alias John Woodroffe), *Shakti and Shakti* (New York: Dover Publications, reprinted, 1978), pp. 188ff.
9. Gopi Krishna, *Kundalini: Evolutionary Energy in Man* (London: Robinson & Watkins, 1971), pp. 12–13.
10. See Lee Sannella, *The Kundalini Experience: Psychosis or Transcendence?* (Lower Lake, Calif.: Integral Publishing, 1987).
11. Gopi Krishna, *Kundalini: The Biological Basis of Religion and Genius* (New Delhi: Kundalini Research and Publication Trust, 1978), p. 88. The book has a lengthy introduction by the German physicist and philosopher Carl Friedrich Freiherr von Weizsäcker.
12. Swami Rama, Rudolph Ballentine, and Swami Ajaya (Allan Weinstock), *Yoga and Psychotherapy: The Evolution of Consciousness* (Glenview, Ill.: Himalayan Institute, 1976), p. 151.
13. See Agehananda Bharati, *The Tantric Tradition* (London: Rider, 1965), pp. 111ff.
14. Swami Satyananda Saraswati, *Sure Ways to Self Realization* (Monghyr, India: Bihar School of Yoga, 1980), p. 45.
15. Cited after the transliterated Sanskrit given in Sudhakar Chattopadhyaya, *Reflections on the Tantras* (Delhi: Motilal Banarsidass, 1978), p. 16, fn. 20.
16. Gopi Krishna, *Kundalini: Evolutionary Energy in Man* (London: Robinson & Watkins, 1971), p. 88.

13 YOGA AS SPIRITUAL ALCHEMY: HATHA–YOGA

1. F. Capra, *The Tao of Physics* (New York: Bantam Books, 1977, pp. 228–229).
2. This image is found in the Agni-Purana (LI.15f). The whole passage reads: "An ascetic (yati) regards his body at best as an inflated bladder of skin, surrounded by muscles, sinew, and flesh, filled with ill-smelling urine, feces, and dirt, a dwelling-place of illness and suffering, and an easy victim of old age, sorrow, and death, more transient than a dew drop on a blade of grass, nothing more or less than the product of the five elements."
3. M. Eliade, *Yoga: Immortality and Freedom* (Princeton, N.J.: Princeton University Press, 1973), p. 227.
4. K. V. Zvelebil, *The Poets of the Powers* (London: Rider, 1973), p. 125.
5. Agehananda Bharati, *The Tantric Tradition* (London: Rider, 1965), p. 28.
6. Kamil V. Zvelebil, op. cit., pp. 29–30; 63.
7. Ibid., p. 87.
8. According to the Indian scholar Mohan Singh, Goraksha's real teaching was not Hatha-Yoga but a form of Mantra-Yoga, called nada-anusamdhana, "practice of the (inner) sound"; he believes that we must study the Samnyasa-Upanishads (dealing with renunciation) for Goraksha's views. However, this interpretation is based on a misunderstanding of Hatha-Yoga, which definitely places considerable emphasis on the inner sound in the higher stages of practice, as is obvious from the Hatha-Yoga-Pradipika.
9. George Weston Briggs, *Gorakhnath and the Kanphata Yogis* (Delhi: Motilal Banarsidass, reprinted 1973), p. 23. This informative, if not always unbiased, ethnographic study was first published in 1938.
10. The meaning of the Sanskrit phrase *dasha-adi* ("states and so on") is not clear. The word *dasha* (with a short final *a*) also means "ten," and hence the phrase could also

signify "the ten and so on," where it remains open what set of ten is being referred to.

11. A. Avalon [John Woodroffe], *The Serpent Power* (London: Luzac, 1919), p. 269.
12. There appears to be another work of this title, by Nityanatha, which has a summary entitled Siddha-Siddhanta-Samgraha by Balabhadra. There is also the seventeenth-century Goraksha-Siddhanta-Samgraha, which draws from about sixty other works.
13. S. L. Katre, "Ānandasamuccaya: A Rare Work on Hatha-Yoga," *Journal of the Oriental Institute (Baroda)*, vol. XI (1961–62), p. 409.
14. P. C. Divanji, *Yoga-Yājñavalkya: A Treatise on Yoga as Taught by Yogi Yajñavalkya* (Bombay, 1954).
15. Other works of the seventeenth century are the Hatha-Samketa-Candrika ("Moonlight Assignation of Hatha-[Yoga]") of Sundaradeva, the Shiva-Yoga-Pradipika ("Torch on Shiva-Yoga") of Sadashiva Brahmendra, a Telegu brahmin, and the Yoga-Cinta-Mani ("Thought-Gem of Yoga") of Shivananda.

Bibliography

This bibliography is intended solely for the nonspecialist who wishes to follow up on some of the themes broached in this volume. A comprehensive bibliography, which covers a good portion of the scholarly literature, can be found in Mircea Eliade, *Yoga: Immortality and Freedom* (Princeton, N.J.: Princeton University Press, 1973). This work complements the present publication in many respects, though *Yoga: The Technology of Ecstasy* has a broader scope and updated information, and also bears in mind the needs of the lay reader.

There are also several bibliographies specifically dedicated to Yoga, notably Howard R. Jarrell, *International Yoga Bibliography, 1950 to 1980* (Metuchen, N.J.: Scarecrow Press, 1981), which includes a whole range of more popular works on the subject.

The following titles will prove useful to those wishing to explore the rather considerable English literature on Yoga and Indian thought in general. Titles marked with an asterisk (*) are especially recommended for the beginning student.

Avalon A. (John Woodroffe). *The Serpent Power: The Secrets of Tantric and Shaktic Yoga.* New York: Dover Publications, reprinted 1974. (First published in 1919.)

Ayyangar, T. R. S. *The Yoga Upaniṣads.* Adyar: Adyar Library, 1952. (Contains renderings of all the Yoga-Upanishads.)

Basham, A. L. *The Wonder That Was India: A Survey of the History and Culture of the Indian Sub-Continent Before the Coming of the Muslims.* New York: Grove Press, 1954.

*Berry, T. *Religions of India: Hinduism, Yoga, Buddhism.* New York: Bruce Publishing Co., 1971.

Bharati, A. *The Tantric Tradition.* London: Rider, 1965.

Bhattacharya, B. *Śaivism and the Phallic World.* New Delhi: Oxford & IBH Publishing, 1975. 2 vols.

*Danielou, A. *Yoga: The Method of Re-Integration.* London: Christopher Johnson, 1954.

Deussen, P. *Sixty Upaniṣads of the Veda.* Delhi: Motilal Banarsidass, 1980. 2 vols. (First published in German in 1897.)

*Eliade, M. *Patanjali and Yoga*. New York: Schocken Books, 1975.

*Feuerstein, G. *The Bhagavad-Gita: Its Philosophy and Cultural Setting*. Wheaton, Ill.: Quest Books, 1983.

Feuerstein, G. *The Yoga-Sutra of Patanjali*. Rochester, VT: Inner Traditions, 1990. (Contains a rendering of the Yoga-Sutra, with brief comments.)

Funderburk, J. *Science Studies Yoga: A Review of Physiological Data*. Glenview, Ill.: Himalayan International Institute, 1977.

Ghosh, S. *The Original Yoga*. New Delhi: Munshiram Manoharlal, 1980. (Contains renderings of the Shiva-Samhita, Gheranda-Samhita, and Yoga-Sutra.)

Goswami, S. S. *Layayoga: An Advanced Method of Concentration*. London: Routledge & Kegan Paul, 1980. (Contains renderings of passages from many Yoga-Upanishads and Tantras.)

Iyengar, B. K. S. *Light on Yoga*. New York: Schocken Books, 1976.

Jaini, Padmanabh S. *The Jaina Path of Purification*. Delhi: Banarsidass, 1979.

*Krishna, Gopi. *Kundalini: The Evolutionary Energy in Man*. London: Robinson & Watkins, 1971.

Larson, Gerald James, and Ram Shankar Bhattacharya, eds. *Sāmkhya: A Dualist Tradition in Indian Philosophy*. Princeton, N.J.: Princeton University Press, 1987.

McDermott, Robert A. *The Essential Aurobindo*. New York: Schocken Books, 1973.

Radhakrishnan, S. *Indian Philosophy*. New York: Macmillan, reprinted 1951. 2 vols.

Radhakrishnan, S. *The Bhagavadgītā*. London: Routledge & Kegan Paul, 1960. (Contains a rendering of the Gita, with a commentary.)

Renou, L. *Hinduism*. New York: Washington Square Press, 1963.

Sangharakshita, Bhikshu. *A Survey of Buddhism*. Boulder, Colo.: Shambhala, 1980.

*Sannella, L. *The Kundalini Experience: Psychosis or Transcendence?* Lower Lake, Calif.: Integral Publishing, 1987.

Schumann, Hans Wolfgang. *Buddhism: An Outline of Its Teaching and Schools*. London: Rider, 1973.

Stutley, M. *Ancient Indian Magic and Folklore: An Introduction*. Boulder, Colo.: Great Eastern Book Co., 1980.

*Varenne, J. *Yoga and the Hindu Tradition*. Chicago: University of Chicago Press, 1976. (Contains a rendering of the Yoga-Darshana-Upanishad.)

Venkatesananda, Swami. *The Concise Yoga Vāsiṣṭha*. Albany, N.Y.: SUNY Press, 1984. (A rendering of important passages from the Yoga-Vasishtha.)

*Walker, B. *Tantrism: Its Secret Principles and Practices*. Wellingborough, England: Aquarian Press, 1982.

Woods, J. H. *The Yoga-System of Patañjali*. Delhi: Motilal Banarsidass, reprinted 1966. (First published in 1914. Contains renderings of the Yoga-Sutra, the Yoga-Bhashya, and the Tattva-Vaisharadi.)

Zimmer, H. R. *Myths and Symbols in Indian Art and Civilization*. Ed. by Joseph Campbell. Princeton, N.J.: Princeton University Press, reprinted 1963.

Index